HUMAN DISEASES AND CONDITIONS

Supplement 2:
Infectious Diseases

HUMAN
DISEASES AND
CONDITIONS

Supplement 2: Infectious Diseases

Neil Izenberg, M.D. • Steven A. Dowshen, M.D.
Editors in Chief

Stephen C. Eppes, M.D. • Joseph Masci, M.D.
Volume Editors

Published in Association with the
Center for Children's Health Media,
The Nemours Foundation

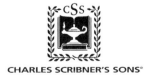

CHARLES SCRIBNER'S SONS®

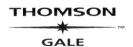

THOMSON
GALE

New York • Detroit • San Diego • San Francisco • Cleveland • New Haven, Conn. • Waterville, Maine • London • Munich

The information in *Human Diseases and Conditions Supplement 2: Infectious Diseases* is not intended to take the place of medical care by physicians and other health care professionals. This book does not contain diagnostic, treatment, or first aid recommendations. Readers should obtain professional advice in making all health care decisions.

Library of Congress Cataloging-in-Publication Data

Human diseases and conditions / Neil Izenberg, editor in chief.
      p. cm.
      "Published in association with the Center for Children's Health Media, the
         Nemours Foundation."
    Contents: V. 1. Abscess-Dysrhythmia.
    Includes bibliographical references and index.
    Summary: present articles dealing with all kinds of diseases and disorders, from acne
      and brain tumor to tobacco-related diseases and yellow fever.
    ISBN 0-684-80543-X (set: alk. paper) —ISBN 0-684-80541-3 (v.1 : alk. paper)
    1. Medicine, Popular—Encyclopedias Juvenile. [1. Diseases—Encyclopedias. 2.
      Health—Encyclopedias.] I. Izenberg, Neil.

RC81.A2 H75 2000
                                              99-051442
    ISBN 0-684-80542-1 (vol. 2)
    ISBN 0-684-80621-5 (vol. 3)
    ISBN 0-684-80643-6 (supp. 1)
    ISBN 0-684-31260-3 (supp. 2)

3 5 7 9 11 13 15 17 19 20 18 16 14 12 10 8 6 4 2

Printed in Canada

The paper used in this publication meets the minimum requirements of the American National Standard for Information Services—Permanence of Paper for Printed Library Materials, ANSI Z39.48-1992.

Editorial and Production Staff

Project Editors
Stacey Blachford • Sarah Feehan

Writers
Kate Barrett • Jennifer Brooks • Joel Ciovacco • Paula Edelsack
Mary Lou Jay • Jennifer Lynch • Elizabeth Merrick • Karen Riley • Eugénie Seifer
Sharon Sexton • Hennie Shore • Shaynee Snider • Amy Sutton

Editors, Researchers, Proofreaders
Lynn M. L. Lauerman • Marcia Merryman Means

Artists
Molly Blessington • Frank Forney

Photo Researcher
Martin Levick

Indexer
Julia Marshall, Marshall Indexing Services

Production Manager
Evi Seoud

Designer
Pamela Galbreath

Senior Editor
John Fitzpatrick

Publisher
Frank Menchaca

Contents

Contents

Preface

Infectious Diseases, the second supplement to *Human Diseases and Conditions*, includes more than 100 topics relating to the organisms that cause infections, the diseases they cause, the laboratory tests used to help understand them, and how specialists track down their spread. Why a volume on infectious diseases? Although the field of medicine has been around, in various forms, for as long as there have been people, it was when scientists began to understand germs and infections that progress in human health accelerated dramatically.

The human body is marvelously complex. Our immune system, those parts of the body that work together to prevent and fight off infections, is a wonderful example of that complexity. Despite the incredibly large number of infectious organisms in the world, most of the time our defenses are able to prevent disease and maintain health without our even thinking about it. Unfortunately, though, some infectious organisms do get through. The stories of these organisms, how they create illness, and what we can do about them are some of the most important stories of humanity.

In this volume, you'll learn about a number of the infections that changed history, like the "Black Death" that wiped out one third of Europe's population in the fourteenth century, and common infections like measles that, though now almost eliminated in the United States through immunizations, still destroys thousands of lives in other countries.

But, the story of infectious diseases is not just about the past. It's about the present—and the future—of humanity. Infections still cause many millions of deaths every year throughout the world and leave behind countless injuries and disabities, affecting ability to see, hear, think, breathe, and move. In many parts of the world, economies are too impoverished to provide adequate sanitation, antibiotics, and life-preserving immunizations. Inadequate diets and starvation diminish the ability to fight infections. In every country, ill-advised behaviors and lack of knowledge help organisms spread and prevent people from seeking help in time.

As humans, we have made tremendous strides in learning how bacteria, viruses, and other organisms do their work. We have made impressive progress in preventing and treating a large number of infectious diseases. But there is so much more to learn and so much more to do in translating knowledge into practical ways to help promote human health.

We hope that *Infectious Diseases* sparks your interest in this important area. Who knows, maybe you will be part of a team that makes a great scientific breakthrough about infections that will change the future for the better.

Neil Izenberg, M.D.
Steven A. Dowshen, M.D.
Editors in Chief
Nemours Center for
Children's Health Media
The Nemours Foundation
www.KidsHealth.org

Acknowledgments

For this supplement, we have worked with volume editors Stephen C. Eppes, M.D., and Joseph Masci, M.D. Both are physicians with special training in the diagnosis and treatment of infectious diseases. Their great expertise and love of teaching has greatly enriched this volume—and we appreciate their efforts.

We also wish to thank Frederick Meier, M.D., for sharing his insights into how infectious diseases have helped shape the course of history and for lending a hand with the medical review of these chapters. At the Nemours Center for Children's Health Media, thanks go to Shirley Morrison and Alesha Pagan for their dependable support.

Introduction

The Impact of Infectious Diseases

Diseases caused by microorganisms* have afflicted humankind since the beginning of our species. Today, infectious diseases remain the number one cause of death in the world, despite steady advances in medical knowledge of how microorganisms cause disease and how to best prevent and treat these illnesses. Important advances have included:

 Edward Jenner's 1796 discovery that inoculation with fluid from a cowpox sore provided protection against smallpox, a contagious and often fatal infection caused by the variola virus*. The success of this first vaccine* set the foundation for the development of other life-saving immunizations.

Louis Pasteur's 1857 development of the germ theory, which concluded that infectious diseases were caused by microorganisms, or germs.

Alexander Fleming's 1928 discovery that a mold could kill bacteria* the cause of many infectious diseases. The active substance from the mold, known as penicillin, was later produced on a large scale for widespread use.

Public health programs that improved sanitation and sewers and encouraged basic principles of cleanliness have helped to prevent the spread of infectious diseases. Epidemiology (eh-pih-dee-me-AH-luh-jee), the study of the occurrence, distribution, and control of disease, has also played an important role in preventing disease and providing better care.

However, despite these successes, pathogens* continue to have a strong impact on the health of humans. One simple reason is that many microorganisms (or microbes) adapt to new environments much more swiftly and effectively than do people. For example, some bacteria have changed into new strains* that can resist the antibiotics* that previously killed them.

Climate also plays a large role when it comes to the impact of diseases. Many of the most stubborn infections, such as malaria*, occur in sub-Saharan Africa, where high temperatures and moisture combine to make an ideal environment for the growth of mosquitoes and other vectors* of many infectious agents. In addition, the lack of a harsh winter climate in these regions means that infectious agents are not regularly

KEYWORDS
for searching the Internet and other reference sources

Alexander Fleming

Edward Jenner

Epidemiology

Infectious diseases

Louis Pasteur

Microbiology

Molecular biology

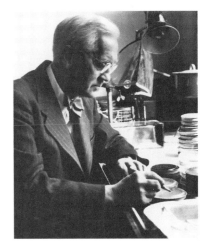

▲

After witnessing the infections that killed soldiers during World War I, the Scottish scientist Alexander Fleming searched for chemicals that could fight bacteria. His discovery of the antibiotic penicillin, which was used during World War II and revolutionized the treatment of infections, earned him the Nobel Prize in 1945. *Corbis Corporation (Bellevue)*

* **microorganisms** are tiny organisms that can only be seen using a microscope. Types of microorganisms include fungi, bacteria, and viruses.

* **virus** (VY-rus) is a tiny infectious agent that can cause infectious diseases. A virus can only reproduce within the cells it infects.

* **vaccine** (vak-SEEN) is a preparation of killed or weakened germs, or a part of a germ or product it produces, given to prevent or lessen the severity of the disease that can result if a person is exposed to the germ itself. Use of vaccines for this purpose is called immunization.

* **bacteria** (bak-TEER-e-uh) are microscopic organisms, some types of which can cause disease.

* **pathogens** (PAH-tho-jens) are microorganisms that can cause disease in another living organism.

* **strains** are various subtypes of organisms, such as viruses or bacteria.

* **antibiotics** (an-tie-by-AH-tiks) are drugs that kill or slow the growth of bacteria.

* **malaria** (mah-LAIR-e-uh) is a disease spread to humans by the bite of an infected mosquito.

* **vectors** (VEK-tors) are animals or insects that carry diseases and transfer them from one host to another.

killed off. Disease-carrying insect vectors, such as mosquitoes, remain active throughout the year.

People are also responsible for the spread of infectious diseases from one population to another. Individuals and groups (such as refugees) travel from place to place bringing infectious diseases and microorganisms with them. Methods of food production and food handling can also spread infections, such as contamination caused by *E. coli*, dangerous bacteria that can multiply in undercooked meat. Similarly, impure water may carry bacteria or parasites that can sicken and even kill those who drink it.

The conditions of poverty, which include poor nutrition, poor sanitation, and overcrowding, contribute to the spread of infectious diseases. Poverty also increases the incidence of infectious diseases by limiting efforts to prevent them. The differences in health care available in developed versus developing countries are often significant. In many developing countries, a lack of funding for basic health education and prevention, too few doctors, nurses, and other caregivers, and limited money for medicines, equipment and vaccinations, can result in increased illness and shortened life spans. Where there is extreme poverty, even simple prevention methods can be too expensive. For example, in certain areas of the world, using mosquito netting to cover a sleeping area can prevent deaths from mosquito-related diseases such as malaria. But poverty prevents some families from spending even the few dollars it would take to buy the netting—and so malaria spreads. In many cases, these issues are made worse by the difficulties in reaching people in rural or isolated areas.

Infections Throughout History

Infectious diseases appear in written histories that date back to ancient times:

■ Thucydides, in early fifth century B.C. Greece, described how a disease decimated the Athenian army and much of the population of Athens, contributing to the fall of this greatest of Greek city-states; students of infectious diseases have argued for years about what infection may have caused this pivotal epidemic.

■ Smallpox killed millions of people over thousands of years before officially being eradicated in 1977 by a worldwide vaccination program supervised by the World Health Organization (WHO) and the U.S. Centers for Disease Control and Prevention (CDC).

■ Malaria, a tropical disease spread by the *Anopheles* mosquito, is mentioned in ancient Egyptian hieroglyphics and sickened invaders of the Roman Empire. In contrast to smallpox, efforts to eliminate malaria have been fully unsuccessful in the tropical

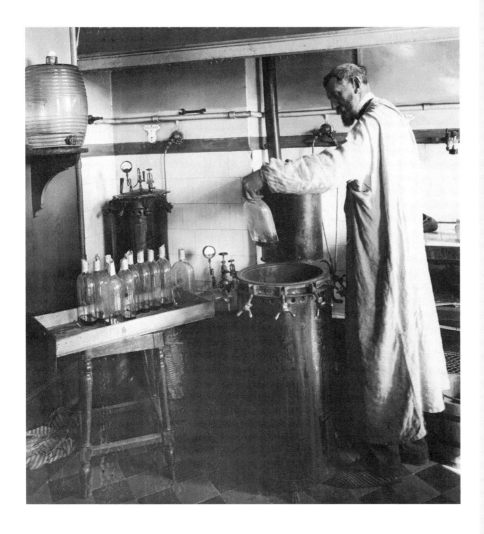

The French chemist Louis Pasteur proposed the "germ theory" while studying alcohol fermentation, which he found was a biological process carried out by microorganisms. He went on to link microbes, or germs, to contagious diseases. His name lives on in the process of "pasteurization," by which milk and other food is heated to prevent the growth of bacteria. *Corbis Corporation (Bellevue)*

◀

and subtropical countries where it has been most common. No successful vaccine has yet been developed to prevent malaria.

In the fourteenth century, a bacterium later identified as *Yersinia pestis* (yer-SIN-e-uh PES-tis) caused the bubonic plague*, or Black Death. Carried into Europe and Africa by infected rodents and fleas that accompanied traders and marauding armies from Mongolia, Black Death ran through Europe, Africa, and the Middle East. The bubonic plague killed one third of the population in Europe. People contracted the plague through bites from fleas that had picked up the bacteria after feeding on infected rats.

Viruses have also influenced history:

In the Cook Islands, explorers unknowingly carried a number of diseases (including measles*) that proved to be disastrous to native island dwellers.

From 1918 to 1919, an influenza* pandemic* spread worldwide, causing between 20 and 40 million deaths.

* **plague** (PLAYG) is a serious bacterial infection that is spread to humans by infected rodents and their fleas.

* **measles** (ME-zuls) is a viral respiratory infection that is best known for the rash of large, flat, red blotches that appear on the arms, face, neck, and body.

* **influenza** (in-floo-EN-zuh), also known as the flu, is a contagious viral infection that attacks the respiratory tract, including the nose, throat, and lungs.

* **pandemic** (pan-DEH-mik) is a worldwide outbreak of disease, especially infectious disease, in which the number of cases suddenly becomes far greater than usual.

* **epidemic** (eh-pih-DEH-mik) is an outbreak of disease, especially infectious disease, in which the number of cases suddenly becomes far greater than usual. Usually epidemics that involve worldwide outbreaks are called pandemics.

* **tetanus** (TET-nus) is a serious bacterial infection that affects the body's central nervous system.

* **diphtheria** (dif-THEER-e-uh) is an infection of the lining of the upper respiratory tract (the nose and throat). It is a serious disease that can cause breathing difficulty and other complications, including death.

* **meningitis** (meh-nin-JY-tis) is an inflammation of the meninges, the membranes that surround the brain and the spinal cord. Meningitis is most often caused by infection with a virus or a bacterium.

* **typhoid** (TIE-foyd) **fever** is an infection with the bacterium *Salmonella typhi* that causes fever, headache, confusion, and muscle aches.

* **yellow fever** is an infectious disease caused by a virus that is transmitted to humans by mosquitoes.

* **hepatitis** (heh-puh-TIE-tis) **A** is inflammation of the liver that is caused by an infection with the hepatitis A virus.

* **cholera** (KAH-luh-ruh) is an infection of the small intestine that can cause severe diarrhea.

* **rabies** (RAY-beez) is a viral infection of the central nervous system that usually is transmitted to humans by the bite of an infected animal.

* **tuberculosis** (too-ber-kyoo-LO-sis) is a bacterial infection that primarily attacks the lungs but can spread to other parts of the body.

■ The AIDS epidemic*, first noted in the early 1980s, has spread throughout the world and led to millions of deaths, most of them in Africa.

Preventing the Spread of Infectious Diseases

When it comes to preventing infections, immunizations have played a major role in reducing and, in the case of smallpox, eradicating infectious diseases. Vaccines are routinely given to young children to prevent once common childhood infections including mumps, measles, and chicken pox. Adults and adolescents also now receive regular booster vaccinations to remain protected against tetanus* and diphtheria*, and adults who never received immunizations during childhood or never had certain diseases such as chicken pox or measles can now receive these vaccinations.

Certain vaccinations for diseases more common outside the United States are recommended when traveling. Immunizations for travel may include those that prevent meningococcal infection (which can cause meningitis*), typhoid fever*, yellow fever*, hepatitis A*, cholera*, rabies*, or other viral or bacterial diseases.

At the start of the twentieth century, infectious diseases were widespread in the United States; in fact, tuberculosis* was the most frequent cause of death. But vaccines played a part in changing that. By 1985, 18 years after the mumps vaccine was introduced, the number of cases dropped by 98 percent. *Haemophilus influenzae* type b (Hib) was once the most frequent cause of fatal bacterial meningitis in children, as well as pneumonia, deafness, and other ailments. Since Hib vaccinations began in 1987, the number of cases of Hib infection has dropped by more than 99 percent and most young pediatricians have never seen a case.

In some instances when rates of vaccination have dropped, the rate of disease has jumped correspondingly. A concern that the pertussis (whooping cough) vaccine was unsafe led to a decrease in immunizations for the disease in Japan and the United Kingdom in the 1970s, which resulted in steep rises in the number of cases and deaths from the disease during the 1980s. Similarly, between 1989 and 1991 an epidemic of measles hit the United States and killed more than 120 people, mainly those who had not been vaccinated or were inadequately vaccinated.

Hospitals, daycare centers, nursing homes, and other institutions must be particularly careful about controlling the spread of disease. In these settings, people are at greater risk of infection and infection-control measures are routinely taught and practiced. The CDC has instituted programs for hospitals to report and monitor instances of hospital-related infections.

BIOLOGICAL WARFARE

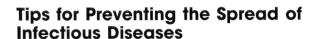

The smallpox virus may have been the first infectious agent to be used in biological warfare* during the French and Indian Wars, when British troops gave Native Americans smallpox-contaminated blankets. Epidemics and widespread death followed.

The plague bacterium has also been used in biological warfare, and great concern exists that other infectious agents (such as those that cause anthrax*, botulism, tularemia*, viral hemorrhagic fevers, and smallpox) may become agents of biological warfare and bioterrorism in the future.

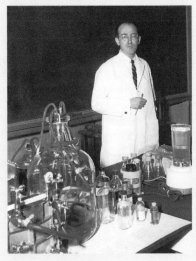

▲

During the first half of the twentieth century, epidemics of polio took their toll in the developed world, causing paralysis and death. In 1955 Dr. Jonas Salk developed the first effective vaccine against the devastating disease. *AP Wide World Photos*

* **biological warfare** is a method of waging war by using harmful microorganisms to purposely spread disease to many people.

* **anthrax** (AN-thraks) is a rare infectious disease caused by the bacterium *Bacillus anthracis.*

* **tularemia** (too-lah-REE-me-uh), sometimes called rabbit fever, is an infection caused by bacteria that can be spread to humans by wild animals.

Tips for Preventing the Spread of Infectious Diseases

Hand washing is a basic, important, and easy way to prevent contracting or passing on many germs. Experts recommend scrubbing hands for at least 15 seconds with soap and water, particularly before working around food, after coughing or sneezing, and after changing a diaper or using the bathroom.

Preparing food safely at home also can help prevent contamination. Experts recommend using caution when purchasing and storing food; washing raw fruits and vegetables before eating; defrosting frozen food either in a refrigerator or in a microwave; and cooling and storing leftovers immediately after food has been served. Disinfecting areas where there is a high concentration of dangerous germs, including the kitchen and bathroom, with a cleaning product that contains bleach can help destroy bacteria or other germs.

Resources

Organizations

U.S. Centers for Disease Control and Prevention (CDC), 1600 Clifton Road, Atlanta, GA 30333. The CDC is the United States government authority for information about infectious and other diseases. The CDC offers information on specific infectious diseases and recommended treatments at its website.
Telephone 800-311-3435
http://www.cdc.gov

U.S. National Library of Medicine, 8600 Rockville Pike, Bethesda, MD 20894. The National Library of Medicine has a website packed with information on diseases and drugs, consumer resources, dictionaries and encyclopedias of medical terms, and directories of doctors and helpful organizations.
Telephone 888-346-3656
http://www.nlm.nih.gov

World Health Organization (WHO), Avenue Appia 20, 1211 Geneva 27, Switzerland. WHO tracks disease outbreaks around the world and offers information about various infectious diseases at its website.
Telephone 011-41-22-791-2111
http://www.who.int

Website

KidsHealth.org. KidsHealth is a website created by the medical experts of the Nemours Foundation and is devoted to issues of children's health. It contains articles on a variety of health topics, including infectious diseases.
http://www.KidsHealth.org

▶ *See also*
Body Defenses
Public Health
The Nature of Germs and Infection

KEYWORDS
for searching the Internet and other reference sources

Bacteria

Fungi

Germs

Immune system

Infections

Infestations

Microbes

Microorganisms

Parasites

Pathogens

Prions

Viruses

*syphilis (SIH-fih-lis) is a sexually transmitted disease that, if untreated, can lead to serious lifelong problems throughout the body, including blindness and paralysis.

The Nature of Germs and Infection

What Is a Germ?

A germ is a microscopic organism that can cause disease. The term "microscopic organism" means that it is so small it can be seen only with a microscope. Sometimes also called microbes (MY-krobes), germs can exist just about anywhere on Earth. They can be found in and on animals, plants, and the human body. Some microscopic organisms actually keep people healthy, by helping in the body's digestion and other functions, but others can cause illness.

It was not until the seventeenth century that a Dutch scientist named Antonie van Leeuwenhoek, using an early microscope, was able to describe the existence of these previously unseen creatures. In the mid-nineteenth century the German doctor Jacob Henle advanced a coherent argument that tiny organisms caused disease. His student and fellow German physician, Robert Koch, some decades later used Henle's sequence of evidence to prove that different organisms cause specific diseases. As the nature of germs became more widely understood, scientists began to appreciate that germs cause many common diseases, such as tuberculosis, pneumonia, and syphilis*. By the end of the twentieth century, researchers began to understand how germs can play a role in many chronic* diseases and disorders, including some forms of cancer, disease of the coronary arteries*, peptic ulcer* disease, and chronic lung diseases, which had not been thought of as infections at all.

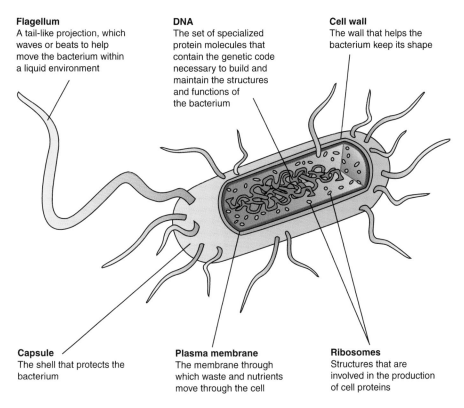

Flagellum
A tail-like projection, which waves or beats to help move the bacterium within a liquid environment

DNA
The set of specialized protein molecules that contain the genetic code necessary to build and maintain the structures and functions of the bacterium

Cell wall
The wall that helps the bacterium keep its shape

Capsule
The shell that protects the bacterium

Plasma membrane
The membrane through which waste and nutrients move through the cell

Ribosomes
Structures that are involved in the production of cell proteins

The outer "shell" of these one-celled organisms is made up of layers, including the cell membrane, cell wall, and in some cases an outer capsule. The flagellum is a whiplike structure on the cell's surface that helps the organism move. Structures inside the bacterium include DNA, which is the molecule that contains the genetic material necessary to build and maintain the organism, and ribosomes, which play a key role in the production of cell proteins.

Microbes generally are classified into three types:

- Commensals (ko-MEN-suls) are organisms that live harmlessly on or in another organism.
- Symbiotes (SIM-be-oatz) are organisms that help each other and, in many cases, need each other for survival, such as bacteria located in the human intestines* that play a crucial role in digesting food.
- Pathogens (PAH-tho-jens) are microbes that can cause damage or disease. This volume on infectious diseases naturally focuses more on pathogens than on commensals or symbiotes.

Germs can be divided into four large groups:

- Bacteria (bak-TEER-e-uh) are single-cell organisms that do not have a nucleus. Aerobic (air-O-bik) bacteria need oxygen to survive, whereas anaerobic (ah-nuh-RO-bik) bacteria do not. But all forms of bacteria, like all living things, require food for energy and building materials. Although countless bacteria exist, less than 1 percent of all bacteria are pathogens.

* **chronic** (KRAH-nik) means continuing for a long period of time.

* **coronary arteries** (KOR-uh-nair-e AR-tuh-reez) are the blood vessels that directly supply blood to the heart.

* **ulcer** is an open sore on the skin or the lining of a hollow body organ, such as the stomach or intestine. It may or may not be painful.

* **intestines** are the muscular tubes that food passes through during digestion after it exits the stomach.

This diagram shows the structure of a virus, the smallest infectious agent. Depending on the type of virus, DNA or RNA is wrapped in a protein coat. Because viruses cannot convert food into energy and cannot reproduce on their own, some scientists do not consider them a life form. ▶

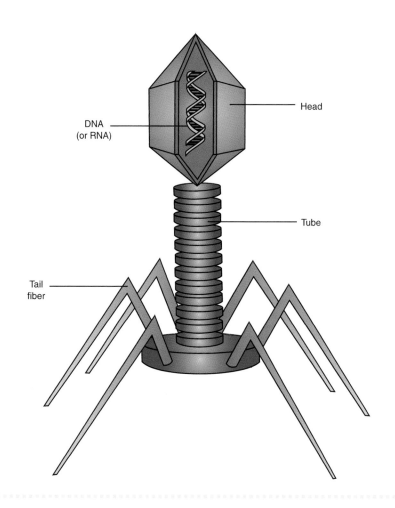

DNA
(or RNA)

Head

Tube

Tail
fiber

* **DNA**, or deoxyribonucleic acid (dee-OX-see-ry-bo-nyoo-klay-ik AH-sid), is the specialized chemical substance that contains the genetic code necessary to build and maintain the structures and functions of living organisms.

* **RNA**, or ribonucleic acid (ry-bo-nyoo-KLAY-ik AH-sid), is the chemical substance through which DNA sends genetic information to build new cells.

* **genes** (JEENZ) are chemical structures composed of deoxyribonucleic acid (DNA) that help determine a person's body structure and physical characteristics. Inherited from a person's parents, genes are contained in the chromosomes found in the body's cells.

* **host** is an organism that provides another organism (such as a parasite or virus) with a place to live and grow.

▓ Viruses (VY-ruh-sez) are particles containing DNA* or RNA*, which make up the virus's genes*, and are wrapped with a protein coat. Because viruses on their own are not alive, they must invade a living cell and then take over some of the machinery within the host* cell in order to reproduce. Without the living cell, a virus cannot reproduce.

▓ Parasites (PAIR-uh-sites) are organisms that feed and live on or within another living being. Many parasites enter the body through the intestines or the skin. Single-cell parasites include those that cause malaria (mah-LAIR-e-uh), a disease spread to humans by the bite of an infected mosquito. Parasites with more than one cell include roundworms, flatworms, and so-called flukes. Some parasites, most notably tapeworms, can reach enormous sizes (20 feet or more) inside the human intestines.

▓ Fungi (FUNG-eye) are more complicated organisms that live in air, in soil, on plants, and in water. Thousands, maybe millions, of species thrive on Earth. Some live in the human body without causing illness. In fact, only a small number are capable of causing disease in humans.

Germs may include other particles as well, like prions (PRE-ons). Prions are transmissible viral-like proteins and are thought to play a role in Creutzfeldt-Jakob (KROYTZ-felt YAH-kub) disease and bovine spongiform (SPUN-jih-form) encephalopathy (en-seh-fuh-LAH-puh-thee), or BSE. Both of these disorders damage the tissues of the brain, causing a rapid decline in mental function and muscle coordination. BSE, commonly known as mad cow disease, only infects cattle. Prions, which were discovered only recently, are not well understood. Because they lack DNA and RNA, which are common to all other forms of life, it is not clear whether they should be considered to be alive.

What Are Infections?

The word "infection" means something different from "disease," although the two terms sometimes are confused. Disease is a general word that describes any abnormality of the human condition or something that interferes with the normal, healthy functioning of the body. Diseases include infections and infestations, among others. Infection is a term that refers specifically to any abnormal condition caused by a microbe, such as a bacterium, virus, or parasite, that has invaded another organism (like a human) and interfered with some aspect of its function. An infestation is similar to an infection. It refers to any abnormal condition caused by an organism larger than a microbe, such as an insect, louse, or worm. The phrase "infectious diseases" is used to refer to both infections and infestations, regardless of the severity of the condition. An infection beneath a fingernail and a serious case of hepatitis* C both are considered infectious diseases.

The hallmark of many infections is inflammation (in-flah-MAY-shun), which is largely a result of the immune system's* response to infection, irritation, or injury. The characteristics of inflammation include redness, warmth, swelling, and pain. Important players in the immune reaction are the white blood cells. In response to germs, white cells race to the area of infection to fight off the invader; the word "pus" refers to a thick fluid produced by the body in response to an infection that contains these white cells along with other substances resulting from the reaction.

If a disease is contagious (kon-TAY-jus), it can be transmitted from person to person through some form of contact. Not all infectious diseases are contagious, and being exposed to an infectious agent does not mean that a person necessarily will contract an infection. Some people exposed to a contagious organism may not become sick. For example, they might have immunity* to a certain infection because they have had it before or because they had a vaccine* against it.

Infections vary in both how long they last and how severe their signs and symptoms are. Acute infections usually appear quickly and may improve quickly (with or without treatment), but often they can cause immediate discomfort, including extreme tiredness (fatigue), body aches, or coughing. Once the immune system has defeated an acute viral infection,

* **hepatitis** (heh-puh-TIE-tis) is an inflammation of the liver. Hepatitis can be caused by viruses, bacteria, and a number of other noninfectious medical conditions.

* **immune system** is the system of the body composed of specialized cells and the substances they produce that helps protect the body against disease-causing germs.

* **immunity** (ih-MYOON-uh-tee) is the condition of being protected against an infectious disease. Immunity often develops after a germ is introduced to the body. One type of immunity occurs when the body makes special protein molecules called antibodies to fight the disease-causing germ. The next time that germ enters the body, the antibodies quickly attack it, usually preventing the germ from causing disease.

* **vaccine** (vak-SEEN) is a preparation of killed or weakened germs, or a part of a germ or product it produces, given to prevent or lessen the severity of the disease that can result if a person is exposed to the germ itself. Use of vaccines for this purpose is called immunization.

Restless in retirement, Robert Koch (seated center) traveled to Africa, where he made invaluable contributions to the study of trypanosomiasis, or sleeping sickness, a disease transmitted by the tsetse fly. To fight the disease, he recommended a program of deforestation to kill the tsetse fly by eliminating its habitat. ▶

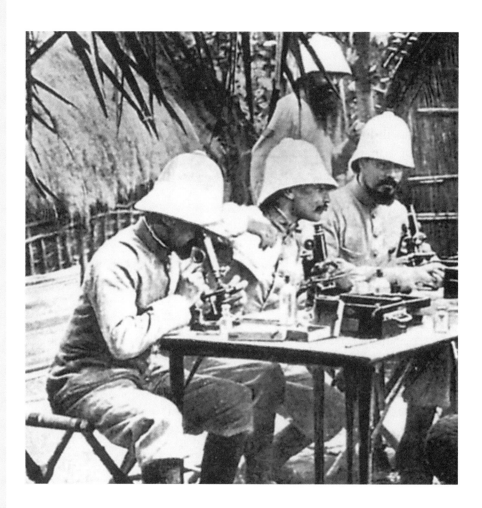

* **cirrhosis** (sir-O-sis) is a condition that affects the liver, involving long-term inflammation and scarring, which can lead to problems with liver function.

* **antibody** (AN-tih-bah-dee) is a protein molecule produced by the body's immune system to help fight a specific infection caused by a microorganism, such as a bacterium or virus.

such as the common cold, the illness probably will not return, unless the person becomes infected with a different virus that can cause the same infection. Because many different viruses can cause a "cold," it often looks as if the same cold keeps coming back, but it is really a different one.

Chronic infections are those infections that last a longer time—weeks, months, or even years. A chronic infection can develop from an acute infection that does not clear up. Some chronic infections continue to have signs and symptoms, causing discomfort and interfering with life for long periods of time. Other chronic infections may have few or no signs. People who have a chronic infection may not be aware that they still have an active infection and may still be capable of passing the infectious microbe to others. One example is hepatitis C, a disease that can have few symptoms but also can cause cirrhosis*, chronic liver disease, or liver cancer. People with hepatitis C may not be aware that they have it without taking an antibody* test that shows that the body is fighting the virus. Serious signs of liver damage may not show up until 20 years after the initial infection. Latent, or hidden, infections can turn on and off for months or years. One example is the herpes simplex (HER-peez SIM-plex) virus, which can cause infections of the skin, mouth, and genitals*, including cold sores and genital herpes. When the infection is "on," a person can spread it to others.

Many infectious organisms live naturally in and on the human body, often without causing harm, but they can produce disease if they travel to another part of the body. The bacterium *Staphylococcus aureus* (stah-fih-lo-KAH-kus ARE-ree-us), also known as "staph," normally lives on the skin and sometimes in the mouth and nose of a healthy person. If staph enters the bloodstream, however, it can cause serious and sometimes fatal illness, such as pneumonia or heart infections. Healthy people sometimes can carry germs that cause infections while never contracting the disease themselves. The most famous example was Mary "Typhoid Mary" Mallon, a young cook who unknowingly passed on *Salmonella typhi* (sal-muh-NEH-luh TIE-fee) bacteria in the food she cooked while working for several New York families in the early 1900s. Many people fell ill with typhoid fever*, but Mary never became sick. Another common example is group B streptococcal (strep-tuh-KAH-kul) bacteria, which can exist in the birth canal of a pregnant woman without causing illness to the mother but can be transmitted to the baby during delivery. Meningococcus (muh-nin-guh-KOH-kus) bacteria, too, can live harmlessly in one person's nose and throat but can cause deadly disease in another. When a person without symptoms has a germ that can be transmitted to others, that person is called a carrier.

In other cases, people may have an immune system that is not working completely, a condition known as a compromised immune system. This problem is most common among the elderly, newborns, and those patients with certain chronic illnesses, diseases that affect the immune system directly, or some genetic* factors. Such people may become sick from an infection because their body defenses cannot fight off the germs as well.

How Germs Spread

Germs can spread through a number of ways. Examples include:

- aerosol spread, such as when tiny droplets of fluid are coughed, laughed, or sneezed into the air and are inhaled by another person or when fungal spores* are stirred up by wind or construction and are breathed in by people in the area
- sexual and intimate contact, sometimes including kissing
- direct contact, such as touching a fungal infection on a person's body or stepping on a parasite while walking barefoot outside
- contact with fomites (surfaces or non-living objects), such as when an infected child sneezes on a toy and then another child plays with the toy and places it in his or her own mouth
- blood contact during intravenous* drug use or, rarely, transfusions*

* **genitals** (JEH-nih-tuls) are the external sexual organs.

* **typhoid** (TIE-foyd) **fever** is an infection with the bacterium *Salmonella typhi* that causes fever, headache, confusion, and muscle aches.

* **genetic** (juh-NEH-tik) refers to heredity and the ways in which genes control the development and maintenance of organisms.

* **spores** are a temporarily inactive form of a germ enclosed in a protective shell.

* **intravenous** (in-tra-VEE-nus) or IV, means within or through a vein. For example, medications, fluid, or other substances can be given through a needle or soft tube inserted through the skin's surface directly into a vein.

* **transfusions** (trans-FYOO-zhunz) are procedures in which blood or certain parts of blood, such as specific cells, are given to a person who needs them because of illness or blood loss.

KOCH'S POSTULATES

Robert Koch (1843–1910), a German scientist and bacteriologist*, was the first researcher to use microscopic examinations and scientific methods to identify germs as the causes of specific diseases. Koch's postulates (POS-chuh-lits), which Koch had learned from his teacher Jacob Henle, are used to prove that an organism is responsible for a certain illness. These are the four criteria:

1. The germ should be present at the site of infection for all animals that have the disease in question.

2. The germ should be isolated from the sick animal; that is, grown in a pure culture* from a sample from the infected site.

3. When the pure culture is introduced into a healthy animal, the germ should trigger the same disease.

4. It should be possible to recover the germ from the experimentally infected animal.

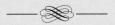

* **bacteriologist** (bak-teer-e-OL-o-jist) is a scientist who studies bacteria.

* **culture** (KUL-chur) is a test in which a sample of fluid or tissue from the body is placed in a dish containing material that supports the growth of certain organisms. Typically, within days the organisms will grow and can be identified.

* **vector** (VEK-tor) is an animal or insect that carries diseases and transfers them from one host to another.

▶ *See also*

AIDS and HIV Infection

Common Cold

Creutzfeldt-Jakob Disease

Helicobacter Pylori Infection (Peptic Ulcer Disease)

Hepatitis, Infectious

Herpes Simplex Virus Infections

Immune Deficiencies

Malaria

Pneumonia

Sexually Transmitted Diseases

Staphylococcal Infections

Tuberculosis

Vaccination (Immunization)

- contaminated foods and water, which can transmit harmful bacteria, viruses, and parasites when people eat the food or drink, swim, or play in the water

- the fecal-oral route, which spreads germs when people come into contact with feces (FEE-seez, or bowel movements) from someone who is infected and then touches the mouth, such as when day-care workers pass diarrhea (dye-uh-REE-uh)-causing rotavirus (RO-tuh-vy-rus) from one infant to the next between diaper changes

- pregnancy, birth, and breast-feeding, which can spread some infections from mother to baby

- animal or insect bites, such as those of mosquitoes (the most common insect vector*), fleas, and ticks

Resources

Organization

U.S. Centers for Disease Control and Prevention (CDC), 1600 Clifton Road, Atlanta, GA 30333. Through the website of the National Center for Infectious Diseases, the CDC provides information on the spread of germs and the prevention of infectious diseases, along with information about specific diseases.

Telephone 800-311-3435
http://www.cdc.gov

Website

KidsHealth.org. KidsHealth is a website created by the medical experts of the Nemours Foundation and is devoted to issues of children's health. It contains articles on a variety of health topics, including the nature and spread of germs and how to avoid infectious diseases. http://www.KidsHealth.org

Body Defenses

Physical Barriers

The human body constantly faces attack from foreign invaders that can cause infection and disease. These invaders range from living microbes (MY-krobes), such as bacteria*, fungi*, parasites*, and viruses*, to non-living toxins, chemicals, and drugs. Fortunately, the body has a number of external and internal safeguards that prevent most dangerous invaders from entering and causing harm. The physical barriers that keep them at bay commonly are referred to as the body's first line of defense. Skin, the largest body organ, provides both a physical and a chemical barrier against the outside world. The skin forms a protective layer that completely wraps around the body, shielding blood vessels, nerves, muscles, organs, and bones. When cuts or tears in the surface of the skin provide an entrance for infective agents, glands beneath the skin produce an enzyme* that helps kill bacteria.

Areas of the body not covered with skin do not go unprotected. Mucous membranes, the moist linings of the respiratory system, produce mucus (MYOO-kus), a sticky substance that traps irritants that enter through the nose. Structures like tiny hairs, called cilia (SIH-lee-uh), line the body's airways and constantly wave foreign particles and mucus away from the lungs to where they can be swallowed safely. Most harmful microbes that make it to the stomach are destroyed by stomach acids. In addition, tears and saliva both contain enzymes that destroy invaders. Another important defense mechanism is the brain-blood barrier, a specialized "filter" that surrounds the brain and spinal cord and acts as a physical barrier to keep out proteins, toxins, and most microbes, while letting in glucose, the source of the brain's nutrients.

The Immune System

A second line of defense is housed within the body: a finely tuned immune system that recognizes and destroys foreign substances and organisms that enter the body. The immune system can distinguish between the body's own tissues and outside substances called antigens*.

KEYWORDS
*for searching the Internet
and other reference sources*

Autoimmune diseases

Gamma globulin

Immune system

Immunodeficiency

Immunoglobulins

Lymph nodes

Lymphatic system

Lymphocytes

Phagocytes

* **bacteria** (bak-TEER-e-uh) are microscopic organisms, some types of which can cause disease.

* **fungi** (FUNG-eye) are microorganisms that can grow in or on the body, causing infections of internal organs or of the skin, hair, and nails.

* **parasites** (PAIR-uh-sites) are organisms such as protozoa (one-celled animals), worms, or insects that must live on or inside a human or other organism to survive. An animal or plant harboring a parasite is called its host. Parasites live at the expense of the host and may cause illness.

* **viruses** (VY-ruh-sez) are tiny infectious agents that can cause infectious diseases. A virus can only reproduce within the cells it infects.

13

* **enzyme** (EN-zime) is a protein that helps speed up a chemical reaction in the body.

* **antigens** (AN-tih-jens) are substances that are recognized as a threat by the body's immune system, which triggers the formation of specific antibodies against the substance.

* **bone marrow** is the soft tissue inside bones where blood cells are made.

* **lymphatic** (lim-FAH-tik) **system** is a system that contains lymph nodes and a network of channels that carry fluid and cells of the immune system through the body.

* **immunity** (ih-MYOON-uh-tee) is the condition of being protected against an infectious disease. Immunity often develops after a germ is introduced to the body. One type of immunity occurs when the body makes special protein molecules called antibodies to fight the disease-causing germ. The next time that germ enters the body, the antibodies quickly attack it, usually preventing the germ from causing disease.

This allows cells of the immune army to identify and destroy only those enemy antigens. The ability to identify an antigen also permits the immune system to "remember" antigens the body has been exposed to in the past, so that the body can mount a better and faster immune response the next time any of these antigens appear.

Lymphocytes (LIM-fo-sites), white blood cells that develop in bone marrow* and circulate throughout the body in the lymphatic system*, are a vital part of the immune system. Lymphocytes can be divided into two subgroups: B lymphocytes and T lymphocytes. B lymphocytes (or B cells) produce immunoglobulins (ih-myoo-no-GLAH-byoo-lins), also called antibodies (AN-tih-bah-deez). These protein molecules attach themselves to specific antigens and work with another type of white blood cell, called phagocytes (FAH-go-sites)—scavenger cells that surround and digest infected cells or microorganisms—to destroy the invaders. T lymphocytes (or T cells) help control the immune response and destroy foreign antigens directly.

The activity of B cells and T cells targets specific antigens. This means that each time a new kind of antigen invades the body, the immune system must produce a new round of B cells and T cells, which attack only that antigen. It is estimated that the immune system can create more than 100 million types of antibodies. As B cells and T cells mature, they begin to recognize which tissues belong in the body and which do not. These cells become "memory" cells that remember a particular antigen, so that the next time it appears, the immune response can mobilize quickly. In some cases, people have permanent immunity* to a disease; for example, people who contract chicken pox usually will not have it again—or, if they do, they will have a much more mild case.

The immune system works with amazing complexity. When a B cell encounters a foreign invader, it starts to produce immunoglobulins, or antibodies. Like a key designed to fit only a specific lock, an antibody "locks" onto a single type of antigen like an identifying marker. Once the antibody attaches to an antigen, one class of T cells called helper T cells alerts other white blood cells to head toward the site, while another class called killer T cells begins to destroy the antigen marked by the antibody. At the same time, millions of antibodies swarm through the bloodstream to attach to any more of that type of antigen and mount a larger attack.

The immune system also includes other proteins and chemicals that assist antibodies and T cells in their work. Among them are chemicals that alert phagocytes to the site of the infection. The complement system, a group of proteins that normally float freely in the blood, move toward infections, where they combine to help destroy microorganisms and foreign particles. They do this by changing the surface of bacteria or other microorganisms, causing them to die.

In some instances, people receive antibodies from another person to help their own immunity. This is known as passive immunity. Infants are born with immature immune systems and receive important anti-

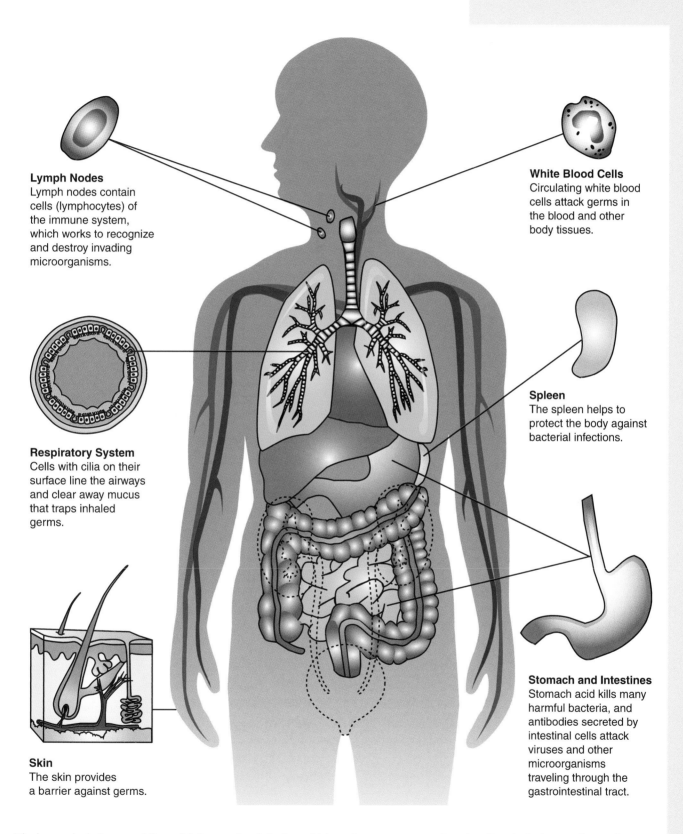

Lymph Nodes
Lymph nodes contain cells (lymphocytes) of the immune system, which works to recognize and destroy invading microorganisms.

White Blood Cells
Circulating white blood cells attack germs in the blood and other body tissues.

Respiratory System
Cells with cilia on their surface line the airways and clear away mucus that traps inhaled germs.

Spleen
The spleen helps to protect the body against bacterial infections.

Skin
The skin provides a barrier against germs.

Stomach and Intestines
Stomach acid kills many harmful bacteria, and antibodies secreted by intestinal cells attack viruses and other microorganisms traveling through the gastrointestinal tract.

The human body has several lines of defense against infection, which work to prevent germs from invading the body or to destroy them once they find their way in.

* **placenta** (pluh-SEN-ta) is an organ that provides nutrients and oxygen to a developing baby; it is located within the womb during pregnancy.

* **pneumonia** (nu-MO-nyah) is inflammation of the lung.

* **bronchitis** (brong-KYE-tis) is a disease that involves inflammation of the larger airways in the respiratory tract, which can result from infection or other causes.

* **influenza** (in-floo-EN-zuh), also known as the flu, is a contagious viral infection that attacks the respiratory tract, including the nose, throat, and lungs.

* **vaccine** (vak-SEEN) is a preparation of killed or weakened germs, or a part of a germ or product it produces, given to prevent or lessen the severity of the disease that can result if a person is exposed to the germ itself. Use of vaccines for this purpose is called immunization.

* **histamine** (HIS-tuh-meen) is a substance released by the body during inflammation. It causes blood vessels to expand and makes it easier for fluid and other substances to pass through vessel walls.

bodies from their mothers, both during pregnancy (across the mother's placenta*) and after birth from breast milk. These antibodies usually disappear within 6 to 12 months, but until then they help protect the infant against a range of infections, including pneumonia*, bronchitis*, influenza*, and ear infection. Doctors also can give people gamma globulin (GAH-muh GLAH-byoo-lin), an antibody preparation that offers temporary immunity to patients who might need this protection. When a person gets an immunization, or vaccine*, the body's immune system learns to recognize that particular bacteria or virus. If, sometime later, the person is exposed to the germ again, the body can fight it off and not come down with the disease.

Other Defenses

Along with physical barriers and the immune system, the body has several other mechanisms that fight antigens. Coughing or sneezing is an automatic reflex that can rid the body of irritants. Interferon (in-ter-FEER-on), a naturally occurring substance in the body that fights infection or tumors, is produced automatically when the immune system is called into action.

The inflammatory response, or inflammation (in-flah-MAY-shun), is an important body response to injury. When bacteria, toxins, burns, or other culprits damage tissue, the injured tissues leak chemicals, including histamine* and other substances. This chemical cocktail causes blood vessels around the damaged area to leak fluid into the injured tissues and make them swell. The increased flow of blood and fluid to the area also brings phagocytes and other infection-fighting cells to take care of any toxins or other antigens in the area. Pus, which is a fluid containing dead body cells and tissue, dead bacteria, dead toxins, and dead and living phagocytes, sometimes forms at the site of inflammation. To the eye, inflamed skin may appear red and swollen, and the area may feel slightly warm to the touch. Ancient physicians used the Latin terms "dolor," "rubor," "calor," and "tumor" to refer, respectively, to pain, redness, heat, and swelling, the hallmarks of inflammation. Inflammation also may cause a fever. The increase in body heat can help kill bacteria or viruses at the site of the infection.

Immune Responses and Disease

Strong and healthy immune systems successfully ward off many diseases, particularly infections, but weakened immune responses can permit various diseases to develop. Age can influence the immune system's effectiveness. Newborns and the elderly may have a weak or impaired immune response to antigens. Newborns' immune systems are not fully developed at birth but typically become stronger during the first year of life. To strengthen their immune response, newborns can benefit from breastfeeding.

Immune systems that work but react incorrectly to the antigens within a person's body can lead to a number of immunological (ih-myoo-no-LAH-jih-kul) disorders. These are called autoimmune (aw-toh-ih-MYOON) diseases. In autoimmune diseases, the body cannot distinguish between itself and foreign particles and may turn its disease-fighting powers on its own tissues, blood, and organs. Although no specific cause for this imbalance has been uncovered, hormones* may be involved.

Gender factors into who might experience an autoimmune disease. According to the American Autoimmune Related Diseases Association, of the more than 80 chronic autoimmune diseases, about 75 percent of cases occur in women, and women appear to be most vulnerable to these diseases during their childbearing years, when the levels of hormones are highest in their bodies. Heredity seems to play a part as well. A person may inherit the tendency to have an autoimmune disorder but might not have the same disease a close relative has. For example, a grandmother may have rheumatoid arthritis*, and the granddaughter may have lupus*. These conditions are related in many ways, but they are different diseases.

Some common medical conditions can put people at increased risk for infections. People with diabetes* are especially prone to infection, in part because high levels of sugar in the blood can interfere with the functions of certain white blood cells. Patients with chronic lung disease are often at a high risk for pneumonia and bronchitis. Urinary tract infections tend to occur more frequently among people born with abnormal urinary tracts or those who experience an obstruction, such as a kidney stone*. People with certain types of heart disease, particularly of the heart valves, are more likely to have endocarditis (en-do-kar-DYE-tis), an inflammation of the inner lining of the heart (called the endocardium, en-doh-KAR-dee-um), after dental procedures or surgery. Chronic malnutrition that causes a protein deficiency in the body also can lead to immune problems, because immunoglobulins and other parts of the immune system are made up largely of proteins.

Compromised Immune Systems

Chronic diseases can wear down the immune system and make people more susceptible to infection. An immune system that is weakened in this way is said to be compromised. Sickle-cell anemia*, for instance, causes damage to the spleen*. Because the spleen helps protect against bacterial infections, this leaves the body more vulnerable to infections, such as those involving the lungs, bone, and blood. As human immunodeficiency virus (HYOO-mun ih-myoo-no-dih-FIH-shen-see) (HIV) infection damages and weakens the immune system, many kinds of infectious diseases that take advantage of a poor immune response can appear. In many cases, prompt diagnosis of such "opportunistic" infections and treatment with combinations of antiviral drugs have been able to slow this process.

Certain drugs and therapy regimens also can undermine the work of the immune system. Chemotherapy drugs, a term for several kinds

* **hormones** are chemical substances that are produced by various glands and sent into the bloodstream carrying messages that have certain effects on other parts of the body.

* **rheumatoid arthritis** (ROO-mah-toyd ar-THRY-tis) is a chronic disease characterized by painful swelling, stiffness, and deformity of the joints.

* **lupus** (LOO-pus) is a chronic, or long-lasting, disease that causes inflammation of connective tissue, the material that holds together the various structures of the body.

* **diabetes** (dye-uh-BEE-teez) is a condition in which the body's pancreas does not produce enough insulin or the body cannot use the insulin it makes effectively, resulting in increased levels of sugar in the blood. This can lead to increased urination, dehydration, weight loss, weakness, and a number of other symptoms and complications related to chemical imbalances within the body.

* **kidney stone** is a hard structure that forms in the urinary tract. This structure is composed of crystallized chemicals that have separated from the urine. It can obstruct the flow of urine and cause tissue damage and pain as the body attempts to pass the stone through the urinary tract and out of the body.

* **sickle-cell anemia**, also called sickle-cell disease, is a hereditary condition in which the red blood cells, which are usually round, take on an abnormal crescent shape and have a decreased ability to carry oxygen throughout the body.

* **spleen** is an organ in the upper left part of the abdomen that stores and filters blood. As part of the immune system, the spleen also plays a role in fighting infection.

In severe combined immunodeficiency, a person's ability to fight infections is severely impaired. This condition has been dubbed "bubble boy disease" and became widely known during the 1970s with the case of David Vetter, who lived for 12 years sealed in a plastic, germ-free environment. *Visuals Unlimited* ▶

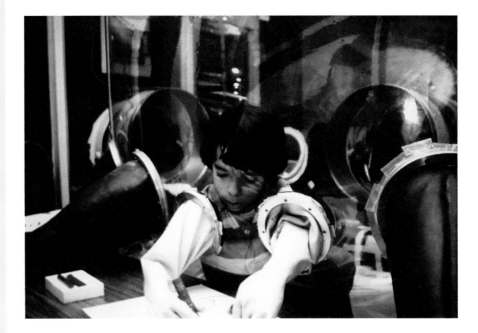

* **genetic** (juh-NEH-tik) refers to heredity and the ways in which genes control the development and maintenance of organisms.

* **sepsis** is a potentially serious spreading of infection, usually bacterial, through the bloodstream and body.

* **meningitis** (meh-nin-JY-tis) is an inflammation of the meninges, the membranes that surround the brain and the spinal cord. Meningitis is most often caused by infection with a virus or a bacterium.

* **lymph** (LIMF) **nodes** are small, bean-shaped masses of tissue that contain immune system cells that fight harmful microorganisms. Lymph nodes may swell during infections.

of drugs that destroy cancer cells, often kill the beneficial white blood cells in the bone marrow as well. Patients who have organ transplants are given high dosages of drugs called corticosteroids (kor-tih-ko-STIR-oyds) to suppress their immune systems and try to keep their bodies from rejecting the transplanted tissue, which typically is recognized as "foreign."

Some people's immunity is weakened from the beginning, because they are born with components missing from their immune systems. Primary immune deficiencies are genetic* conditions that impair the immune system. Hypogammaglobulinemia (hi-po-gah-muh-gloh-byoo-lih-NEE-me-uh), a condition that arises when the body has fewer antibodies than normal, can result in more bacterial respiratory illnesses. Agammaglobulinemia (a-gah-muh-gloh-byoo-lih-NEE-me-uh), a complete lack of antibodies in the blood, can cause severe, often fatal infections. Other primary immune disorders include these:

▪ Severe combined immune deficiency syndrome, in which an infant is born with a significant lack of both B cells and T cells, often leads to serious immunity problems; it occurs in one in a million births. During the first 3 months of life, babies with this condition can experience life-threatening infections and diseases, particularly sepsis*, pneumonia, and meningitis*. Common childhood diseases, such as chicken pox, can easily overwhelm these patients' immune systems.

▪ Chronic granulomatous (gran-yoo-LO-muh-tus) disease occurs in males when the body's phagocytes are ineffective against certain bacteria and fungi. Patients develop recurrent and unusual skin, lymph node*, and other infections. Repeated infections can lead to granulomas (gran-yoo-LO-muhs), masses that develop in the skin, lungs, liver*, lymph nodes, and bones. They can be slow to heal and drain.

Other Influences

Numerous other influences can affect the health of the immune system as well. In societies where smoking is acceptable, for example, people are more at risk for lung cancer and respiratory ailments, both of which can lead to various secondary infections, including bronchitis. Second-hand smoke, or passive smoking, increases respiratory infections for both infants and children. Children who are exposed to second-hand smoke may be predisposed to pneumonia, allergies*, and asthma* as well as repeated irritations of the eyes, nose, and mouth.

Nutrition, too, has an impact on the immune system. Malnutrition, with diets deficient in a variety of nutrients, such as certain vitamins, minerals, or protein, can cause increased vulnerability to infection.

Resources

Organizations

American Autoimmune Related Diseases Association, 22100 Gratiot Avenue, E. Detroit, MI 48021. The American Autoimmune Related Diseases Association offers information on many autoimmune diseases. Telephone 586-776-3900
http://www.aarda.org

Genetic Alliance, 4301 Connecticut Avenue NW, Suite 404, Washington, D.C., 20008. The Genetic Alliance offers information about genetic diseases, including autoimmune disorders, and links to support groups.
Telephone 800-336-4363
http://www.geneticalliance.org

Website

KidsHealth.org. KidsHealth is a website created by the medical experts of the Nemours Foundation and is devoted to issues of children's health. It contains articles on a variety of health topics, including information about the immune system and related topics, such as urinary tract infections, bronchitis, immunization, lupus, the spleen and lymphatic system, fungal infections, diabetes, genetic disorders, and many others.
http://www.KidsHealth.org

* **liver** is a large organ located beneath the ribs on the right side of the body. The liver performs numerous digestive and chemical functions essential for health.

* **allergies** are immune system–related sensitivities to certain substances, for example, cat dander or the pollen of certain plants, that cause various reactions, such as sneezing, runny nose, wheezing, or swollen, itchy patches on the skin, called hives.

* **asthma** (AZ-mah) is a condition in which the airways of the lungs repeatedly become narrowed and inflamed, causing breathing difficulty.

▶ See also

AIDS and HIV Infection

Bronchitis, Infectious

Endocarditis, Infectious

Fungal Infections

Immune Deficiencies

Meningitis

Pneumonia

Sepsis

Urinary Tract Infections

Vaccination (Immunization)

Varicella (Chicken Pox) and Herpes Zoster (Shingles)

Signs and Symptoms

What Is a Sign and What Is a Symptom?

Although the words may sound interchangeable, doctors use the word "symptom" to mean something different from the word "sign." A symptom is anything a patient experiences or feels, such as a headache, dizziness, or the sensation of nausea (NAW-zee-uh). A sign, on the other hand, is something that can be noted by a doctor during a physical examination, such as elevated blood pressure, fever, or swollen elbow. Doctors, when they see a patient, typically ask about symptoms that the person might be experiencing and check the body for signs of disease. By carefully evaluating symptoms and signs of a patient's illness, by taking a thorough history, and, if necessary, by ordering laboratory tests, doctors can determine the nature of a patient's problem (that is, they can make a diagnosis).

Common Signs and Symptoms

Modern medicine uses all sorts of advanced laboratory testing and imaging techniques, such as X rays, computerized tomography* scans, and magnetic resonance imaging*. Most of the time, however, doctors make a correct diagnosis in the same basic way as physicians have for hundreds of years—by talking with patients about what hurts or what seems different about how they feel, and by examining patients to see whether an illness or problem can be seen, heard, felt, or even smelled. Certain bacterial infections, for example, have characteristic odors—such as the sweet smell caused by the bacteria* *Pseudomonas aeruginosa.* Just as with detective work, reaching the proper medical conclusion involves a lot of careful listening and observing.

People with infectious diseases, whether caused by viruses*, bacteria, or other agents, often have many of the same signs and symptoms. The following examples are some of the most common:

- Fever, which many patients recognize when they feel warm or hot, is described as any body temperature that exceeds about 100 degrees Fahrenheit. Fevers generally are described as falling into two categories: low grade, about 102 degrees or less, and high grade, about 103 degrees or more. A fever may spike, where it soars and then drops quickly, or cycle, where the person's temperature rises and falls at regular intervals. Chills and shivering sometimes appear with a fever, especially during a temperature spike.

- Coughs often accompany airway irritations—for example, the inflammation that comes with an airway infection, such as a cold, or with the postnasal drip of allergies. One purpose of the cough reflex is to protect the body by expelling irritants from the airway. When confronted with a cough in a physical exam, a

KEYWORDS
for searching the Internet
and other reference sources

Congestion

Cough

Fever

Jaundice

Malaise

Medical examination

Medical history

Nausea

Rash

Sore throat

* **computerized tomography** (kom-PYOO-ter-ized toe-MAH-gruh-fee) or CT, also called computerized axial tomography (CAT), is a technique in which a machine takes many X rays of the body to create a three-dimensional picture.

* **magnetic resonance imaging (MRI)** uses magnetic waves, instead of X rays, to scan the body and produce detailed pictures of the body's structures.

* **bacteria** (bak-TEER-e-uh) are microscopic organisms, some types of which can cause disease.

* **viruses** (VY-ruh-sez) are tiny infectious agents that can cause infectious diseases. A virus can reproduce only within the cells it infects.

By identifying the precise signs (objective information that a doctor gathers from physical examination and tests) and symptoms (the patient's subjective physical feelings and experiences), physicians can determine the nature of an illness or injury. In this case, the signs and symptoms indicate that this girl has a broken bone in her arm.

Signs

Swelling of the wrist

Wrist area warm to the touch

Rapid heartbeat in response to pain

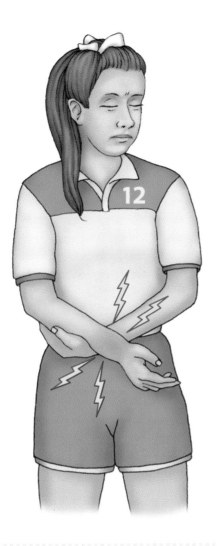

Symptoms

Pain in the hand and arm

Dizziness

Nausea

physician tries to discover as much about it as possible, through talking with and examining the patient. Observing breathing patterns and listening through a stethoscope are important parts of such an exam.

Congestion, otherwise known as a stuffy nose, may be caused by a viral infection, an allergy, or another problem that affects mucus* production in the airway or causes swelling and blockage of nasal and airway tissues.

Nausea is the feeling that the patient is queasy or needs to vomit. People also may describe this sensation as an upset stomach. Some instances of nausea may be due to eating food contaminated with bacteria (such as *Salmonella*, sal-muh-NEH-luh, in chicken that was not cooked thoroughly), but other medical problems, such as a concussion* or kidney* failure, also can result in nausea. Vomiting or diarrhea (dye-uh-REE-uh) often accompany nausea.

* **mucus** (MYOO-kus) is a thick, slippery substance that lines the insides of many body parts.

* **concussion** (kon-KUH-shun) is an injury to the brain, produced by a blow to the head or violent shaking.

* **kidney** is one of the pair of organs that filter blood and remove waste products and excess water from the body in the form of urine.

* **autoimmune** (aw-toh-ih-MY-OON) **diseases** are diseases in which the body's immune system attacks some of the body's own normal tissues and cells.

* **lupus** (LOO-pus) is a chronic, or long-lasting, disease that causes inflammation of connective tissue, the material that holds together the various structures of the body.

* **immune system** is the system of the body composed of specialized cells and the substances they produce that helps protect the body against disease-causing germs.

* **lymphatic** (lim-FAH-tik) **system** is a system that contains lymph nodes and a network of channels that carry fluid and cells of the immune system through the body.

* **mononucleosis** (mah-no-nu-klee-O-sis) is an infectious illness caused by a virus that often leads to fever, sore throat, swollen glands, and tiredness.

* **mucous membranes** are the moist linings of the mouth, nose, eyes, and throat.

* **bilirubin** (bih-lih-ROO-bin) is a substance that the body produces when hemoglobin, an iron-containing component of the blood, is broken down.

* **liver** is a large organ located beneath the ribs on the right side of the body. The liver performs numerous digestive and chemical functions essential for health.

* **bile duct** is a passageway that carries bile, a substance that aids the digestion of fat, from the liver to the gallbladder (a small pouch-like organ where the bile is temporarily stored) and from the gallbladder to the small intestine.

Sore throats (called pharyngitis, fair-un-JY-tis) are characterized as pain, discomfort, or a scratchy feeling, often when swallowing. The most common cause of sore throat is a viral infection, though there are many other causes.

Muscle aches often accompany infections, but they also can stem from a variety of other causes, ranging from overuse of a muscle during work or exercise to autoimmune diseases*. Aches may occur over much of the body, or they may be confined to one area.

Rashes are temporary changes in the skin's color and texture. They may erupt suddenly, and many are marked by inflammation. Some infectious diseases, such as chicken pox or Lyme disease, can be identified by their distinctive rashes. Rashes also can be caused by many noninfectious conditions, such as lupus* or allergies.

Swollen lymph (LIMF) glands, or lymph nodes, may appear when the immune system* is fighting an infection. Lymph nodes contain cells that fight harmful microorganisms and are part of a system (the lymphatic system*) that helps protect the body against infections. During certain infections these protective nodes, which are usually the size of peas, can swell and become tender. Lymph nodes may be swollen near the site of infection (for example, in the neck with strep, a bacterial infection of the throat) or more generally at different sites of the body (for example, in the groin, under the armpits, and in the neck with mononucleosis* and certain other viral illnesses).

Jaundice (JON-dis) is a yellow hue to the skin, the whites of the eyes, and the mucous membranes*. A buildup of excess bilirubin* in the blood causes the color change. While jaundice in newborn infants often is harmless and easily resolved, in older children or adults, this symptom may signal a problem with the liver*, a blocked bile duct*, or an abnormal breakdown of red blood cells. Hepatitis B (heh-puh-TIE-tis), an infectious disease caused by a virus that inflames the liver, often results in jaundice.

Malaise describes a general feeling of illness and exhaustion that can accompany various diseases. A patient with malaise will typically "just feel sick."

Fatigue is a sensation of weariness or tiredness that may suggest too little sleep, too much physical activity, poor nutrition, stress, infection, or other medical or emotional problem. Patients who experience fatigue may or may not want to sleep.

Weakness can be described as a loss of muscle strength. This symptom can be subjective, meaning that a patient feels the symptom but there is no measurable loss of strength, or it can be objective, meaning that a decrease in strength can be measured.

▨ Swelling is an enlargement of a part of the body, such as an area of skin or an organ. Swelling often stems from a buildup of fluid or tissue. It can occur in one specific area or throughout the body. Infections are just one possible cause of swelling.

▨ Irritability is a word often used to describe young infants who act extremely fussy and cannot be comforted as they usually would be. Irritability may signal any of a number of problems, including the start of an illness, even before other signs and symptoms appear.

What Is the Doctor's Role?

To arrive at an accurate diagnosis of an infectious illness, doctors take a "history." This means they ask patients about their symptoms, any medications they are taking, their past medical problems, and their family's medical problems. Then they examine patients and sometimes order laboratory and other diagnostic tests, as necessary. Putting together all this information, doctors then can consider the possibilities.

The questions posed to a patient in the course of the medical history are tailored to that person's particular symptoms. The doctor may ask for a description of the symptoms, such as how and when they occur. He or she may ask how long the symptoms last and what makes them better or worse. The doctor also may ask what sorts of illnesses the patient has had previously and whether anyone in the patient's family has similar problems or if certain diseases run in the family.

Once the doctor completes a medical history and a family history, the interview moves on to a complete physical examination. As the doctor examines different parts of the body, four basic techniques are used:

▨ Inspection is simply observing the affected body area or part.

▨ Palpation involves touching the area with the hands to check for size, texture, or tenderness.

▨ Auscultation describes the technique of using a stethoscope to listen to the sounds made by the heart, lungs, and intestines.

▨ Percussion is tapping the skin over organs with fingers or small instruments to produce different sounds. These sounds can reveal whether the organ is filled with fluid. Lungs, for example, should have a "hollow" sound, because they are filled with air, whereas the abdomen (the area below the ribs and above the hips that contains the stomach, intestines, and other organs) may have a duller, flatter sound because it contains some fluid.

To confirm a diagnosis or to gather additional clinical information, the doctor may also order laboratory tests. With test results in hand, the doctor combines this information with the knowledge gained from the

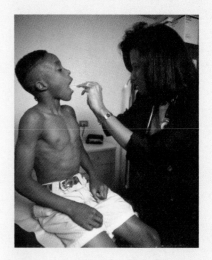

▲

A sample of the discharge from an infection can be swabbed from the throat and placed in a culture medium, a jelly-like substance that aids bacterial growth. If the cause of a sore throat is bacterial, the bacteria will grow and multiply in the medium and then can be identified. *Custom Medical Stock Photo, Inc.*

23

▶ *See also*
Laboratory Tests
Sore Throat

KEYWORDS
*for searching the Internet
and other reference sources*

Blood tests

Complete blood count (CBC)

Computerized tomography (CT) scan

Echocardiogram

ELISA

Erythrocyte sedimentation rate (ESR)

Gram stain

Laboratory culture

Magnetic resonance imaging (MRI)

Nucleic acid test (NAT)

Serology testing

Ultrasound

Urinalysis

X rays

* **pus** is a thick, creamy fluid, usually yellow or greenish in color, that forms at the site of an infection. Pus contains infection-fighting white cells and other substances.

history and the physical exam to arrive at a possible explanation for the patient's symptoms.

Resource

Organization

U.S. National Library of Medicine, 8600 Rockville Pike, Bethesda, MD 20894. The National Library of Medicine has a website packed with information on diseases and drugs, consumer resources, dictionaries and encyclopedias of medical terms, and directories of doctors and helpful organizations.
Telephone 888-346-3656
http://www.nlm.nih.gov

Laboratory Tests

What Are Laboratory Tests?

Before doctors can treat someone, they have to understand what is causing the illness. By talking with the patient ("taking the history"), examining the patient, and, when necessary, ordering tests (often called laboratory or lab tests), a doctor is better able to determine the illness. Most of the time, a doctor will be able to make the diagnosis without needing to order any tests. Thousands of possible tests exist, ranging from simple, inexpensive tests, such as looking at the color of urine, to much more complicated and expensive ones, such as certain types of X rays. Through training and experience, doctors learn when to order lab tests, which ones to order, and how to interpret the results.

Tests are meant to help identify the cause of a person's illness. Sometimes a test reveals the specific organism or cause and the diagnosis will be made relatively easily. For example, a person with a high fever, painful sore throat, and pus* on the tonsil* area may have a positive throat culture for *Streptococcus* (strep-tuh-KAH-kus) bacteria. The lab test, in this case a throat culture, confirms the diagnosis of strep throat.

Sometimes a lab test will only suggest the possibility of a specific cause and making the diagnosis will require much more judgment. For example, an elderly person feeling short of breath may have an X ray that could mean a type of heart disease, but more tests would be necessary to confirm that diagnosis.

A lab test also can eliminate a suspected cause, shortening the list of diagnoses to be considered. For example, a person with anemia* might have been tested for the amount of iron in the blood. A normal (or "negative") test would help eliminate the diagnosis of "iron-deficiency" anemia and help guide the evaluation toward other possibilities.

The History of Laboratory Testing

The existence of microbes has been known since Antonie van Leeuwenhoek first described "little animals in rain water" in 1674, but it was Robert Koch, the "father of modern bacteriology" (the study of bacteria), who proved that a specific organism caused a specific disease. His first discovery was with anthrax (AN-thraks), an infectious disease caused by the bacterium *Bacillus anthracis.* In 1876, Koch described the life cycle of the bacillus as it went from spore* to infectious agent. In 1881 Louis Pasteur took it one step further and was able to develop an effective vaccine against anthrax for sheep and cattle.

Following his work with anthrax, Koch set out to find a better way of growing and isolating microorganisms*. Previously, he had used liquid cultures, which were easily contaminated with other organisms, and he needed live animals as incubators to grow the bacteria he was studying. Based on his observations of colonies (groups visible to the naked eye) of microorganisms growing on a boiled potato, he set out to develop a solid substance (a nutrient medium) on which he could grow bacteria. With the help of his assistant Julius Richard Petri, who is remembered for the invention of the petri dish, he developed methods for isolating colonies of microorganisms.

The method for culturing bacteria that Koch developed over a century ago became the commonly accepted standard for use by labs. Since that time, culture methods have improved—and laboratories now also culture yeast, fungi*, and viruses*. How is that done? First, a sample of the infected fluid or tissue is obtained. This can be as simple as a swab of fluid taken from the throat or a urine sample, or it may be pus drained from an abscess* or a piece of tissue removed from an infected area (a procedure called a biopsy, BI-op-see). Then, under special conditions, the organisms are allowed to grow and are identified under the microscope. Additional testing may be done to determine whether the microorganism would be killed by various commonly used antibiotics*. This is how the doctor knows that the right antibiotic has been chosen to eliminate the organism. This step has become increasingly important because some bacteria that were once successfully treated with a certain antibiotic are now becoming resistant to it.

Culture results usually take 24 to 48 hours, but some bacteria take a long time to grow, and those results may take a week or longer. In the meantime, doctors may use other tests that yield immediate results, such as looking at the organism under a microscope and staining techniques. These tests can help doctors make a diagnosis and decide on treatment while they are waiting for the final culture results. For example, the thrashing tail movements of the protozoa* *Trichomonas vaginalis,* the cause of trichomoniasis*, are easily seen on a slide under a microscope in the doctor's office. Staining (adding certain colors, or dyes) an organism allows the doctor to identify the organism based on its appearance. This is

* **tonsils** are paired clusters of lymph tissues in the throat that help protect the body from bacteria and viruses that enter through a person's nose or mouth.

* **anemia** (uh-NEE-me-uh) is a blood condition in which there is a decreased amount of oxygen-carrying hemoglobin in the blood and, usually, fewer than normal numbers of red blood cells.

* **spore** is a temporarily inactive form of a germ enclosed in a protective shell.

* **microorganisms** are tiny organisms that can be seen only using a microscope. Types of microorganisms include fungi, bacteria, and viruses.

* **fungi** (FUNG-eye) are microorganisms that can grow in or on the body, causing infections of internal organs or of the skin, hair, and nails.

* **viruses** (VY-ruh-sez) are tiny infectious agents that can cause infectious diseases. A virus can only reproduce within the cells it infects.

* **abscess** (AB-ses) is a localized or walled-off accumulation of pus caused by infection that can occur anywhere in the body.

* **antibiotics** (an-tie-by-AH-tiks) are drugs that kill or slow the growth of bacteria.

* **protozoa** (pro-tuh-ZOH-uh) are single-celled microorganisms (tiny organisms), some of which are capable of causing disease in humans.

* **trichomoniasis** (trih-ko-mo-NYE-uh-sis) is a common sexually transmitted disease caused by the parasite *Trichomonas vaginalis.*

Julius Richard Petri, an assistant to Robert Koch, gave his name to the petri dish. In 1887 he developed a way of growing bacteria in a shallow glass dish with a cover. This method made it easier to separate and identify the specific organisms that cause various infectious diseases. *Photo Researchers, Inc.*

▶

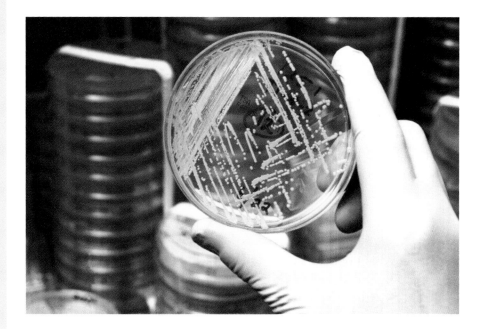

* **meningitis** (meh-nin-JY-tis) is an inflammation of the meninges, the membranes that surround the brain and the spinal cord. Meningitis is most often caused by infection with a virus or a bacterium.

* **diabetes** (dye-uh-BEE-teez) is a condition in which the body's pancreas does not produce enough insulin or the body cannot use the insulin it makes effectively, resulting in increased levels of sugar in the blood. This can lead to increased urination, dehydration, weight loss, weakness, and a number of other symptoms and complications related to chemical imbalances within the body.

especially helpful when rapid diagnosis is required, as in cases of meningitis*. A stain of a sample of spinal fluid can help distinguish between the purple stained, round streptococcal bacteria and the red stained, rod-shaped *E. coli*. Other rapid tests can lead to the right diagnosis, such as those looking for the antibodies produced during infection or for particles of the disease-causing microorganism. Many times the health of a patient will depend on how fast doctors can make the right diagnosis and start the right treatment.

Types of Laboratory Tests

Urinalysis   Urinalysis, or urine tests, allows for the rapid analysis of the urine. Special strips react by turning colors when dipped into a urine sample testing for blood, glucose (sugar), and other substances that may indicate infection. These "dipsticks" are a quick screen for possible urine infections, as well as other diseases such as diabetes* and problems with the kidneys. The urine also is examined under a microscope to look for bacteria, and the urine sample is sent to the lab to be cultured for bacteria if a urinary infection is suspected.

Stool tests   Just as doctors can examine and test the urine, they are able to examine the stool by a number of methods. Doctors can test for the presence of illness-causing bacteria, pus, blood, or unusual chemicals. Stool can be cultured for the bacteria that may cause diseases such as typhoid fever. The color of the stool may give evidence as to the cause of the problem. For example, very light stools could suggest a type of hepatitis.

Blood tests   Blood tests may be used to look for general signs of infection or to diagnose a specific infection. A complete blood count (CBC) measures the different parts that make up blood, including the numbers of red blood cells, white blood cells, and platelets*; the total amount of hemoglobin* in the blood; and even the size of red blood cells. During a bacterial infection, the number of white cells is often increased because they help fight off infection. If a person has anemia, this suggests the infection is attacking the red blood cells, as is seen with malaria*. A long-standing infection may also cause anemia. The platelets are involved in clotting* the blood, and their numbers may drop in some serious and overwhelming infections, such as meningitis. A CBC screen often is ordered when an infectious disease is suspected. Although it is not used to diagnose the cause, it is helpful for seeing how the body is reacting to an infection.

Spinal tap (lumbar puncture)   Sometimes, when an infection involving the brain or the coverings of the brain is suspected, doctors need to test the fluid that surrounds the brain. That type of infection, known as meningitis (the coverings of the brain are the meninges), can be life-threatening—and needs to be diagnosed and treated right away. One of the ways doctors can make the diagnosis is by a spinal tap (also known as a lumbar puncture or LP). This occurs when a doctor places a very thin hollow tube through a space between the bones (the vertebrae) in the lower back and then takes out a small amount of spinal fluid. Spinal fluid is the liquid that surrounds the brain and the spinal cord. By testing spinal fluid for bacteria and other substances, doctors can tell whether an infection is the cause of the person's illness.

Antibody and antigen tests   Antibody tests are commonly used to diagnose many infectious diseases. These tests measure the body's response to an infectious disease. Antibodies* are produced by the immune system* in response to antigens* found on the surface of the invading organism. It takes some time for the body to mount an antibody response to a new infection, so this test may not be useful when an illness is starting. The test is often repeated weeks later to measure any increase in antibodies. Once they are formed, many antibodies are present long after the infection is gone. This often (but not always) gives a person immunity, or protection, from future infection. Many infections are diagnosed using antibody testing, including hepatitis, Lyme disease, and HIV infection.

Unlike antibody tests (which indirectly measure the body's response to an infection), antigen tests directly detect the presence of the organism by identifying the specific proteins that the infectious organism has on its surface. Unlike antibody tests (which might indicate that there was an infection in the past), the presence of antigens most likely means the infection is present at that moment. Examples of antigen testing include rapid strep tests, chlamydia* tests, and some HIV testing.

Nucleic acid tests   Nucleic acid tests (NATs) are methods to identify tiny amounts of infectious organisms by multiplying (or amplifying) a small amount of that organism's DNA* to create a larger sample that

* **platelets** (PLATE-lets) are tiny disk-shaped particles within the blood that play an important role in clotting.

* **hemoglobin** (HE-muh-glo-bin) is the oxygen-carrying pigment of the red blood cells.

* **malaria** (mah-LAIR-e-uh) is a disease spread to humans by the bite of an infected mosquito.

* **clotting** is the body's way of thickening blood to stop bleeding.

* **antibodies** (AN-tih-bah-deez) are protein molecules produced by the body's immune system to help fight specific infections caused by microorganisms, such as bacteria and viruses.

* **immune system** is the system of the body composed of specialized cells and the substances they produce that helps protect the body against disease-causing germs.

* **antigens** (AN-tih-jenz) are substances that are recognized as a threat by the body's immune system, which triggers the formation of specific antibodies against the substances.

* **chlamydia** (kla-MIH-dee-uh) are microorganisms in the *Chlamydia* family that can infect the urinary tract, genitals, eye, and respiratory tract, including the lungs.

* **DNA**, or **deoxyribonucleic acid** (dee-OX-see-ry-bo-nyoo-klay-ik AH-sid), is the specialized chemical substance that contains the genetic code necessary to build and maintain the structures and functions of living organisms.

* *Helicobacter pylori* (HEEL-ih-ko-
bak-ter pie-LOR-eye) is a bacterium that causes inflammation
and ulcers, or sores, in the lining
of the stomach and the upper
part of the small intestine, also
known as peptic ulcer disease.

* pneumonia (nu-MO-nyah) is inflammation of the lung.

* radiotracer is a substance that
contains radioactive material.

can then be analyzed. They are a new and valuable tool in the identification of infectious agents, particularly those that are difficult to culture.
NATs are currently used in the diagnosis of hepatitis C and HIV and
are useful in making the diagnosis in infants because antibody testing is
not reliable at such a young age. NATs have also been used in the diagnosis of *Helicobacter pylori** infection, and tests are being developed
for the rapid diagnosis of many serious infectious diseases.

Imaging tests   Imaging tests, using a variety of technologies, give
physicians pictures of the inside of the body.

X RAYS   The use of X rays helps physicians "see" into the body without
opening it. In general, X rays involve aiming a controlled amount of radiation at a specific area of the body. When the radiation passes through
that part, it exposes a sort of photographic plate on the other side. If the
part of the body that the radiation passes through is dense (like bone) or
has a high water content (for example, lungs infected with pneumonia*),
the image on the plate will appear whiter. On occasion, doctors use a
special liquid to improve the contrast between light and dark, which helps
them better distinguish between different organs or see things in greater
detail. This contrast dye may be injected into veins or swallowed.

BONE SCANS   A bone scan is a type of X ray that helps doctors locate areas of infection or cancer deep within the bone. It does this by revealing spots of increased or decreased bone cell activity. First, a radiotracer*,
which can illuminate certain areas when scanned, is injected into a vein.
The scan is performed hours later, once the radiotracer has had time to
circulate in the body. A computer records the data from the scan and
translates it into an image. By comparing places on the image where the
tracer has (or has not) collected, doctors can pick out problem areas where
bones may be damaged or infected.

COMPUTERIZED TOMOGRAPHY   Computerized tomography (kom-PYOO-ter-
ized toe-MAH-gruh-fee), or CT, scans X ray the body from a variety of
angles. A scanner detects the X ray beams and transmits those data to a
computer, which shapes the data into a series of images or photographs.

MAGNETIC RESONANCE IMAGING   Magnetic resonance imaging (MRI) uses a
super-strong magnetic field, rather than X rays, to help create images.
The magnetic field causes the protons in the body's water to vibrate a
certain way, and the MRI machine records those vibrations and develops images based on them.

ULTRASOUND   In ultrasound, ultra-high-frequency waves are beamed into
the body, where they bounce off various structures. Somewhat similar in
principle to sonar in submarines, ultrasound is painless and cannot be
heard by the human ear. The machine records where the waves strike and
bounce back and interprets this data, creating images. Ultrasound is widely

used to help make diagnoses. One of the most common uses is part of regular prenatal care, when ultrasound is used to look at a baby in the womb to make sure it is developing normally. Ultrasound can be used to check specific organs, such as the liver* or kidneys, to look for unusual masses (tumors) or for abnormal size or density, such as might be seen with an abscess. An ultrasound image may appear as a single image, somewhat like a photograph, or as a moving image, like a video or movie.

ECHOCARDIOGRAM An echocardiogram (eh-ko-KAR-dee-uh-gram) is a specific type of ultrasound that sends sound waves into the chest to "paint a picture" of the heart's structure. This test can be used to see the size of the heart's valves and chambers, how well they move, and other qualities that a physician would need to know.

Other tests Other techniques also are used to identify infections. Some are very complex and expensive. Others are simple and cost almost nothing. For example, smell can sometimes help identify certain bacteria. *Pseudomonas* (which can cause urinary tract* infections and ear infections) smells sweet and fruity. The "whiff test" is a technique for diagnosing bacterial vaginosis, an overgrowth of vaginal bacteria. The chemical potassium hydroxide (KOH) is added to a small sample of fluid from the vagina. If the sample contains large numbers of bacteria, the KOH will make it smell fishy. A doctor also might add a few drops of KOH to a slide with scrapings from a suspected fungal infection, which will highlight the fungus. Using an ultraviolet or black light is another easy way to diagnose some fungal infections: the infected area glows when the light shines on it. Once the diagnosis of bacterial vaginosis is made, it is easily treated by a doctor.

Resources

Organization

U.S. National Library of Medicine, 8600 Rockville Pike, Bethesda, MD 20894. The National Library of Medicine has a website packed with information on diseases and drugs, consumer resources, dictionaries and encyclopedias of medical terms, and directories of doctors and helpful organizations.
Telephone 888-346-3656
http://www.nlm.nih.gov

Website

KidsHealth.org. KidsHealth is a website created by the medical experts of the Nemours Foundation and is devoted to issues of children's health. It contains articles on a variety of health topics, including why doctors order laboratory tests.
http://www.KidsHealth.org

* **liver** is a large organ located beneath the ribs on the right side of the body. The liver performs numerous digestive and chemical functions essential for health.

* **urinary tract** (YOOR-ih-nair-e TRAKT) is the system of organs and channels that makes urine and removes it from the body. It consists of the urethra, bladder, ureters, and kidneys.

▶ *See also*
Signs and Symptoms
The Nature of Germs and Infection
Treatments

Treatments

What Are Treatments?

Throughout life, every person will have at least one infection and more than likely, dozens of them. Fortunately, in many cases these infections will be relatively minor and will not require special treatment. However, some infections will need treatment to prevent them from spreading further and causing complications.

When you think about treating an infection, antibiotics (an-tie-by-AH-tiks) come to mind. Antibiotics are medicines aimed at halting the growth and spread of bacteria*, and they are a relatively new development in the history of medicine. None of the antibiotics we know today existed before the twentieth century. Before that time, people had to try to fight serious bacterial infections with other, mostly ineffective, treatments.

For thousands of years, it was not known what caused infections. However, it was known that once certain infections began, they could spread, sometimes with deadly results. Early physicians noticed that how an infection was treated could affect how a person recovered. Celsus, physician to the Roman gladiators, both observed the changes that we now call inflammation* and commented that keeping wounds dry, clean, and warm had beneficial effects. Yet it would be about a thousand years before it was fully understood why. Through the centuries, wounds and infections were treated with a variety of poultices, compounds, and elixirs. These substances, which might be made of herbs, various acids or caustic liquids, and even mud, were among the treatments used to prevent infections from spreading. Some of these treatments may have had some beneficial effects, though many probably did not.

Before the development of antibiotics, one of the primary treatments for a significant bacterial infection was cutting open the infected tissue and draining any pus* before the bacteria could spread further. Opening, or lancing, boils* and abscesses* was among the most common medical procedures. Physicians at a battlefield would amputate (AM-pyoo-tayt), or remove, limbs to prevent infections in wounds from spreading further in the injured soldiers. In fact, more soldiers died of infections during the American Civil War than died of bullet wounds. Dentists would travel from town to town to yank out infected teeth, and their patients would be glad to rid themselves of the pain. To make matters worse, treatment of pain was not very advanced either.

Nevertheless, many people survived their infections. Fortunately, the human body evolved with an immune system* that is able to fight off infection much of the time. The surgeries of the past worked partly because removing the infected tissue (an infected toe, for example) gave the body enough time to mount a successful defense against the infection. Still, before antibiotics and before doctors understood the need for

KEYWORDS
*for searching the Internet
and other reference sources*

Antibiotic resistance

Antibiotics

Antimicrobials

* **bacteria** (bak-TEER-e-uh) are microscopic organisms, some types of which can cause disease.

* **inflammation** (in-flah-MAY-shun) is the body's reaction to irritation, infection, or injury that often involves swelling, pain, redness, and warmth.

* **pus** is a thick, creamy fluid, usually yellow or greenish in color, that forms at the site of an infection. Pus contains infection-fighting white cells and other substances.

* **boils** are skin abscesses, or collections of pus in the skin.

* **abscesses** (AB-seh-sez) are localized or walled off accumulations of pus caused by infection that can occur anywhere within the body.

* **immune system** is the system of the body composed of specialized cells and the substances they produce that helps protect the body against disease-causing germs.

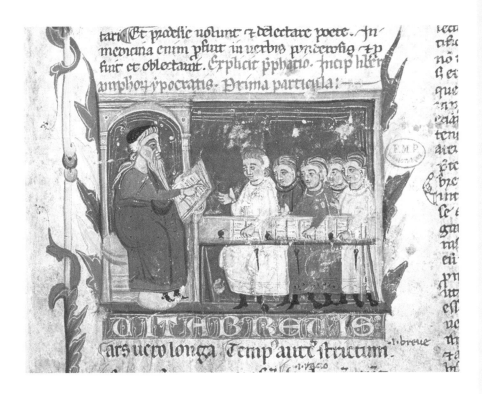

The Greek physician Hippocrates (ca. 460–370 B.C.) is considered the founder of clinical medicine. His descriptions of case histories of patients and comments on the symptoms of various diseases show the emerging rational and scientific approach to the diagnosis of disease, though his treatments had limited success. *Photo Researchers, Inc.*

complete cleanliness (sterility) during surgical procedures, treating a bacterial infection was often painful and destructive. Many infections that are successfully treated today, such as bacterial infections of the throat, lungs, heart, or nervous system, once were disabling or fatal.

Even though there is little need today for amputations to treat infections, the use of surgery to help combat certain types of infections is still important. This is particularly true for infections that are deep within the body—and where pockets of pus need to be removed (or drained). Other types of infections, like those involving bone, may also need surgery to help the healing process. Surgery often is required to prevent the spread of infection when a foreign object such as a bullet enters the body and needs to be removed.

Antibiotics and Bacterial Infections

Although today's antibiotics have only been around for two or three generations, herbs and other naturally occurring substances were among the treatments used to fight bacterial infection for thousands of years. In the fifteenth century, arsenic and mercury were used to treat syphilis*. These deadly compounds did have some success in killing the tiny bacterium that caused syphilis, but they unfortunately often poisoned the patient as well.

The era of modern antibiotics began in the 1890s when a German physician, Paul Ehrlich, began experimenting to develop methods to fight germs. He had noted that bacteria could be stained with dyes (colored chemicals) to be better seen through a microscope. Ehrlich believed that dyes could be created that would poison only the bacteria and not

* **syphilis** (SIH-fih-lis) is a sexually transmitted disease that, if untreated, can lead to serious lifelong problems throughout the body, including blindness and paralysis.

people. This idea of creating chemicals that would selectively kill bacteria (and other germs) and not their human hosts is the basis for modern antibiotics.

In 1928, Alexander Fleming, a Scottish scientist, first observed that the mold *Penicillium notatum* interfered with the growth of *Staphylococcus* (stah-fih-lo-KAH-kus) bacteria on a culture plate. Fleming's student, Cecil Paine, successfully used a crude extract of the mold to treat eye infections.

The job of purifying the extract to make the medicinal use of penicillin more practical was left to two British scientists, Howard Florey and Ernst Chain. By the end of World War II (1939-1945), the drug penicillin was produced for general use. Penicillin, the "wonder drug," transformed medical care, wiping out serious infections ranging from strep throat to pneumonia* to syphilis and from tuberculosis* to infections from war wounds. Penicillin gave birth to the wave of antibiotics that swept into the medical field throughout the twentieth century. Today a wide variety of antibiotics work by various means to prevent the growth and kill a wide range of disease-causing bacteria.

Different antibiotics work in different ways, but in general, these medicines work by interfering with key aspects of the life cycle of bacteria and limiting their growth. Others work to kill the bacteria by damaging their structure. In the future, antibiotics will work by a number of other mechanisms, including interfering with how bacteria attach to cells.

Antibiotics not only treat infections but also may be used in certain situations to prevent some infections from starting. For example, patients who have certain types of heart defects may be at risk for bacterial endocarditis (en-do-kar-DYE-tis), an inflammation of the inner membranes of the heart. They receive preventive (or prophylactic, pro-fih-LAK-tik) antibiotics to ward off bacterial infections when they undergo procedures that could involve minor bleeding, such as dental procedures. Preventive antibiotics also are given when someone is exposed to meningococcal meningitis (meh-nin-JY-tis); meningitis causes an inflammation of the membranes (or meninges; meh-NIN-jeez) that surround the brain and spinal cord and can be fatal if not treated promptly. People who have been exposed to pertussis (per-TUH-sis), or whooping cough, receive preventive antibiotics as well; whooping cough, a disease caused by the *Bordetella pertussis* bacterium, is a serious infection that can be fatal, especially in infants.

People who are at increased risk for developing bacterial infections may take daily antibiotics to help prevent infections. Among those who benefit from these preventive antibiotics are people with sickle-cell disease*, those who have had their spleen* removed, some children with chronic ear infections (otitis, o-TIE-tis), and people with HIV* infection.

How are antibiotics given?
For antibiotics to work, they have to get to the bacteria, and that can happen in a number of ways. Topical

* **pneumonia** (nu-MO-nyah) is inflammation of the lung.

* **tuberculosis** (too-ber-kyoo-LO-sis) is a bacterial infection that primarily attacks the lungs but can spread to other parts of the body.

* **sickle-cell disease** is a hereditary condition in which the red blood cells, which are usually round, take on an abnormal crescent shape and have a decreased ability to carry oxygen throughout the body.

* **spleen** is an organ in the upper left part of the abdomen that stores and filters blood. As part of the immune system, the spleen also plays a role in fighting infection.

* **HIV**, or **human immunodeficiency** (HYOO-mun ih-myoo-no-dih-FIH-shen-see) **virus**, is the virus that causes AIDS (acquired immunodeficiency syndrome).

antibiotics are placed directly on the involved area; oral medicine is swallowed as a pill or liquid; intravenous (in-tra-VEE-nus) antibiotics are injected into a vein using a liquid form; and intramuscular medication enters the body through a shot (or injection) into a muscle. Which form of medication and way it is given depends on the type of infection, where in the body the infection is, how severe the infection is, how much medication is needed, and the method that is most effective for the particular type of antibiotic. Some medications cannot be taken by mouth because the stomach acids would destroy them, for example.

Although antibiotics have saved and improved the lives of millions, like all medications they still have risks as well as benefits. Some antibiotics can react negatively with other medications or treatments a person is taking. Sometimes antibiotics can cause side effects that may be unpleasant, such as an upset stomach or a rash. Less commonly, the use of antibiotics can lead to damage to the body, dangerous allergic reactions, and other undesirable effects. Physicians, pharmacists, and other medical providers are trained to make choices regarding which antibiotics to use and when to use them.

Bacterial resistance In recent years, many bacteria have become resistant to antibiotics. That means bacteria that once would have been easily killed by certain antibiotics now require greater and greater doses of antibiotics before they are destroyed. Some bacteria now even survive the antibiotic completely. Why have certain bacteria become resistant? A number of factors are involved, including overuse and misuse of antibiotics for non-bacterial infections such as colds, influenza*, and other viral infections; widespread use of antibiotics with animals; and the ability of many bacteria to pass resistance on to new generations of bacteria. Together they have contributed to drug-resistant forms of bacteria.

Antibiotic resistance tends to increase as strains* of hardy bacteria reproduce and pass from one person (or other host) to the next. Those that are killed or sensitive to the antibiotic are wiped out, leaving the resistant ones to reproduce. Because bacteria multiply rapidly, there is concern among researchers that these drug-resistant forms of the organism may become increasingly responsible for human disease and be ever more difficult to treat. Tuberculosis, malaria*, and even ear infections are just a few diseases that have become more difficult to treat because of drug-resistant germs.

Drug-resistant infections prove particularly problematic in hospitals, where there are high numbers of microbes and wide use of antibiotics and other drugs. Strains of *Staphylococcus aureus* (stah-fih-lo-KAH-kus ARE-ree-us) in U.S. hospitals have recently proved increasingly resistant to vancomycin, a powerful antibiotic that was believed to be able to kill off any *Staphylococcus* bacteria. Viruses* may also become resistant to medications used to combat them. For example, recent studies have shown an apparent drug resistance developing in the HIV virus.

* **influenza** (in-floo-EN-zuh), also known as the flu, is a contagious viral infection that attacks the respiratory tract, including the nose, throat, and lungs.

* **strains** are various subtypes of organisms, such as viruses or bacteria.

* **malaria** (mah-LAIR-e-uh) is a disease spread to humans by the bite of an infected mosquito.

* **viruses** (VY-rus-sez) are tiny infectious agents that can cause infectious diseases. A virus can only reproduce within the cells it infects.

Soup for the Soul?

Mom was right. Chicken soup is good for a cold or the flu. While a steaming mug will not drive the virus away, the warm fluid can ease symptoms of illness such as dehydration*, a stuffy nose, or a sore throat. Chicken soup is also easy on the stomach, which can be appealing if a person is not feeling very hungry.

* **dehydration** (dee-hi-DRAY-shun) is a condition in which the body is depleted of water, usually caused by excessive and unreplaced loss of body fluids, such as through sweating, vomiting, or diarrhea.

* **enzyme** (EN-zime) is a protein that helps speed up a chemical reaction in the body.

* **fungi** (FUNG-eye) are microorganisms that can grow in or on the body, causing infections of internal organs or of the skin, hair, and nails.

* **parasites** (PAIR-uh-sites) are organisms such as protozoa (one-celled animals), worms, or insects that must live on or inside a human or other organism to survive. An animal or plant harboring a parasite is called its host. Parasites live at the expense of the host and may cause illness.

To fight drug resistance, the National Center for Infectious Diseases recommends that people:

- not take antibiotics to treat anything but a bacterial infection
- not save antibiotics that were prescribed for one illness to use for a future illness
- not share another person's medication
- take all prescriptions precisely according to a doctor's instructions.

The problem of drug resistance has made doctors and others in the health care field increasingly careful about prescribing, and over-prescribing, medications. To deal with drug-resistant bacteria, new types of antibiotics are being developed, and new knowledge from scientists throughout the world points to ways that disease-causing microscopic organisms can be dealt with.

Treating Infections Caused by Viruses and Other Organisms

Not all infections are caused by bacteria; in fact, most infections are not. Viruses cause many infections, such as the common cold, influenza, various types of pneumonia, and most types of encephalitis (en-seh-fuh-LYE-tis, inflammation of the brain). With only a few exceptions, there are no specific medications that kill or slow the growth of most viruses. Take the common cold, for example, which is caused by any one of a number of respiratory viruses. When people get colds, there is little they can do to make them go away faster. Resting, drinking plenty of fluids (maybe even chicken soup), and taking medications to lower fever can help people feel better, but it will usually still take 5 to 10 days for the cold to run its course. It was that way a thousand years ago, and it is that way today.

A few viruses do respond to medications developed to fight them. One example is the herpes (HER-peez) virus, which can cause a number of infections, including cold sores and infections of the newborn central nervous system. The antiviral medication used against the herpes virus does not kill it, but it can slow the virus growth and shorten the length of an outbreak. Human immunodeficiency virus (HIV) can be suppressed with antiviral medications that interfere with an enzyme* critical for the functioning of the HIV virus. These special anti-HIV medications have helped people with HIV/AIDS live longer, more symptom-free lives.

As described elsewhere in this volume, a number of fungi* also cause significant human disease worldwide. Parasites*, too, are widespread, particularly in polluted rivers, ponds, and drinking water, as well as in contaminated meat, such as bears or pigs infested with a parasitic worm known as *Trichinella spiralis*. A large number of medications are available to combat fungi and parasite infections.

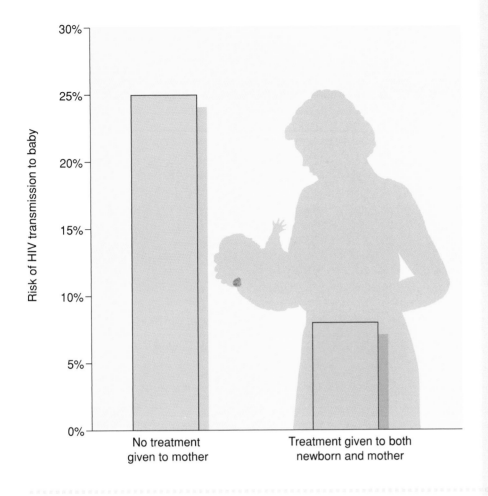

Risk of HIV transmission to baby

No treatment given to mother

Treatment given to both newborn and mother

Many infections require treatment to prevent them from spreading. In fact, in the case of some infections, such as HIV, giving treatment to an infected mother can prevent infection of her baby before it is born. If treatment is given to both the mother and the child, the risk of transmission declines from 25 percent to less than 10 percent.

Immunostimulants

The best disease fighter is, of course, the human body, with its complex array of defenses. As scientists study the human immune system, they learn about substances naturally made by the body that have powerful protective effects. One such substance is interferon (in-ter-FEER-on). Inteferon is a type of immunostimulant, a substance the body's cells produce naturally to increase the immune system's effectiveness in fighting infections and certain types of cancer. Synthetic, or man-made, versions of the drug can be used for a number of diseases, including hepatitis*.

The Future of Treatment

Will humans ever be free of all infections? Perhaps someday, although not in the near future. The answer, of course, is not to wipe out all bacteria. Humans and other complex life forms need bacteria to survive. Our health depends on our better understanding of how bacteria, viruses, fungi, and other organisms almost too small to see can affect human health. It is also vital to increase our understanding of why some people get infections and others do not, how infections move through populations, and

* **hepatitis** (heh-puh-TIE-tis) is an inflammation of the liver. Hepatitis can be caused by viruses, bacteria, and a number of other noninfectious medical conditions.

LET IT BLEED

Before germ theory was understood, physicians and other non-medical practitioners struggled to drain "toxic" substances from the body to cure disease. The preferred treatment was phlebotomy, or bloodletting, in which a lancet or other sharp device was pushed into a vein and used to drain blood. This practice, which dates back to the ancient Egyptians (and perhaps even before), peaked during the eighteenth and nineteenth centuries, when barber-surgeons in Europe and physicians in America enthusiastically pursued bloodletting. In fact, George Washington, the first U.S. president, died after having about 80 ounces of his blood drained within 24 hours for a throat infection. By the end of the nineteenth century, bloodletting had been abandoned. Other treatments once used to cleanse the body of infections included blistering, in which the fluid in induced blisters was believed to drain foul liquids; and purging, in which laxatives were used to empty the bowels.

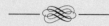

how getting (or resisting) infections is affected by such factors as age, gender, nutrition, genetics*, and even emotions. The development of new types of vaccinations*, antibiotics, immunostimulants, and other methods of fighting infections no doubt will play an increasing role in limiting the spread of certain diseases.

Resources

Organization

U.S. Centers for Disease Control and Prevention (CDC), 1600 Clifton Road, Atlanta, GA 30333. The CDC is the United States government authority for information about infectious and other diseases. The CDC offers information on specific infectious diseases and recommended treatments at its website.
Telephone 800-311-3435
http://www.cdc.gov

Website

KidsHealth.org. KidsHealth is a website created by the medical experts of the Nemours Foundation and is devoted to issues of children's health. It contains articles on a variety of health topics, including different types of treatments for infections.
http://www.KidsHealth.org

* **genetics** (juh-NEH-tiks) is the branch of science that deals with heredity and the ways in which genes control the development and maintenance of organisms.

* **vaccinations** (vak-sih-NAY-shunz), also called immunizations, are the giving of doses of vaccines, which are preparations of killed or weakened germs, or a part of a germ or product it produces, to prevent or lessen the severity of a disease.

▶ See also
Laboratory Tests
Signs and Symptoms
The Nature of Germs and Infection

Public Health

Public Health

People often think of health and illness in terms of a single person contracting an infection such as the flu by being exposed to the virus*, or a person trying to avoid an infection by careful hand washing or getting a shot. However, there are other, broader ways to look at health and illness that go beyond just one individual person. The field of public health looks at a larger view that includes whole populations and health practices. Public health involves the field of medicine devoted to disease prevention and control, environmental health, and health promotion and educational activities to improve general health and safety.

Epidemiology

In the field of public health, the science of epidemiology (eh-pih-dee-me-AH-luh-jee) is an important tool in understanding human diseases. Epidemiology is the study of what causes disease, how it spreads, and all the factors that influence it. Epidemiologists (eh-pih-dee-me-AH-lo-jists), the scientists involved in public health, study epidemics*, or outbreaks, to determine the source of the infection and to prevent its further spread.

Public health officials look at patterns of infections and other diseases to see if changes occur over time. The goal of this monitoring (called surveillance) is to recognize an outbreak early so that something can be done about it. Once an outbreak has been identified, epidemiologists look for the source of infection. Infections are spread through one of four routes:

- direct contact with someone who is infected
- a common source, such as contaminated water
- the air, such as through a contaminated ventilation system
- a vector*, such as a mosquito or a tick that spreads an infection through its bite

In addition, certain factors may increase the risk of becoming sick. Poverty, poor sanitation, crowded living conditions, and malnutrition all contribute to the spread of infections. Climate can also play a role. For example, the hot and humid environments found in the tropics and subtropics can contribute to particularly rapid growth of certain microorganisms* and vectors. Infections happen in every climate and part of the world, however.

Local public health departments coordinate surveillance efforts and are responsible for creating plans to prevent and control outbreaks and for informing and educating the public. The U.S. Centers for Disease Control and Prevention (CDC) is one of the main federal agencies responsible for protecting the health and safety of people in the United

KEYWORDS
for searching the Internet and other reference sources

Environmental safety

Epidemics

Epidemiology

Immunization

Outbreaks

Sanitation

Vaccines

* **virus** (VY-rus) is a tiny infectious agent that can cause infectious diseases. A virus can only reproduce within the cells it infects.

* **epidemics** (eh-pih-DEH-miks) are outbreaks of diseases, especially infectious diseases, in which the number of cases suddenly becomes far greater than usual. Usually epidemics are outbreaks of diseases in specific regions, whereas widespread epidemics are called pandemics.

* **vector** (VEK-tor) is an animal or insect that carries a disease and transfers it from one host to another.

* **microorganisms** are tiny organisms that can be seen only using a microscope. Types of microorganisms include fungi, bacteria, and viruses.

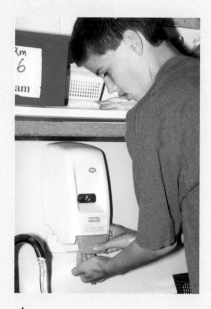

▲

Hand washing is a good way to protect against transmitting the bacteria and viruses that can cause infections. *Field Mark Publications*

* **paralysis** (pah-RAH-luh-sis) is the loss or impairment of the ability to move some part of the body.

* **vaccine** (vak-SEEN) is a preparation of killed or weakened germs, or a part of a germ or product it produces, given to prevent or lessen the severity of the disease that can result if a person is exposed to the germ itself. Use of vaccines for this purpose is called immunization.

* **measles** (ME-zuls) is a viral respiratory infection that is best known for the rash of large, flat, red blotches that appear on the arms, face, neck, and body.

* **mumps** is a contagious viral infection that causes inflammation and swelling in the glands of the mouth that produce saliva.

States and abroad. The CDC provides health information, guidelines for disease prevention and safety, public health policy, and research. The surgeon general, who is part of the U.S. department of health and who is appointed by the president, is the nation's leading spokesperson on public health issues.

Public Health Tools

Public health programs employ a number of tools to prevent disease, to change behaviors that contribute to the spread of disease, and to monitor and control the spread of infections.

Immunization   Most people do not like the idea of getting shots. However, widespread immunization programs have saved millions of lives and have proven to be an incredible public health success story. Take the example of polio (paralytic poliomyelitis, po-lee-o-my-uh-LYE-tis). Polio, a viral infection that causes paralysis* in approximately 1 in 200 people infected, reached a peak in the United States in 1952 with over 20,000 cases of paralytic polio reported. Following the introduction of polio vaccines* in 1955 and 1961, there were only 61 cases in 1965. The last cases of naturally occurring (wild) polio in the United States were reported in 1979. The World Health Organization (WHO) hopes to eradicate polio throughout the world by providing vaccination in areas where polio still occurs, primarily in India and parts of Africa and the eastern Mediterranean.

Immunization programs also have been successful in preventing smallpox, a disfiguring, often fatal infection caused by the variola (ver-e-O-luh) virus. Following a worldwide immunization program, in 1980 WHO declared that smallpox had been eradicated. In developed countries, vaccinations have reduced the number of cases and the severity of many childhood diseases that were once common and feared, including measles*, mumps*, and diphtheria*.

Conditions in developing countries are very different, however. Many diseases that are preventable with routine vaccination continue to occur in large epidemics in many areas because these countries lack the money required for immunizations. Worldwide immunization rates have been declining in recent years. By 2000, 37 million children throughout the world were not immunized during their first year of life. Giving these children vaccines that are part of normal health care in the developed world could save 5,000 children's lives every day.

After 10 years, these careful measures paid off: the last natural case of smallpox was reported in Somalia in 1977. One fatal case of smallpox occurred in the United Kingdom in 1978 following a laboratory accident. In 1980, after careful confirmation, WHO certified that smallpox had been completely erased.

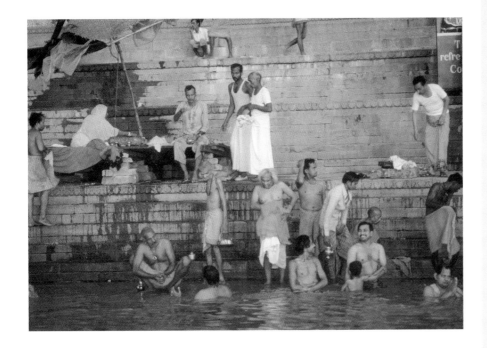

Controlling the spread of disease Efforts to control the spread of infectious diseases include insect control programs and improved sanitation. For example, malaria (mah-LAIR-e-uh), a tropical disease carried by mosquitoes, once was found along the coast of the southeastern United States but was wiped out following insect control programs during the 1940s. Worldwide, however, cases of malaria and malaria deaths are on the rise because of difficulty in eliminating mosquito breeding places and the lack of medical resources to treat the disease.

To prevent the spread of disease through contaminated water, widespread sanitation practices also are monitored, including sewage disposal, water treatment plants, and solid waste (such as trash) disposal. In addition, safety standards for processing, packaging, and selling food protect people from contaminated foods.

The effectiveness of well-organized public health efforts is easy to see in a country such as the United States where public health programs can be carried out. It is a sad fact, however, that about one sixth of the world's population does not have access to clean drinking water. WHO also estimates that one third of the world's population does not have access to essential medications. Unfortunately, the lack of resources has hindered progress in developing countries where public health initiatives would have the most benefits.

Other public health campaigns In addition to working to control the spread of infectious diseases, public health programs are aimed at preventing injuries, reducing the risk of environmental hazards, promoting healthy lifestyles, and making health care available to as many

* **diphtheria** (dif-THEER-e-uh) is an infection of the lining of the upper respiratory tract (the nose and throat). It is a serious disease that can cause breathing difficulty and other complications, including death.

SARS: A New Virus

Severe acute respiratory syndrome (SARS) first appeared in November 2002 and soon caused fear as the number of cases climbed into the thousands. What was causing this flulike illness? How serious was the threat?

It took years to identify the virus behind another frightening illness—AIDS. But thanks to advances in medical science and epidemiology, scientists identified a coronavirus as the probable culprit behind SARS within a matter of weeks.

Symptoms of SARS include fever, cough, headache, body aches, and chills. In some cases, SARS can cause breathing difficulty and, rarely, death. The vast majority of people survive, and with the rapid response of public health officials and quarantine methods, SARS can be contained.

This new virus is not alone. Public health officials believe that the way we live—and travel around the world—may play a significant role in the spread of many new diseases. For example, feeding animal remains to livestock helped spur Creutzfeldt-Jakob disease (CJD).

As some diseases are wiped out, like polio, others will continue to emerge. With medical advances, however, we are well equipped at identifying their causes and ways that they can be treated and prevented.

* **chronic** (KRAH-nik) means continuing for a long period of time.

* **biological warfare** is a method of waging war by using harmful microorganisms to purposely spread disease to many people.

STAMPING OUT SMALLPOX

Smallpox was eliminated through a global immunization campaign conducted by the World Health Organization (WHO). Believed to have originated in Egypt or India, the 3,000-year-old disease regularly rampaged across continents, causing devastating epidemics that often cut into populations and changed history. No effective treatment was ever found for the disease, which, in addition to causing blindness, killed close to a third of its victims.

In the early 1950s, about 50 million cases of smallpox were tracked around the globe each year. By 1967 that number had dropped to 10 to 15 million cases due to vaccination, and that year WHO began a plan to rid the world of smallpox. The organization used surveillance techniques to monitor outbreaks of the disease. When the typical rash was observed, often on the face and hands, workers quarantined (or isolated) the patient and then tracked down everyone who had been in close contact with the person so that they could be vaccinated.

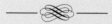

people as possible. Mandatory seatbelt and bike helmet laws are the result of public health campaigns. Public health efforts to reduce lead in the environment by banning lead-based paint and leaded gasoline have decreased the number of children ages 1 to 5 who have elevated levels of lead in their blood by more than 90 percent since the late 1970s. Education through advertisements and public information programs, such as car seat safety, hand-washing, safer-sex, and stop-smoking campaigns, is another way to change behavior and prevent diseases.

Public health agencies also promote healthy living in local communities by providing access to health care. Examples include setting up school health programs and providing medical insurance programs for the uninsured. The National Health Service Corps and the Indian Health Service provide medical care where it would not otherwise be available.

Public Health in the Twenty-First Century

With the increased success of infection control measures, routine vaccination, and advances in the treatment of infectious diseases, there has been a shift in the focus of public health toward chronic* diseases, injury prevention, and environmental safety. However, with the appearance of new infections, emerging resistance to some medications, and the concern about biological warfare*, combating infectious diseases will continue to be an important challenge within the field of public health.

Resources

Organizations

National Institute of Allergy and Infectious Diseases (NIAID), Building 31, Room 7A-50, 31 Center Drive MSC 2520, Bethesda, MD 20892. The NIAID, part of the National Institutes of Health, posts information about infectious diseases and public health at its website. http://www.niaid.nih.gov

U.S. National Library of Medicine, 8600 Rockville Pike, Bethesda, MD 20894. The National Library of Medicine has a website packed with information on infectious diseases and public health, consumer resources, dictionaries and encyclopedias of medical terms, and directories of doctors and helpful organizations.
Telephone 888-346-3656
http://www.nlm.nih.gov

U.S. Centers for Disease Control and Prevention (CDC), 1600 Clifton Road, Atlanta, GA 30333. The CDC offers information on

---

TOP PUBLIC HEALTH ACHIEVEMENTS, 1900 TO 1999

During the 1900s, Americans added on average 30 years to their life span, with 25 years of this gain coming from advances in public health programs, according to the U.S. Centers for Disease Control and Prevention. The most notable public health achievements in the 1900s include:

- vaccinations
- increased motor vehicle safety
- safer workplaces
- greater control of infectious diseases
- fewer deaths from heart disease and stroke*
- safer and healthier foods
- healthier mothers and babies
- widespread fluoridation* of drinking water
- recognition of tobacco as a health hazard

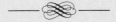

---

*stroke is a brain-damaging event usually caused by interference with blood flow to the brain. A stroke may occur when a blood vessel supplying the brain becomes clogged or bursts, depriving brain tissue of oxygen. As a result, nerve cells in the affected area of the brain, and the specific body parts they control, do not properly function.

*fluoridation is the process of adding fluoride to drinking water to help prevent tooth decay.

infectious diseases and public health efforts to control them on its website.
Telephone 800-311-3435
http://www.cdc.gov

World Health Organization (WHO), Avenue Appia 20, 1211 Geneva 27, Switzerland. WHO tracks disease outbreaks around the world and offers information about infectious diseases and public health programs around the world at its website.
Telephone 011-41-22-791-2111
http://www.who.int

Website

The Johns Hopkins infectious diseases website provides information about numerous infectious diseases and other public health issues.
http://hopkins-id.edu

KEYWORDS
for searching the Internet and other reference sources

Active immunity

Antibodies

Antigens

DTaP vaccine

Edward Jenner

Herd immunity

Hib vaccine

Immune response

IPV vaccine

Louis Pasteur

MMR vaccine

Passive immunity

Smallpox

Td vaccine

Vaccination (Immunization)

Vaccination (vak-sih-NAY-shun) is a way of producing immunity* to certain diseases by giving a person a small amount of an inactive, altered, or weakened form of a microorganism*.

What Are Vaccinations?

Before about 1800, a dangerous disease known as smallpox killed millions of people throughout the world. All that was soon to change as the result of an observation made by Edward Jenner, an English country doctor, in 1796. Jenner reported that milkmaids who milked cows infected with an animal disease called cowpox did not contract smallpox. Instead, the milkmaids had a mild case of a similar rash-producing disease. Jenner concluded that cowpox must somehow protect these milkmaids against the smallpox infection.

As an experiment, Jenner deliberately gave people the mild cowpox infection to protect them against the more dangerous smallpox infection. Jenner was experimenting with vaccination, or immunization. He discovered that the body's natural defense system can be stimulated to become more protective against a specific infection after being exposed to a similar or weakened version of that infection. In the late nineteenth century, the French scientist Louis Pasteur further developed the concept and named it vaccination, a word derived from the Latin word for cow, *vacca*. The first vaccine Pasteur developed was against sheep anthrax (AN-thraks).

Since Jenner's time, scientists have developed many types of lifesaving vaccinations, including ones against polio, measles, diphtheria, and pertussis (whooping cough). These vaccinations have prevented disease and saved hundreds of millions of lives. Vaccinations activate the body's immune response to protect against certain diseases. Small amounts of weak antigens*, substances found in disease-causing organisms such as bacteria and viruses, are given to a person, usually by injection (a shot). When they enter the body, those antigens train infection-fighting white blood cells to recognize the antigen quickly in the future and respond if the real bacteria or viruses enter the body. When the body's immune system* can respond rapidly and effectively to fight off the infection so that it cannot spread and cause disease within the body, the person has developed resistance to the illness.

Booster doses of vaccines (further doses given months or years after the first immunization dose) take advantage of the immune cells' "memory" of specific antigens from the first vaccinations to build even greater immunity. When the white cells that recognize the antigen are exposed to it again after a booster dose, their memory of the infectious agent is strengthened and reinforced. Some vaccinations require booster doses, whereas others do not.

Immunizations protect more than just the people who receive them. They also protect people around those who have been vaccinated, a concept called herd immunity. A vaccination protects a person from contracting and then spreading an infection. When enough people have been immunized in one area, the infectious germ has difficulty spreading. It is much less likely to be passed on, even to the few people who are not protected against it. It is estimated that this herd effect occurs when about 95 percent of the people in a given community receive immunizations.

Vaccinations boost immunity through a so-called active process, meaning that in response to an antigen, the body's immune system reacts actively. This is not the only form of immunity boosting our bodies receive. Infants are born with a passive natural immunity that protects them from some diseases. This immunity comes from the protective antibodies* passed from a mother to her baby in the womb and, later, through breast milk. A mother who has immunity against tetanus (lockjaw), for example, will pass this immunity along to her baby through antibodies while she is pregnant. This immunity is only temporary, however. An infant's passive immunity (those antibodies from the mother) disappears in the months after birth. The infant later will make his or her own antibodies after being exposed to an infectious agent or receiving a vaccine.

Historical Success

Vaccinations are one of the greatest success stories of public health programs in the twentieth century. Widespread use of immunizations has brought about dramatic decreases in the number of cases of certain potentially deadly and disabling childhood diseases. Before measles vaccination began in 1963, for example, an average of 500,000 measles cases and 500 measles-associated deaths were reported each year, according to

* **immunity** (ih-MYOON-uh-tee) is the condition of being protected against an infectious disease. Immunity often develops after a germ is introduced to the body. One type of immunity occurs when the body makes special protein molecules called antibodies to fight the disease-causing germ. The next time that germ enters the body, the antibodies quickly attack it, usually preventing the germ from causing disease.

* **microorganisms** are tiny organisms that can be seen only using a microscope. Types of microorganisms include fungi, bacteria, and viruses.

* **antigens** (AN-tih-jenz) are substances that are recognized as a threat by the body's immune system, which triggers the formation of specific protective antibodies against the substances.

* **immune system** is the system of the body composed of specialized cells and the substances they produce that helps protect the body against disease-causing germs.

* **antibodies** (AN-tih-bah-deez) are protein molecules produced by the body's immune system to help fight specific infections caused by microorganisms, such as bacteria and viruses.

the U.S. Centers for Disease Control and Prevention (CDC). Compare those high numbers with the number of cases after immunizations began. In the year 2000, only 86 cases occurred in the United States, and there were no deaths.

In the 1920s, before vaccination for diphtheria was available, 150,000 cases occurred annually in the United States, on average. Diphtheria is a particularly frightening and painful disease. The thick mucus* produced in the course of the disease closes the airway and can lead to suffocation. Since the introduction of diphtheria immunization, millions of people have been protected from this disease.

Polio is another disease that once provoked fear. Tens of thousands of people who had polio needed leg braces to walk, because the poliovirus damages the nerves of the leg muscles. As a result of this viral infection, paralysis* could progress, and patients could die of respiratory failure* through paralysis of the diaphragm (DYE-uh-fram), the chief muscle used for breathing. In 1952, there were more than 21,000 cases of paralytic (pair-uh-LIH-tik) polio in the United States. Since the introduction of polio vaccine in 1955, the incidence of this disease steadily declined, and there have been no naturally occurring cases in the United States since 1979.

Around the globe, smallpox is the only disease that has been eradicated through an aggressive international immunization program. This highly infectious disease once could kill as many as 1 of every 3 infected people, but the last known naturally occurring case was reported in Somalia, Africa, in 1977.

Vaccines Today

The twentieth century saw not only the tremendous success of vaccines but advances in vaccine technology as well. Some old vaccines have been improved, and new vaccines have been introduced. There are four different types of vaccines currently available.

Attenuated (ah-TEN-yoo-a-tid), or weakened, types of vaccine contain live but weaker forms of a virus. These weakened viruses usually do not cause disease symptoms, but they do stimulate the body to develop immunity to the virus. Examples of attenuated vaccines include the combined vaccine for measles, mumps*, and rubella* (German measles), known as the MMR vaccine, and the vaccine for varicella (var-uh-SEH-luh), or chicken pox. Although these immunizations last longer than others, they occasionally create serious infections in people, particularly those with weakened immune systems, sometimes called compromised immune systems. Killed, or inactivated, viruses or bacteria are used in other vaccines, such as the one for influenza*. These organisms are not live, but they do cause an immune response in the body. These vaccines are considered safe for people with weakened immune systems.

Toxoid (TOX-oyd) vaccines contain a toxin* produced by the infecting bacterium or virus. When faced later on with the toxins created

*mucus (MYOO-kus) is a thick, slippery substance that lines the insides of many body parts.

*paralysis (pah-RAH-luh-sis) is the loss or impairment of the ability to move some part of the body.

*respiratory failure is a condition in which breathing and oxygen delivery to the body is dangerously altered. This may result from infection, nerve or muscle damage, poisoning, or other causes.

*mumps is a contagious viral infection that causes inflammation and swelling in the glands of the mouth that produce saliva.

*rubella (roo-BEH-luh) is a viral infection that usually causes a rash and mild fever.

*influenza (in-floo-EN-zuh), also known as the flu, is a contagious viral infection that attacks the respiratory tract, including the nose, throat, and lungs.

*toxin is a poison that harms the body.

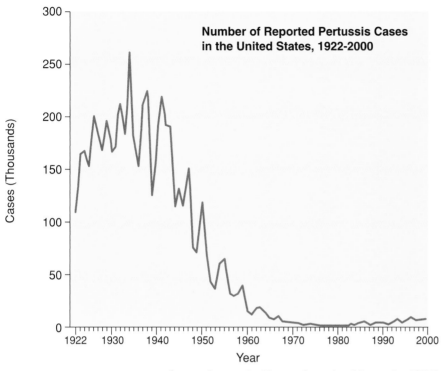

Number of Reported Pertussis Cases in the United States, 1922-2000

Cases (Thousands) / Year

Source: Centers for Disease Control and Prevention (CDC)

The policy of vaccinating children against pertussis, or whooping cough, has caused a dramatic drop in the number of annual cases in the United States.

by an infecting organism, the body's immune system responds. Diphtheria and tetanus vaccines are both of the toxoid type.

Biosynthetic vaccines include man-made substances. One example is the Hib (*Haemophilus influenzae* type B*) vaccine, which contains two antigens that scientists have combined to make something called a conjugate molecule. Subunit vaccines contain the parts of a particular microorganism that trigger the immune response, but not the whole microorganism itself. The acellular (meaning it contains no whole cells) vaccine for pertussis is an example of a subunit vaccine.

What Are the Recommended Vaccinations?

Vaccines can be used to protect people against more than a dozen diseases, though most people do not get every possible immunization. On a regular basis, a number of national organizations (such as the CDC and the American Academy of Pediatrics) review the list of available immunizations and make recommendations concerning who should get them, how often, and under what circumstances. There are several well-known immunizations available now.

Hepatitis* B vaccine (HBV) protects against hepatitis B, a virus that infects the liver. People who are infected can develop long-term illness such as cirrhosis* of the liver or liver cancer. Hepatitis B infection is one

* *Haemophilus influenzae* **type B** refers to bacteria that can cause serious illnesses, including meningitis, pneumonia, and other infections.

* **hepatitis** (heh-puh-TIE-tis) is an inflammation of the liver. Hepatitis can be caused by viruses, bacteria, and a number of other noninfectious medical conditions.

* **cirrhosis** (sir-O-sis) is a condition that affects the liver, involving long-term inflammation and scarring, which can lead to problems with liver function.

* **pneumonia** (nu-MO-nyah) is inflammation of the lung.

* **meningitis** (meh-nin-JY-tis) is an inflammation of the meninges, the membranes that surround the brain and the spinal cord. Meningitis is most often caused by infection with a virus or a bacterium.

* **sepsis** is a potentially serious spreading of infection, usually bacterial, through the bloodstream and body.

* **diabetes** (dye-uh-BEE-teez) is a condition in which the body's pancreas does not produce enough insulin or the body cannot use the insulin it makes effectively, resulting in increased levels of sugar in the blood. This can lead to increased urination, dehydration, weight loss, weakness, and a number of other symptoms and complications related to chemical imbalances within the body.

* **sickle-cell disease** is a hereditary condition in which the red blood cells, which are usually round, take on an abnormal crescent shape and have a decreased ability to carry oxygen throughout the body.

* **rabies** (RAY-beez) is a viral infection of the central nervous system that usually is transmitted to humans by the bite of an infected animal.

of the most common causes of cancer worldwide. HBV usually is given as a series of three injections: one shortly after birth, another at 1 or 2 months of age, and the third at 6 to 18 months of age.

Pneumococcal (nu-moh-KAH-kal) conjugate vaccine (PCV) offers protection against many infections caused by pneumococcus (nu-moh-KAH-kus) bacteria, including pneumonia*, meningitis*, and sepsis*. PCV immunizations are given as a series of four shots when an infant is 2, 4, 6, and 12 to 15 months old.

The vaccine for diphtheria, tetanus, and pertussis protects against these three diseases. DTaP, as it is called, is a series of five shots, usually administered when a child is 2 months, 4 months, 6 months, 15 to 18 months, and 4 to 6 years old (or before starting school). Five years after these immunizations, generally at age 11 or 12, children receive a booster shot for tetanus and diphtheria, called Td. Doctors recommend that people receive Td boosters once every ten years after that, throughout adulthood.

Hib vaccine for *Haemophilus influenzae* type B bacteria, which were once a leading cause of meningitis in children, is given by injection at ages 2, 4, and 6 months. A booster dose is delivered at 12 to 15 months.

The inactivated poliovirus vaccine (IPV) for polio is given by injection at ages 2 months, 4 months, 6 to 18 months, and 4 to 6 years (or before entering school).

MMR vaccine protects against measles, mumps, and rubella. The vaccine is administered in two doses, the first at age 12 to 15 months and the second before a child starts school, generally at age 4 to 6 years.

Varicella vaccine provides protection against chicken pox, a common childhood viral illness. Children are immunized with a shot of varicella vaccine between the ages of 12 and 18 months; older children and adults who have never had chicken pox also can receive the vaccine.

Children who travel or those with special conditions may need other types of vaccines as well. An influenza vaccine, or "flu shot," is particularly recommended for children with certain conditions, including diabetes* and sickle-cell disease*, that could put them at risk of serious infection. Recent recommendations advise that children between 6 months and 2 years of age receive the flu shot, because they are also at risk of serious problems associated with the infection. Vaccination for hepatitis A, a disease that particularly affects the liver, may be necessary for people who visit or live in certain areas where the disease is prevalent. A rabies* vaccine typically is administered after a person is bitten by an animal that could have the disease or when a person plans to spend more than 30 days in a place where rabies is common.

Children are not the only people who are immunized routinely. Adults sometimes require vaccines too. For example, adults generally need a tetanus booster every 10 years, and older adults or those with certain medical problems are advised to get a flu shot every year. Adults who did not undergo immunization as children, those who have emigrated from a country where vaccines are not readily available, or those who travel to areas where there is a higher risk for certain infectious diseases also receive vaccinations.

Vaccination Fears and Answers

Vaccinations have been shown to lessen the incidence of certain diseases and even to wipe some of them out. Still, some parents are reluctant to vaccinate their children because they fear that the injection will be too painful or they worry about possible reactions. Other parents mistakenly believe that with lower rates of certain diseases in the United States, regular vaccinations are no longer necessary. A dramatic example proves otherwise. The United Kingdom, Japan, and Sweden cut back their use of pertussis vaccine in the 1970s, when some people feared that it was unsafe. Between 1971 and 1979, the United Kingdom experienced more than 100,000 cases of the disease and 36 pertussis-related deaths. From 1974 to 1979, Japan's vaccination coverage dropped from 80 percent to 20 percent, while the annual number of pertussis cases rose from a low of 393 in 1974, with no deaths, to a 1979 epidemic* high of 13,000 cases and 41 deaths. In Sweden, the annual incidence of pertussis per 100,000 children up to age 6 leapt from 700 in 1981 to 3,200 in 1985.

Another common belief is that vaccines cause the infectious diseases that they are trying to protect against. In fact, killed vaccines or those made from only a component of the infectious agent, such as a protein, cannot cause the infectious disease. In addition, constant efforts are made to minimize the possibility of contracting a disease from a live vaccine. For example, in January of 2000, the Advisory Committee on Immunization Practices recommended that the polio vaccine be switched from an attenuated oral version to a killed vaccine, to eliminate the tiny risk of contracting vaccine-associated paralytic polio. Although the live oral vaccine was largely responsible for ridding the United Sates of polio, it caused polio in 1 of every 1.4 million people who received their first dose of the vaccine. The killed version, however, cannot cause polio.

What Are the Side Effects?

Although immunizations prevent many cases of serious, and even fatal, illness, some people experience side effects after receiving an immunization. Relatively common side effects for a number of immunizations may include low fever; mild pain, tenderness, and redness at the site of the injection; a rash; and irritability. Less common, but more serious reactions include seizures*, usually as a result of fever, and an allergic reaction to parts of the vaccine. Reports that link childhood vaccinations to autism*, sudden infant death syndrome*, and brain damage have not been proved, though research continues.

Why Is It Important to Vaccinate?

Vaccination provides the best protection against certain childhood diseases, and preventing the spread of such infections is vital to public health.

* **epidemic** (eh-pih-DEH-mik) is an outbreak of disease, especially infectious disease, in which the number of cases suddenly becomes far greater than usual. Usually epidemics are outbreaks of diseases in specific regions, whereas widespread epidemics are called pandemics.

* **seizures** (SEE-zhurs) are sudden bursts of disorganized electrical activity that interrupt the normal functioning of the brain, often leading to uncontrolled movements in the body and sometimes a temporary change in consciousness.

* **autism** (AW-tih-zum) is a developmental disorder in which a person has difficulty interacting and communicating with others and usually has severely limited interest in social activities.

* **sudden infant death syndrome**, or SIDS, is the sudden death of an infant less than a year old that is not explained even after an autopsy or examination of the death scene. Most cases occur while the otherwise well baby is asleep on its stomach.

Not only do vaccines protect the people who receive them, they also keep the illness from spreading to people who have not been vaccinated. Modern technology has led to the development of many effective vaccines. Technology also has made travel from region to region and country to country much easier than in previous centuries. As diseases that once were rarely seen in the United States are now more readily "imported" from other parts of the world, it is even more important to get immunizations. If people start to believe that they or their children do not need immunizations or if they depend on others to be vaccinated, overall vaccination levels might drop. That could lead to the return of diseases that can be prevented by vaccination.

Future Vaccinations

Medical researchers are working to develop more vaccines for a wide range of illnesses, including HIV/AIDS. In general, however, such research takes years and is expensive to carry out. Because almost all vaccinations carry some risk, an important part of their development is to assess how effective they are and whether the benefits of a new vaccine outweigh the risks.

Resources

Organization

U.S. Centers for Disease Control and Prevention (CDC), 1600 Clifton Road, Atlanta, GA 30333. The CDC provides information on vaccinations and the diseases they can help prevent at its website. Telephone 800-311-3435
http://www.cdc.gov

Website

KidsHealth.org. KidsHealth is a website created by the medical experts of the Nemours Foundation and is devoted to issues of children's health. It contains articles on a variety of health topics, including vaccinations. http://www.KidsHealth.org

A

Abscesses

Abscesses (AB-seh-sez) are localized or walled off accumulations of pus* caused by infection that can occur anywhere within the body. Furuncles (FYOOR-ung-kulz), which are also known as boils, and carbuncles (KAR-bung-kulz) are types of abscesses that involve hair follicles* and occur on the skin.

What Are Abscesses?

An abscess develops when the body's immune system isolates an area of body tissue that has been infected by an invading microorganism* (usually bacteria) to prevent the infection from spreading further into the body. It does this by sending infection-fighting leukocytes (LOO-kuh-sites) to the infected area; leukocytes are specialized white blood cells that can destroy infectious microorganisms such as bacteria, parasites, and viruses.

As the bacteria and white blood cells clash at the site of infection, pus begins to form within the involved tissue. As the infection progresses, a wall of tissue develops surrounding the infection site, forming an abscess. A growing abscess on the skin is usually warm, red, painful, and swollen with pus.

Abscesses that grow inside the body are rare in healthy people but can be very serious. Internal abscesses can occur anywhere within the body, but some of the more common areas where they form include the appendix* (as when someone has appendicitis, ah-pen-dih-SY-tis, an inflammation of the appendix), surrounding one of the tonsils* (a peritonsillar, per-ih-TON-sih-lar, abscess), and in the gums or jaw (a dental abscess). They may also form in the liver, spinal cord, or on or in the brain. People who have weak immune systems, such as those who need chemotherapy for cancer or someone with diseases such as long-standing diabetes or HIV/AIDS, are more at risk for developing internal abscesses.

Furuncles (boils) are a type of skin abscess most commonly found on the face, neck, armpit, groin, buttocks, and thighs. Carbuncles are larger areas of skin infection made up of several boils that have formed close together and then joined. They take longer to form and are often located on the back and the nape of the neck. Men are more likely to

KEYWORDS
for searching the Internet and other reference sources

Boils

Carbuncles

Furuncles

Job syndrome

Skin infections

***pus** is a thick, creamy fluid, usually yellow or greenish in color, that forms at the site of an infection. Pus contains infection-fighting white cells and other substances.

***hair follicles** (FAH-lih-kuls) are the skin structures from which hair develops and grows.

***microorganism** is a tiny organism that can be seen only by using a microscope. Types of microorganisms include fungi, bacteria, and viruses.

***appendix** (ah-PEN-diks) is the narrow, finger-shaped organ that branches off the part of the large intestine in the lower right side of the abdomen. It has no known function.

***tonsils** are paired clusters of lymphatic tissue in the throat containing cells of the immune system that help protect the body from bacteria and viruses that enter through a person's nose or mouth.

A carbuncle is a deep-seated infection of the skin and underlying tissue that typically forms in closely placed hair follicles. *Photo Researchers, Inc.* ▶

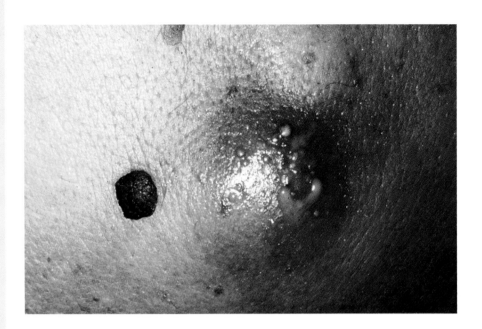

develop carbuncles than are women. Fever and a general feeling of illness are often associated with carbuncles.

What Causes Abscesses?

Bacteria that are commonly found on the skin, such as *Staphylococcus aureus* (stah-fih-lo-KAH-kus ARE-ree-us) and Group A β-hemolytic *Streptococcus* (he-muh-LIH-tik strep-tuh-KAH-kus) typically cause most abscesses, furuncles, and carbuncles.

Much of the skin's surface is covered by hair. At the base of each hair is a hair follicle, a sac-like pit in which the hair shaft develops and grows. If the skin around a hair follicle has been damaged in some way, such as with a cut or a nick on the skin from shaving, bacteria on the skin's surface can enter and start to cause an infection. This alerts the body's immune system, which walls off the area around the infected hair follicle. As the body's defenses go to work, the area fills with pus and becomes inflamed. When an area of skin contains infected, inflamed hair follicles, the condition is known as folliculitis (fuh-lih-kyoo-LYE-tis).

A boil usually starts out within an area of folliculitis. The growing pus inside the boil creates pressure and swelling around the infected spot, often forming a drainage point at the surface of the skin called a head. A carbuncle typically has many small areas where pus has collected and formed heads.

Abscesses that appear inside the body, such as within the abdomen, may be caused by types of bacteria different than those that cause skin infections. For example, an abscess that forms with appendicitis may be caused by a blockage in the appendix (known as a stone). These abscesses usually contain bacteria normally found inside the intestine and in bowel movements. A liver abscess can occur when an infection in the abdomen spreads or when an infectious agent from somewhere else in the body travels through the bloodstream and is deposited in the liver.

Are Abscesses Contagious?

Abscesses are not contagious, but the bacteria that cause them can spread from person to person and can cause other types of infections. Anyone who touches a boil that is draining pus should wash their hands, and cloths or towels that have touched an open or draining boil or carbuncle should not be shared.

How Are Abscesses Treated and Prevented?

Skin abscesses sometimes need to be drained before they can heal, although most of the time they heal on their own without medical treatment. Skin abscesses are often treated at home by applying warm compresses. The abscess usually comes to a head on its own, then begins to drain and heals soon afterward.

Boils and carbuncles that do not drain on their own should not be squeezed or lanced (cut open) to remove pus by anyone but a health care provider. Trying to puncture a boil at home could force the infection deeper into the skin or spread the bacteria. Skin abscesses that do not improve on their own need to be lanced by a doctor to prevent the infection from becoming worse. The area is then thoroughly cleaned, and antibiotics are sometimes prescribed. Most carbuncles require antibiotic treatment.

Internal abscesses are usually treated with surgical drainage and antibiotics. If a dental abscess is not treated with antibiotics it can destroy the root of a tooth, leading to the need for a root canal* procedure or removal of the entire tooth.

Keeping the area around a minor skin wound clean and dry, not sharing razors, and using antibacterial soap can help prevent skin abscesses.

Resources

Book

Turkington, Carol, and Dover, Jeffrey, MD. *Skin Deep: The Encyclopedia of Skin and Skin Disorders.* New York, Facts on File, 2002.

Organization

U.S. National Library of Medicine, 8600 Rockville Pike, Bethesda, MD 20894. The National Library of Medicine has a website packed with information on diseases and conditions (including abscesses), consumer resources, dictionaries and encyclopedias of medical terms, and directories of doctors and helpful organizations. Telephone 888-346-3656
http://www.nlm.nih.gov

Job Syndrome

In the Bible, God tests the faith and devotion of Job by allowing him to become afflicted from head to toe with painful boils. Job syndrome is named for this biblical figure. People who have this rare disease experience recurring cases of severe abscesses on the skin and in the lungs, sinuses*, and bones.

* **sinuses** (SY-nuh-ses) are hollow, air-filled cavities in the facial bones.

* **root canal** is a procedure in which a dentist cleans out the pulp of an infected tooth, removes the nerve, and then fills the cavity with a protective substance.

▶ *See also*
Staphylococcal Infections
Streptococcal Infections

51

African Sleeping Sickness   *See* **Trypanosomiasis**

AIDS and HIV Infection

HIV, or human immunodeficiency (HYOO-mun ih-myoo-no-dih-FIH-shen-see) virus, is a virus that can weaken the body's immune system*. Infection with HIV causes a life-threatening illness called AIDS, or acquired immunodeficiency syndrome.

What Are AIDS and HIV?

AIDS is the disease caused by human immunodeficiency virus type 1, or HIV-1 (usually referred to as HIV). HIV belongs to the retrovirus family, a group of viruses that have the ability to use cells' machinery to replicate (make more copies of the infecting virus).

HIV attacks the immune system by damaging or killing a specific type of white blood cell in the body called a T-lymphocyte (LIM-fo-site), also called a CD4+ or T-helper cell. T-lymphocytes help the immune system perform its important task of fighting disease in the body caused by invading germs. As a result of HIV infection, the immune system becomes weakened and the body has trouble battling certain infections caused by bacteria, viruses, parasites, and fungi. Many of these infections are highly unusual in people with healthy immune systems. They are called opportunistic infections because they take advantage of a weakened immune system. People with HIV disease not only are more likely to contract these infections, they are more likely to have them repeatedly and to become much more sick from them.

Infection with HIV takes about 10 years to develop into full-blown AIDS. During most of this period, people usually look and feel healthy

KEYWORDS
for searching the Internet and other reference sources

Highly active antiretroviral therapy (HAART)

Immunodeficiency

Opportunistic infections

Protease inhibitors

Retroviruses

Sexually transmitted diseases

T-lymphocytes

* **immune system** is the system of the body composed of specialized cells and the substances they produce that helps protect the body against disease-causing germs.

The HIV virus attacks T-helper cells, or CD4+ cells, by fitting itself into the cell like a key in a lock. Once it has invaded, it can use its own RNA as a template to make copies of itself, multiplying and traveling through the body. This process destroys the body's own T cells over time; as the T-cell count falls, the body's resistance to germs and disease declines. ▼

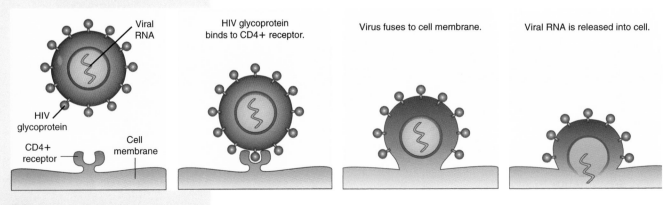

Viral RNA

HIV glycoprotein binds to CD4+ receptor.

Virus fuses to cell membrane.

Viral RNA is released into cell.

HIV glycoprotein

CD4+ receptor

Cell membrane

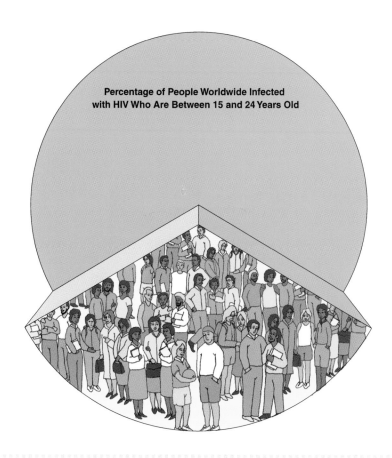

Percentage of People Worldwide Infected
with HIV Who Are Between 15 and 24 Years Old

Worldwide, about one-third of people with HIV/AIDS are between 15 and 24 years of age. Teens and young adults are at particular risk because they are more likely to have unprotected sex.

and are not aware that they are infected unless they are tested for the virus. Currently, experts think that, untreated, people with HIV infection eventually will develop AIDS unless they die first of other causes. Medications for HIV infection improved greatly in the 1990s, and the life expectancy of people receiving proper treatment has been extended dramatically. However, none of these medicines actually cure the infection.

AIDS was first described in the United States in 1981, after many gay men in San Francisco and New York City became ill from an unknown infectious cause. In 1985, it became clear that a retrovirus causes AIDS.

How Common Is HIV Infection?

In some areas of the world, such as in sub-Saharan Africa, rates of HIV infection are extremely high and continue to rise rapidly. Worldwide, it is estimated that 42 million people are living with HIV/AIDS. In 2002 alone, 5 million people became infected with HIV, and more than 3 million died from AIDS. Many infected people live in impoverished areas where medicines and other treatments are not available or affordable.

In the United States, HIV infection is less common. According to the U.S. Centers for Disease Control and Prevention (CDC), by the end of 2001 a total of about 816,000 cases of AIDS had been reported and about 468,000 deaths had been attributed to AIDS since the disease was

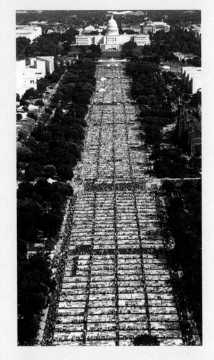

▲

Since 1987 the AIDS Memorial Quilt (shown here on display in Washington, D.C.) has underscored the devastating impact of the disease. Each of the more than 44,000 panels memorializes the life of someone who has died of AIDS.
Paul Margolies

*semen (SEE-men) is the sperm-containing whitish fluid produced by the male reproductive tract.

*vaginal (VAH-jih-nul) refers to the canal in a woman that leads from the uterus to the outside of the body.

*intravenous (in-tra-VEE-nus) means within or through a vein. For example, medications, fluid, or other substances can be given through a needle or soft tube inserted through the skin's surface directly into a vein.

*transfusions (trans-FYOO-zhunz) are procedures in which blood or certain parts of blood, such as specific cells, are given to a person who needs them because of illness or blood loss.

first recognized. More than 9,000 children in the United States under the age of 13 are living with AIDS. The infection is spreading most rapidly among people of African ancestry and people of Latino ancestry, especially among young men. As with other sexually transmitted diseases (STDs), teens and young adults are at higher risk for contracting HIV infection because they are more likely to have unprotected sex. Approximately one-third of people worldwide with HIV or AIDS are 15 to 24 years old.

How Is HIV/AIDS Spread?

HIV/AIDS is contagious from person to person. People can spread the virus before they have developed any symptoms and are unaware they are infected. The HIV virus spreads in certain body fluids, including blood, semen*, breast milk, vaginal* fluid, and any other body fluid that contains blood. HIV can spread in the following ways:

- through vaginal, anal, or oral sexual intercourse
- by sharing needles to inject intravenous* (IV) drugs
- from mother to child in the womb
- during childbirth or breast-feeding
- from any blood-to-blood contact with someone who is infected, such as, in very rare cases, contact with an open wound (though the virus cannot be transmitted unless the skin of both people is broken).

Because it can be difficult to see small breaks in the skin such as hangnails, doctors advise caution when coming into contact with any cut or wound on someone infected with HIV. Medical personnel are at risk of contracting HIV infection through accidental injuries with medical instruments (especially needles and scalpels) that have been contaminated with the blood of an HIV-infected patient.

THE ORIGIN OF AIDS

Evidence suggests that AIDS likely originated in Africa from a virus called simian immunodeficiency virus (SIV) found in monkeys. People probably became infected with SIV from a particular type of chimpanzee when they hunted the chimpanzees for food. Once the virus was in humans, it may have mutated (changed) into the virus known as HIV.

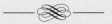

Sharing living space or items such as eating utensils or clothes does not transmit the virus. Neither does casual contact—doing things like hugging or shaking hands—so there is no need to avoid this type of contact with someone who has HIV. Blood donations and blood products in the United States have been screened for HIV since 1985, and today the blood supply is considered safe. The risk of becoming infected through blood transfusions* is extremely low.

What Are the Signs and Symptoms of HIV/AIDS?

Before a person has developed signs of AIDS, it is impossible to tell whether someone is infected with HIV by just looking at that person. People usually develop an illness with symptoms like those of the flu a few weeks after becoming infected with the virus. They may have a fever, a sore throat, muscle aches, and, sometimes, a measles-like rash. This illness usually goes away after a couple of weeks, and other symptoms may not appear for 5 to 15 years. The incubation (ing-kyoo-BAY-shun) period, or amount of time after infection before symptoms appear, varies from person to person.

When symptoms do appear, they might include dry cough, sweating excessively at night, rapid weight loss, recurring fever, pneumonia, white spots or patches on the tongue or throat, headache, persistent diarrhea (dye-uh-REE-uh), memory loss, depression, extreme tiredness, skin rashes, and swollen lymph nodes*.

How Is HIV/AIDS Diagnosed?

In order to diagnose HIV infection, doctors perform a blood test to look for antibodies* to the virus. This test may not show signs of infection until several months after infection occurs. Other tests can detect the presence of the virus in the blood directly. The most common of these uses a technique called the polymerase (pah-LIM-er-ace) chain reaction (PCR). Special cultures* of the blood for HIV or a measurement of p24 antigen (AN-tih-jen), a part of the virus's coat, are available but are used less frequently.

A diagnosis of AIDS is made when a person who is infected with HIV develops certain infections or conditions associated with the disease that indicate a weakening of the immune system. AIDS is also diagnosed when the number of CD4+ T-cells in the body drops below a certain level. The level or "count" of these cells can be measured by taking a blood sample.

About one in four infants born to mothers infected with HIV will be infected with the virus if the mother does not receive treatment during her pregnancy, and the baby after birth, to prevent spread of HIV to the infant. Sometimes infants who are not infected test positive for HIV antibodies in their blood for more than a year because antibodies were passed to the baby through the placenta* from the mother. Other tests must be done to help determine whether an infant is truly infected.

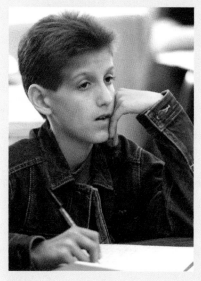

▲

In 1984, at the onset of the AIDS epidemic, Ryan White became infected with the HIV virus through a blood transfusion. His spirited fight to educate the public about the disease and to end prejudice against people with AIDS ended with his death in 1990 at the age of eighteen. *Corbis Corporation (New York)*

* **lymph** (LIMF) **nodes** are small, bean-shaped masses of tissue that contain immune system cells that fight harmful microorganisms. Lymph nodes may swell during infections.

* **antibodies** (AN-tih-bah-deez) are protein molecules produced by the body's immune system to help fight specific infections caused by microorganisms, such as bacteria and viruses.

* **cultures** (KUL-churz) are tests in which a sample of fluid or tissue from the body is placed in a dish containing material that supports the growth of certain organisms. Typically, within a few days the organisms will grow and can be identified.

* **placenta** (pluh-SEN-ta) is an organ that provides nutrients and oxygen to a developing baby; it is located within the womb during pregnancy.

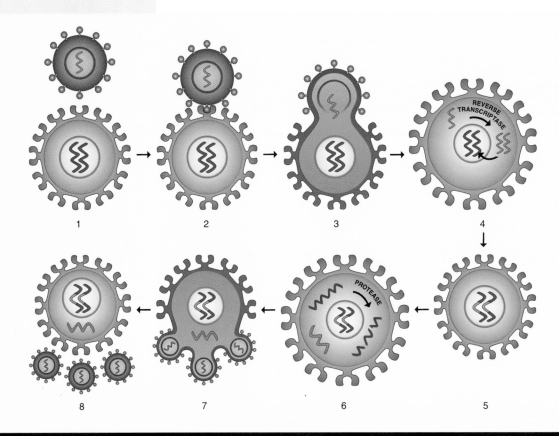

Legend

HIV genetic material (RNA)		RNA "blueprint" for making new HIV		CD4+ (T-helper) lymphocyte
Genetic material (DNA) of CD4+ lymphocyte		Protein to be used to make new HIV		CD4+ lymphocyte infected with HIV
HIV genetic material inserted into cell's genetic material		Human immunodeficiency virus (HIV)		

(1) The human immunodeficiency virus (HIV) particle (top) travels through the bloodstream and (2) attaches to the receptor on the surface of a lymphocyte (bottom), an immune system cell involved in fighting infections. (3) Genetic material (RNA) from the virus enters the lymphocyte and, (4) with the help of an enzyme called *reverse transcriptase*, makes copies of itself to be inserted into the genetic material of the host lymphocyte. Drugs known as *reverse transcriptase inhibitors* act at this step to block the virus' genetic material from copying itself. (5) Copies of the virus' genetic material are inserted into the genetic material of the lymphocyte. (6) This new genetic material in the cell causes the lymphocyte to make the "blueprint" needed for manufacturing new HIV particles. This blueprint contains the code for making virus proteins. An enzyme known as a *protease* acts to clip the large virus protein molecules into smaller pieces so they can be used to make new HIV particles. Drugs known as *protease inhibitors* work at this step by interfering with the processing of virus protein. (7,8) New HIV particles are produced and released from the lymphocyte, which is destroyed. These viruses can then travel through the body and enter and destroy other cells.

How Is HIV/AIDS Treated?

Receiving treatment as early as possible, before the start of symptoms, increases a person's chances of staying healthier and living longer with HIV infection. Advances in treatment have greatly improved the quality of life, and prolonged life, for many people living with HIV and AIDS. Since the 1980s, various types of medications have been developed to treat AIDS. All of these drugs work by interfering with the replication cycle of HIV; they block the action of certain enzymes* that the virus needs in order to make copies of itself. Taking these medicines slows the spread of HIV in a person's body, delaying the onset of AIDS. The class of drugs called protease (PRO-tee-aze) inhibitors (the enzyme that the drug blocks is known as a protease) has proven to be especially effective. These drugs and others are most often used in combinations of three to five medications in a treatment known as highly active antiretroviral (an-tie-REH-tro-vy-rul) therapy (HAART). Other medicines also are used to treat or prevent the opportunistic infections associated with HIV infection. The amount of HIV in the body, called the viral load, is followed with regular blood tests to see how well treatment is working. CD4+ (T-helper) cell counts are followed as well. Over time, the virus can develop resistance to the drugs used to fight it and treatment may have to be changed, so research and development of new medicines is essential.

Taking all medications exactly as they are prescribed is crucial because it can help keep resistance to the medicines from developing. Maintaining general good health, getting enough rest, eating a nutritious diet, not smoking or taking drugs, and visiting the doctor for regular checkups are also important parts of treatment.

Currently there is no cure for HIV and AIDS, so once someone becomes infected that person is infected for life. Experts believe that people with AIDS eventually will die from it, unless death from another cause occurs sooner.

Can HIV/AIDS Cause Other Medical Complications?

Complications include AIDS-related opportunistic infections; invasive bacterial infection; certain cancers such as non-Hodgkin's lymphoma, Kaposi's (kuh-POE-zees) sarcoma, and cervical* cancer; pneumonia; and AIDS dementia (dih-MEN-sha), in which there is impairment of thinking, memory, and concentration. HIV-infected people who use IV drugs are at increased risk for hepatitis* C infection, which can lead to severe liver damage and death. People with AIDS also are more likely to develop more severe symptoms and complications from other infections such as syphilis* and tuberculosis*.

* **enzymes** (EN-zimes) are proteins that help speed up a chemical reaction in a cell or organism.

* **cervical** refers to the cervix (SIR-viks), the lower, narrow end of the uterus that opens into the vagina.

* **hepatitis** (heh-puh-TIE-tis) is an inflammation of the liver. Hepatitis can be caused by viruses, bacteria, and a number of other noninfectious medical conditions.

* **syphilis** (SIH-fih-lis) is a sexually transmitted disease that, if untreated, can lead to serious lifelong problems throughout the body, including blindness and paralysis.

* **tuberculosis** (too-ber-kyoo-LO-sis) is a bacterial infection that primarily attacks the lungs but can spread to other parts of the body.

*vaccine (vak-SEEN) is a preparation of killed or weakened germs, or a part of a germ or product it produces, given to prevent or lessen the severity of the disease that can result if a person is exposed to the germ itself. Use of vaccines for this purpose is called immunization.

How Can HIV/AIDS Be Prevented?

Researchers are working to develop a vaccine* for AIDS. Until one is available, the best means of prevention is avoiding contact with the bodily fluids of someone who is infected. This means:

- avoiding sexual contact; this is the only certain way of preventing HIV infection from heterosexual or homosexual sexual contact

- practicing safer sex (using a latex condom properly every time for vaginal, anal, or oral sex), which reduces but does not eliminate the risk of HIV infection; other forms of birth control such as birth control pills offer no protection against the HIV virus

- avoiding IV drug use and never sharing needles for drugs, steroids, medications, tattooing, or body piercing.

For pregnant women infected with HIV, taking antiretroviral drugs during pregnancy and delivering the infant by cesarean section can greatly reduce the risk of a woman passing the infection to her baby. When

---

UNDERSTANDING OPPORTUNISTIC INFECTIONS

The opportunistic infections associated with HIV disease can affect every system in the body, such as:

- *Pneumocystis carinii* (nu-mo-SIS-tis kah-RIH-nee-eye) pneumonia (PCP): pneumonia caused by an organism that has both parasite and fungus properties. It leads to fever, cough, and trouble breathing and can spread to the liver, spleen, and bone marrow. Untreated, the infection causes death.

- Cryptosporidiosis (krip-toh-spo-rid-e-O-sis) and isosporiasis (eye-so-spuh-RYE-uh-sis): intestinal infections caused by parasites that can cause diarrhea, fever, and stomach cramps.

- Cytomegalovirus (sye-tuh-meh-guh-lo-VY-rus): member of the herpesvirus family. Can cause severe infections in people with weakened immune systems. In people with HIV, it can cause an eye infection that may lead to blindness.

- Histoplasmosis (his-toh-plaz-MO-sis): a fungal infection that usually begins in the lungs and causes symptoms such as fever and cough. In people with HIV infection, it can spread throughout the body

and lead to problems such as nausea (NAW-zee-uh) and vomiting, joint pain, rash, and sores on the skin.

- Cryptococcal meningitis (krip-toh-KAH-kul meh-nin-JY-tis): an infection of the membranes lining the brain and spinal cord caused by a fungus-like organism found in soil. It can cause fever, vomiting, and hallucinations, and can eventually lead to coma or death.

- Cerebral toxoplasmosis (suh-REE-brul tox-o-plaz-MO-sis): an infection caused by an organism that affects the brain, heart, lungs, and other vital organs. It can cause headaches, blurred vision, seizures, and brain damage in people with HIV infection.

- Disseminated mycobacterium avium (my-ko-bak-TEER-e-um A-vee-um) complex (MAC): an infection caused by bacteria found in food, water, and soil. Though these germs usually do not make people sick, in those with weakened immune systems they can cause lung disease, fever, night sweats, weight loss, and diarrhea.

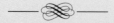

treatment is given to both mother and infant, the risk of HIV transmission drops by about 75 percent. Doctors also advise that HIV-infected mothers feed their infants formula to prevent passing the virus through breast milk.

Resources

Organizations

American Foundation for AIDS Research, 120 Wall Street, 13th Floor, New York, NY 10005. The American Foundation for AIDS Research is a nonprofit organization dedicated to AIDS research, prevention, and education.
Telephone 800-392-6327
http://www.amfar.org

U.S. Centers for Disease Control and Prevention (CDC), 1600 Clifton Road, Atlanta, GA 30333. The CDC is the U.S. government authority for information about infectious and other diseases. It provides information about HIV and AIDS at its website. It also offers the National AIDS Hotline, which provides confidential information and referrals 24 hours a day.
Telephone 800-342-2437
http://www.cdc.gov

Websites

HIVInSite, from the University of California, San Francisco, offers in-depth information about HIV disease, including http://whatudo.org, a site written just for adolescents in easy-to-understand language.
http://hivinsite.ucsf.edu/InSite

KidsHealth.org. KidsHealth is a website created by the medical experts of the Nemours Foundation and is devoted to issues of children's health. It contains articles on a variety of health topics, including HIV and AIDS.
http://www.KidsHealth.org

▶ *See also*
Hepatitis, Infectious
Immune Deficiencies
Pneumonia
Sexually Transmitted Diseases
Syphilis
Tuberculosis

Anthrax

Anthrax (AN-thraks) is a rare infectious disease caused by the bacterium Bacillus anthracis.

What Is Anthrax?

Anthrax is primarily a disease of livestock, such as sheep, cattle, or goats. It is rarely seen in humans, and most cases occur in developing countries. Anthrax is most likely to occur in people whose work regularly

KEYWORDS
for searching the Internet and other reference sources

Bacillus anthracis

Biological warfare

Bioterrorism

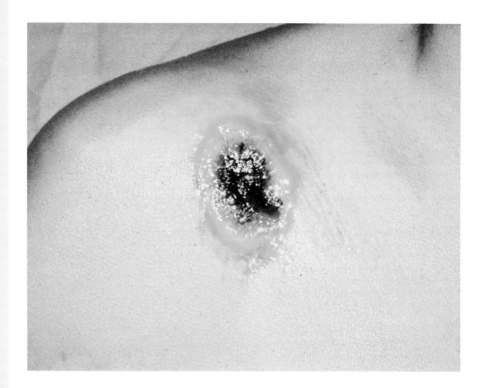

Over the course of a few days, cutaneous anthrax develops into a sore with a coal-black center. *Custom Medical Stock Photo, Inc.* ▶

Anthrax in the News

In 2001, just after the terrorist attacks on the World Trade Center in New York and the Pentagon in Washington, D.C., the threat of biological terrorism arose when anthrax spores were discovered in Florida, New York City, and the offices of the United States Congress. More than 20 people showed signs of either inhalation anthrax or cutaneous anthrax. Several of those with the inhalation form of the disease died. In most of those cases, authorities were able to trace the exposure to letters intentionally contaminated with a highly concentrated, aerosolized form of anthrax spores.

Initially, the anthrax threat was assumed to be part of the same terrorist plot that targeted the World Trade Center. Government investigators now believe that a single person without ties to a specific terrorist organization could have mailed the anthrax-laced letters. Regardless of their origin, the letters proved that anthrax can be used as a weapon. The production and release of highly potent forms of anthrax bacteria—to cause illness deliberately in large groups of people—is a type of potential biological warfare, or bioterrorism, that cannot be ignored. As a result, national, state, and local governments and public health officials are planning responses to possible future attacks with biological weapons.

brings them into contact with animal hides, such as those who cut sheep's wool, livestock handlers, laboratory workers, and veterinarians. The bacterium *Bacillus anthracis (buh-SIH-lus an-THRAY-kus)* is found naturally in the soil of farming regions all over the world, including parts of the United States. It can exist undisturbed for many years as spores, a temporarily inactive form of the organism with a protective, shell-like coating. Grazing animals typically become infected with anthrax if they eat vegetation or feed contaminated with spores. Livestock in the United States rarely get anthrax.

There are three forms of anthrax in humans, each resulting from a different route of infection. Cutaneous (kyoo-TAY-nee-us), or skin, anthrax, the least serious form of the disease, occurs when the bacteria enter a break in the skin. Gastrointestinal* anthrax is caused by eating food contaminated with anthrax bacteria; this form is very rare. The third and deadliest form of the disease, inhalation (in-huh-LAY-shun) anthrax, also called pulmonary anthrax or "woolsorter's disease," is also very uncommon and results from breathing in anthrax spores.

How Common Is Anthrax?

Historians believe that anthrax has been around for thousands of years, at least since the fifth and sixth plagues described in the Bible's Book of Exodus. Cutaneous anthrax, the most common form of the disease (about 95 percent of anthrax cases), occurs most often in agricultural regions in Asia, Africa, South and Central America, southern and eastern Europe, the Middle East, and the Caribbean. Anthrax is rare in the United States: according to the U.S. Centers for Disease Control and Prevention, between 1955 and 1999 only 236 cases of anthrax were reported in the United States, nearly all the cutaneous form. Before 2001 the last case of inhalation anthrax in the United States was reported in 1978.

How Does a Person Get Anthrax?

Scientists do not believe that anthrax can be passed from person to person. Cutaneous anthrax occurs when someone with a cut, sore, or other break in the skin touches an infected animal or the by-product of an infected animal, such as contaminated hide, wool, or goat hair. Gastrointestinal anthrax usually is traced to contaminated foods, especially undercooked meat. Inhalation anthrax stems from breathing anthrax spores into the lungs. Although spores are inactive forms of the bacteria, they germinate, or become activated, in the moist, warm environment of the lungs. Someone has to inhale thousands of spores to contract the disease, and spores found in soil rarely are concentrated enough to cause inhalation anthrax.

What Are the Signs and Symptoms?

Symptoms of the disease usually appear within 1 to 7 days after infection with *Bacillus anthracis* and differ according to the way in which a person became infected with the bacterium. The most visible sign of cutaneous anthrax explains how the disease got its name, which is derived from the Greek word *anthracis,* meaning "coal." An anthrax skin infection typically begins as a raised, itchy bump, and within a few days it develops into a small sore or ulcer* with a black, coal-like center. Gastrointestinal anthrax can cause nausea, loss of appetite, fever, and severe bloody vomiting and diarrhea. The first symptoms of inhalation anthrax often resemble those of a common cold or influenza and include cough, difficulty in swallowing, headache, swollen lymph nodes* in the neck, and tiredness. Within days the symptoms rapidly progress to severe breathing problems and shock*, often leading to heart failure and death.

How Do Doctors Make the Diagnosis?

Bacillus anthracis bacteria sometimes can be seen in a bit of skin from the sore of a person who has cutaneous anthrax or in the coughed-up mucus* of someone with inhalation anthrax when those samples are viewed under a microscope. To help confirm the diagnosis, samples of blood or fluid taken from the nose or sores are cultured* to identify the anthrax bacteria. Blood tests also are used to detect anthrax antibodies*, which indicate that someone has come into contact with anthrax-causing bacteria and may have the disease. Chest X rays can help diagnose inhalation anthrax.

* **gastrointestinal** (gas-tro-in-TES-tih-nuhl) means having to do with the organs of the digestive system, the system that processes food. It includes the mouth, esophagus, stomach, intestines, colon, and rectum and other organs involved in digestion, including the liver and pancreas.

* **ulcer** is an open sore on the skin or the lining of a hollow body organ, such as the stomach or intestine. It may or may not be painful.

* **lymph** (LIMF) **nodes** are small, bean-shaped masses of tissue containing immune system cells that fight harmful microorganisms. Lymph nodes may swell during infections.

* **shock** is a serious condition in which blood pressure is very low and not enough blood flows to the body's organs and tissues. Untreated, shock may result in death.

* **mucus** (MYOO-kus) is a thick, slippery substance that lines the insides of many body parts.

* **cultured** (KUL-churd) means subjected to a test in which a sample of fluid or tissue from the body is placed in a dish containing material that supports the growth of certain organisms. Typically, within a few days the organisms will grow and can be identified.

* **antibodies** (AN-tih-bah-deez) are protein molecules produced by the body's immune system to help fight specific infections caused by microorganisms, such as bacteria and viruses.

* intravenous (in-tra-VEE-nus) means within or through a vein. For example, medications, fluid, or other substances can be given through a needle or soft tube inserted through the skin's surface directly into a vein.

* vaccine (vak-SEEN) is a preparation of killed or weakened germs, or a part of a germ or product it produces, given to prevent or lessen the severity of the disease that can result if a person is exposed to the germ itself. Use of vaccines for this purpose is called immunization.

▶ *See also*

Bioterrorism

Vaccination (Immunization)

What Is the Treatment for Anthrax?

Doctors prescribe antibiotics to fight anthrax infections. Patients with gastrointestinal and inhalation anthrax typically need intensive, round-the-clock care with intravenous* medications and fluids in a hospital. Inhalation anthrax can cause severe breathing problems that may require the use of a respirator, a machine that can assist a person's breathing until he or she recovers.

What to Expect

Untreated, all three forms of anthrax can lead to widespread infection and death. If it is treated, cutaneous anthrax generally is not fatal. Gastrointestinal anthrax results in death in about half of all cases. Even with medical treatment, inhalation anthrax is often fatal.

How Is Anthrax Prevented?

Agricultural and textile workers in developed countries such as the United States are instructed to wash their hands after working in the soil or handling animals and animal by-products. People who live in high-risk areas of the world are advised to avoid contact with livestock and not to eat improperly prepared or undercooked meat. An anthrax vaccine* exists, but this vaccine is not given routinely in the United States, except to people in the military or to scientists who may come into contact with the bacteria through their research. Veterinarians and people whose jobs involve handling livestock typically are vaccinated against the disease if they work in high-risk areas of the world. In the fall of 2001, when anthrax spores contaminated several U.S. post offices and office buildings (see sidebar), public health experts recommended antibiotics for people who had been exposed to anthrax—even if they had no symptoms of the disease. Officials stressed, however, that it was not necessary or advisable for the general public to take antibiotics to prevent anthrax.

Resource

Organization

U.S. Centers for Disease Control and Prevention (CDC), 1600 Clifton Road, Atlanta, GA 30333. The CDC maintains a website that includes information about anthrax, plus notices about public health threats, vaccinations, and antibiotics.
Telephone 800-311-3435
http://www.cdc.gov

Arthritis, Infectious

Infectious arthritis (in-FEK-shus ar-THRY-tis) is a bacterial, fungal, or viral infection of the tissue and fluid within a joint*. The infection causes inflammation and can result in pain, swelling, and limited motion of the joint.

What Is Infectious Arthritis?

Most of the time, bacteria cause infectious arthritis. This form of arthritis is also called septic arthritis, and the infected joint is referred to as a "septic joint." *Staphylococcus* (stah-fih-lo-KAH-kus) or *Streptococcus* (strep-tuh-KAH-kus) bacteria are the culprits in most cases of septic arthritis. Arthritis also can occur in Lyme disease, tuberculosis, and many other infections. Bacteria can be introduced directly into the joint by injury or surgery, but more often the bacteria are carried to the joint through the bloodstream from an infection somewhere else in the body. The most common cause of septic arthritis in young adults is *Neisseria gonorrhoeae* (nye-SEER-e-uh gah-no-REE-eye), the bacterium that causes gonorrhea. These bacteria may spread from infected areas, such as the cervix* and rectum*, and infect joints at the hands, wrists, elbows, and knees. Certain viruses, including those that produce measles, rubella (roo-BEH-luh, a rash-causing viral infection that is also called German measles), and hepatitis B or C, also can cause arthritis. Fungi found in soil, bird droppings, and some plants are uncommon causes of infectious arthritis.

People whose immune systems are weak because they have a disease such as diabetes*, sickle-cell disease*, certain cancers, lupus*, or AIDS are more likely to get infectious arthritis. Alcoholism and intravenous drug use also put people at higher risk. Because a joint that is damaged is more vulnerable to germs, people with existing disease involving the joints (for example, rheumatoid arthritis*) are more likely to develop infectious arthritis. Anyone who has had joint-replacement surgery is at increased risk for infection of that joint in the future.

How Common Is It?

Some places in the world have more cases of infectious arthritis than others. Rates are highest in Africa, Latin America, and Asia. In the United States, about 20,000 cases of infectious arthritis occur each year. Men, women, and children of all ages can get infectious arthritis, but almost half of patients in whom the illness is diagnosed are 65 years or older.

Is Arthritis Contagious?

Infectious arthritis is not contagious, but certain viruses and the bacterium that causes gonorrhea can be transmitted from one person to

KEYWORDS
for searching the Internet
and other reference sources

Bacterial arthritis

Osteoarthritis

Rheumatoid arthritis

Septic arthritis

* **joint** is the structure where two or more bones come together, allowing flexibility and motion of the skeleton.

* **cervix** (SIR-viks) is the lower, narrow end of the uterus that opens into the vagina.

* **rectum** is the final portion of the large intestine, connecting the colon to the anus.

* **diabetes** (dye-uh-BEE-teez) is a condition in which the body's pancreas does not produce enough insulin or the body cannot use the insulin it makes effectively, resulting in increased levels of sugar in the blood. This can lead to increased urination, dehydration, weight loss, weakness, and a number of other symptoms and complications related to chemical imbalances within the body.

* **sickle-cell disease** is a hereditary condition in which the red blood cells, which are usually round, take on an abnormal crescent shape and have a decreased ability to carry oxygen throughout the body.

* **lupus** (LOO-pus) is a chronic, or long-lasting, disease that causes inflammation of connective tissue, the material that holds together the various structures of the body.

* **rheumatoid arthritis** (ROO-mah-toyd ar-THRY-tis) is a chronic disease characterized by painful swelling, stiffness, and deformity of the joints.

another. This does not necessarily mean that someone who gets a particular infection caused by these organisms will also get infectious arthritis.

What Are the Signs and Symptoms of Arthritis?

The symptoms of infectious arthritis vary by type of infection and the particular joint that is affected. With septic arthritis, symptoms usually appear within a few hours or days and include redness, warmth, swelling, pain, and sometimes fever and chills. It is difficult to move the affected joint because of the pain and swelling. Arthritis from a viral infection tends to come on more slowly, often with absence of fever and with less swelling, limitation of movement, and pain at the affected joint. Viruses may infect the joint directly, or sometimes the response of the body's immune system to a virus may cause joint inflammation (called "postinfectious arthritis"). Inflammation stemming from a fungal infection or tuberculosis usually develops very slowly, sometimes over weeks or months. The bacteria that cause Lyme disease can settle in a joint and may lead to recurrent bouts of arthritis. Usually, swelling and limitation of movement of the joint are the main symptoms of this form of arthritis.

How Do Doctors Make the Diagnosis?

A doctor who suspects infectious arthritis based on a patient's symptoms and the findings of a physical examination will want to know the details of the person's medical history. Taking a medical history might include asking questions about whether the patient is sexually active, injects drugs, has been bitten by a tick (which can cause Lyme disease), has had arthritis in the past, or has recently been injured, hospitalized, or exposed to an illness. Laboratory tests can help confirm the diagnosis. A common diagnostic test is aspiration* of some of the synovial fluid* within the affected joint. The doctor inserts a thin, sterile needle through the skin directly into the joint and removes a sample of fluid. The fluid is then examined under a microscope to look for evidence of microorganisms (such as bacteria) and infection-fighting white blood cells. Some of the sample is put in a jelly-like medium containing nutrients that support the growth of bacteria, and this is placed in an incubator for a few days. If bacteria grow, bacterial infectious arthritis is diagnosed. This synovial fluid also can be tested for evidence of viral or fungal infections. In addition, blood tests can help diagnose arthritis caused by a virus or bacterium. If the suspected cause of inflammation is a fungus or tuberculosis, a tissue sample from the infected joint may need to be removed and analyzed. X rays, computerized tomography*, or magnetic resonance imaging* studies can detect excess fluid and sometimes destruction of the tissues within or surrounding an affected joint.

What Is the Treatment for Arthritis?

The type of organism causing arthritis determines which medicines are needed to treat the infection. Antibiotics are prescribed to treat joint in-

* **aspiration** (as-puh-RAY-shun) is the sucking of fluid or other material out of the body, such as the removal of a sample of joint fluid through a needle inserted into the joint.

* **synovial** (sih-NO-vee-ul) **fluid** is the fluid produced in the synovium, the inner lining of the flexible capsule that encloses the joint space between two bones. This fluid lubricates and nourishes the joint.

* **computerized tomography** (kom-PYOO-ter-ized toe-MAH-gruh-fee) or CT, also called computerized axial tomography (CAT), is a technique in which a machine takes many X rays of the body to create a three-dimensional picture.

* **magnetic resonance imaging (MRI)** uses magnetic waves, instead of X rays, to scan the body and produce detailed pictures of the body's structures.

fections caused by bacteria, and anti-fungal medications are given for infection due to a fungus. Doctors also may recommend that a person with infectious arthritis keep the affected joint elevated, or raised up, and avoid moving it. Over-the-counter anti-inflammatory medications, such as ibuprofen, can relieve swelling and pain. Sometimes, to help healing and decrease discomfort, some of the excess synovial fluid is removed from a joint. This procedure may have to be repeated several times. In certain cases, a septic joint might be drained by a surgical procedure to help cure the infection.

How Long Does the Infection Last?

Eliminating the infection can take time. Antibiotics may need to be given intravenously for 3 weeks or more. It may take even longer for someone to be able to use an affected joint without pain. In cases of severe infectious arthritis, physical therapy may be recommended after other treatment has been completed, to help patients recover full movement and function of the joint. Infectious arthritis can be cured with prompt and proper treatment. In cases that are severe or where treatment is delayed, the infection may cause permanent damage to the joint and the bone, sometimes resulting in persistent pain and disability.

Can Infectious Arthritis Be Prevented?

Abstinence (not having sex) will prevent arthritis caused by STDs like gonorrhea. For sexually active people, the use of latex condoms can lessen the risk of exposure to bacteria that can cause arthritis. Doctors may recommend that people who have a high risk of the disease, such as those with artificial joints, take antibiotics to prevent an infection in the joint, even when the person has no symptoms of disease.

Resources

Organizations

The Arthritis Society, 393 University Avenue, Suite 1700, Toronto, Ontario, Canada M5G 1E6. The Arthritis Society details types of arthritis on its website and tracks research on causes and treatment of the disease.
Telephone 416-979-7228
http://www.arthritis.ca

U.S. National Library of Medicine, 8600 Rockville Pike, Bethesda, MD 20894. The National Library of Medicine has a website packed with information on diseases and drugs, consumer resources, dictionaries and encyclopedias of medical terms, and directories of doctors and helpful organizations.
Telephone 888-346-3656
http://www.nlm.nih.gov

▶ See also
Gonorrhea

Hepatitis, Infectious

Immune Deficiencies

Lyme Disease

Measles (Rubeola)

Rubella (German Measles)

Sexually Transmitted Diseases

Staphylococcal Infections

Streptococcal Infections

Tuberculosis

B

Bioterrorism

Bioterrorism is the intentional use of harmful biological, or living, organisms or their toxic products to cause injury or death to people or animals.

What Is Bioterrorism?

Also known as biological warfare, bioterrorism is a form of warfare that uses specific microorganisms*, such as harmful bacteria and viruses, to cause illness or death deliberately in people or animals. When organisms are used in this way, they become weapons.

The History of Bioterrorism

The use of microorganisms to spread disease intentionally is not new to the twenty-first century. In 1346, it is believed that the Tartar army tried to capture the port city of Caffa on the Black Sea in the Crimea by catapulting bodies of plague (PLAYG) victims over the city walls. A plague epidemic* ensued, and Caffa surrendered. During the French and Indian Wars in the eighteenth century in North America, the British were rumored to have given blankets contaminated with smallpox to Native Americans, leading to an epidemic of the disease.

The Tartars and the British troops did not know that certain microorganisms cause disease. They knew only that disease was rumored to have spread from dead bodies or, in the case of smallpox, even from the blankets that touched victims. People were not aware that microorganisms are at the root of infectious disease until the latter part of the nineteenth century, when scientists began to understand the connection. In 1876, the German scientist Robert Koch had proved that anthrax (AN-thraks) bacteria cause anthrax. After World War II the United States and other nations experimented with harmful biological organisms and various methods of transmitting them. In 1972 the Biological Weapons Convention treaty was signed by more than 100 countries around the world, including the United States and the Soviet Union, to stop research and production of biological organisms as weapons of war.

It is likely that some countries in the world today—especially those harboring or supporting known terrorist groups—continue to manufacture and store stockpiles of dangerous microorganisms, such as those that cause anthrax. The use of bioterrorism to wage warfare is favored

KEYWORDS
for searching the Internet and other reference sources

Anthrax

Biological agent

Biological warfare

Bioweapon

Botulism

Plague

Smallpox

Tularemia

Vaccination

* **microorganisms** are tiny organisms that can be seen only using a microscope. Types of microorganisms include fungi, bacteria, and viruses.

* **epidemic** (eh-pih-DEH-mik) is an outbreak of disease, especially infectious disease, in which the number of cases suddenly becomes far greater than usual. Usually epidemics are outbreaks of diseases in specific regions, whereas worldwide epidemics are called pandemics.

among terrorists or fringe groups because it requires few resources compared with traditional warfare and can potentially harm large numbers of people.

How Can Biological Agents Be Spread?

Deadly microorganisms (also known as biological agents or bioweapons) can be spread purposely through air or food and water supplies or by intentionally infecting someone with a highly contagious agent and letting that person circulate in a community, starting a massive wave of disease. But the handling and release of many of these organisms are dangerous and could be deadly for potential terrorists trying to use them.

Some organisms can be aerosolized (AIR-o-suh-lized), meaning that they are processed into the tiniest of particles, in a wet or dry form, that can be sprayed or released into the air so that large numbers of people can inhale them. Aerosolized organisms can be dispersed by aerosol containers, small crop-dusting planes, ventilation systems, or contamination of an object that can carry disease throughout a region, like the anthrax-tainted letters received by various government and media employees in the United States in late 2001.

Some harmful biological organisms become weakened, however, as they spread into water or food supplies, making them less likely to cause significant harm to anyone who comes into contact with them. For example, a person would have to inhale thousands of anthrax spores* to become sick. A terrorist group trying to use anthrax as a bioweapon would have to use a highly concentrated form to be able to harm large numbers of people via contaminated packages or envelopes.

What Are Potential Biological Agents?

The U.S. Centers for Disease Control and Prevention (CDC) separates biological organisms into categories according to their virulence (VEER-uh-lents), or ability to cause disease. The most virulent biological diseases are also the most likely to be used by terrorists. These diseases are anthrax, smallpox, plague, botulism (BOH-chu-lih-zum), and tularemia (too-lah-REE-me-uh).

Anthrax   Anthrax is caused by the bacterium *Bacillus anthracis*. The bacteria can form spores, which have a hard coating that allows them to survive in harsh environments. The spores are found naturally in soil and can infect grazing animals, most often livestock such as cattle, sheep, or horses. The disease is not contagious from person to person, and natural human infection is rare.

There are three types of anthrax, distinguished by the three different ways in which a person becomes infected: cutaneous (kyoo-TAY-nee-us) anthrax, which infects the skin; inhalation (in-huh-LAY-shun) anthrax, which results from breathing in large numbers of concentrated spores;

* **spores** are a temporarily inactive form of a germ enclosed in a protective shell.

and gastrointestinal* (gas-tro-in-TES-tih-nuhl) anthrax, which is caused by ingesting spores. Cutaneous anthrax causes brownish-black ulcers, or sores, that turn into scabs on the skin. Symptoms of inhalation anthrax include rapid onset of fever, chills, headache, nausea, and vomiting, with victims quickly experiencing difficulty in breathing. Gastrointestinal anthrax is very rare and causes severe abdominal* pain, diarrhea (dye-uh-REE-uh), and hemorrhaging* from the gastrointestinal tract.

All forms of anthrax can be treated with antibiotics if they are diagnosed early, but the inhalation and gastrointestinal types of anthrax are extremely deadly if left untreated. Even with treatment, patients with inhalation or gastrointestinal anthrax can die from the disease. There is an anthrax vaccine*, but it is given only to people in the military and people such as veterinarians who routinely handle livestock and are therefore more likely to come into contact with the natural form of the disease.

Smallpox Smallpox is a deadly viral infection that is caused by the variola virus and is found only in humans. In the twentieth century smallpox claimed millions of lives, but in 1980 the World Health Organization (WHO) declared the disease to have been eradicated (eliminated) from the human population following an aggressive worldwide vaccination (vak-sih-NAY-shun) program. Routine vaccination against smallpox in the United States ended in 1972, and the last known natural case of smallpox was in 1977 in Somalia in Africa. Today there are two official facilities that store samples of the virus: the CDC in Atlanta, Georgia, and the Russian State Research Center of Virology and Biotechnology in Koltsovo.

Smallpox is the most contagious disease known and is transmitted through direct contact with the lesions* of an infected person, by inhaling infected droplets of moisture released into the air by coughing patients, and even by handling contaminated clothing that contains fluid from smallpox sores. The symptoms of smallpox are high fever, headache, backache, vomiting, and a painful rash of lesions that covers the face, arms, and body and often leaves scars. The disease is fatal in up to 30 percent of cases, and at this time there is no known medication that can cure smallpox. Vaccination given within 4 days of exposure to the virus sometimes can prevent smallpox or lessen its symptoms, including the rash.

The CDC keeps an emergency supply of smallpox vaccine in the event that bioterrorism attacks with smallpox occur in the United States. In 2002, some vaccine-making companies received approval from the CDC to make an additional supply of the vaccine, should it be needed on a more widespread basis.

In order to protect U.S. citizens against the threat of a bioterrorism attack, President George W. Bush announced in late 2002 that some

* **gastrointestinal** means having to do with the organs of the digestive system, the system that processes food. It includes the mouth, esophagus, stomach, intestines, colon, and rectum and other organs involved in digestion, including the liver and pancreas.

* **abdominal** (ab-DAH-mih-nul) refers to the area of the body below the ribs and above the hips that contains the stomach, intestines, and other organs.

* **hemorrhaging** (HEM-rij-ing) describes a condition in which uncontrolled or abnormal bleeding occurs.

* **vaccine** (vak-SEEN) is a preparation of killed or weakened germs, or a part of a germ or product it produces, given to prevent or lessen the severity of the disease that can result if a person is exposed to the germ itself. Use of vaccines for this purpose is called immunization.

* **lesions** (LEE-zhuns) is a general term referring to sores or damaged or irregular areas of tissue.

* **lymph** (LIMF) **nodes** are small, bean-shaped masses of tissue that contain immune system cells that fight harmful microorganisms. Lymph nodes may swell during infections.

* **shock** is a serious condition in which blood pressure is very low and not enough blood flows to the body's organs and tissues. Untreated, shock may result in death.

* **respiratory tract** includes the nose, mouth, throat, and lungs. It is the pathway through which air and gases are transported down into the lungs and back out of the body.

* **sputum** (SPYOO-tum) is a substance that contains mucus and other matter coughed out from the lungs, bronchi, and trachea.

* **septic shock** is shock due to overwhelming infection and is characterized by decreased blood pressure, internal bleeding, heart failure, and, in some cases, death.

* **toxin** is a poison that harms the body.

* **neurotransmitters** (nur-o-trans-MIH-terz) are chemical substances that transmit nerve impulses, or messages, throughout the brain and nervous system and are involved in the control of thought, movement, and other body functions.

* **paralysis** (pah-RAH-luh-sis) is the loss or impairment of the ability to move some part of the body.

* **respiratory failure** is a condition in which breathing and oxygen delivery to the body are dangerously altered. This may result from infection, nerve or muscle damage, poisoning, or other causes.

members of the U.S. military will be vaccinated against smallpox and he called for health care workers to volunteer to receive the vaccine.

Plague   Plague, caused by the bacterium *Yersinia pestis* (yer-SIN-e-uh PES-tis), has been around for centuries. It can take three forms: bubonic (byoo-BAH-nik), septicemic (sep-tih-SEE-mik), and pneumonic (nu-MOH-nik). Bubonic plague, the most common form, involves the body's lymph nodes*; septicemic plague enters the bloodstream, causing internal bleeding and shock*; and pneumonic plague infects the respiratory tract*. The last form is potentially important in biological warfare because *Yersinia pestis* bacteria can remain alive in the air for up to an hour, making aerosolized transmission possible.

Yersinia pestis is found in rats and other rodents in all parts of the world, including the United States. Plague can spread from infected rats to humans by direct bites or from fleas. The pneumonic form of plague is the only kind that is contagious among humans; transmission takes place by being in close contact with someone who is coughing or sneezing. Symptoms of the plague include fever, chills, headache, abdominal pain, painful and swollen lymph nodes (called buboes, BYOO-boze), chest pain, coughing, bloody sputum*, and septic shock*. There is no vaccine available in the United States, but antibiotics can treat the disease successfully if it is diagnosed early.

Botulism   Botulism is caused by the toxin* produced by the bacterium *Clostridium botulinum.* The bacteria can be inhaled or swallowed, or they can enter the body through a wound, but the disease is not contagious from person to person. The toxin produced by the bacteria affects neurotransmitters* in the body, causing nerve damage and temporary paralysis*, including the muscles for speaking, swallowing, and breathing. Botulism can lead to respiratory failure* and even death. The bacterium and its toxin could be used to produce bioweapons. An antitoxin* against the *Clostridium botulinum* toxin is available from the CDC, but there is currently no vaccine available.

Tularemia   Tularemia is caused by the bacterium *Francisella tularensis* and is highly infectious. It occurs naturally in mice, rabbits, squirrels, and other small mammals. The disease is not contagious among humans, and human infection is rare. Tularemia can be transmitted through contact with infected animals or contaminated water or soil. The disease is potentially dangerous as a biological weapon, because even small numbers (less than 10 to 50) of the aerosolized bacteria can cause serious disease, such as life-threatening pneumonia*. Symptoms include fever, chills, headache, cough, and extreme tiredness. Patients also may have painful ulcers on the skin; swollen, painful eyes; and abdominal pain. Early treatment with antibiotics may prevent or limit the severity of the disease.

What Can We Do to Protect Ourselves?

Following the terrorist incidents and anthrax scare of fall 2001, the U.S. government proposed that billions of dollars be channeled into improving national resources that provide protection against and treatment of the effects of bioweapons. The Office of Homeland Security was formed in late 2001 to oversee the government's preparation for and defense against future acts or threats of bioterrorism that might occur in the United States. The government has authorized an increase in federal stockpiles of antibiotics to treat anthrax, plague, tularemia, and other potential bioweapons, as well as the production of additional supplies of smallpox vaccine. Research continues in the development of better medical treatment and the creation of vaccines for protection against biological agents. Medical professionals and emergency response teams are being trained to diagnose the diseases and respond quickly to the epidemics that could result from bioterrorism. Experts advise that people not stockpile antibiotics out of fear of possible biological warfare, because they could end up using the medicine incorrectly or in the wrong situation. Stockpiling also can lead to a shortage of certain antibiotics and make them unavailable to people who truly need them to treat other diseases.

Resources

Organizations

Center for Civilian Biodefense Strategies, Johns Hopkins University, 111 Market Place, Suite 830, Baltimore, MD 21202. The Center for Civilian Biodefense Strategies carries information about possible bioweapons and posts news updates on the preparedness and response plans of public health agencies and the work of the Department of Homeland Security.
Telephone 410-223-1667
http://www.hopkins-biodefense.org

U.S. Centers for Disease Control and Prevention (CDC), 1600 Clifton Road, Atlanta, GA 30333. The CDC's website carries information about bioterrorism and fact sheets about various biological agents and threats, including anthrax, smallpox, plague, botulism, and tularemia.
Telephone 800-311-3435
http://www.cdc.gov

World Health Organization (WHO), Avenue Appia 20, 1211 Geneva 27, Switzerland. WHO tracks disease outbreaks and emergencies around the world and posts information at its website about potential biological weapons.
Telephone 011-41-22-791-2111
http://www.who.int

* **antitoxin** (an-tih-TOK-sin) counteracts the effects of toxins, or poisons, on the body. It is produced to act against specific toxins, like those made by the bacteria that cause botulism or diphtheria.

* **pneumonia** (nu-MO-nyah) is inflammation of the lung.

▶ *See also*
Anthrax
Botulism
Plague
Smallpox
Tularemia
Zoonoses

Botulism

KEYWORDS
for searching the Internet
and other reference sources

Botulinum toxin

Clostridium botulinum

Food poisoning

Home-canned foods

Neurotoxin

Paralytic illness

* **toxins** are poisons that harm the body.

* **spores** are a temporarily inactive form of a germ enclosed in a protective shell.

* **immune globulins** (ih-MYOON GLAH-byoo-linz), also called gamma globulins, are the proteins of which antibodies are composed.

* **aerosolize** (AIR-o-suh-lize) is to put something, such as a medication, in the form of small particles or droplets that can be sprayed or released into the air.

* **intravenous** (in-tra-VEE-nus) means within or through a vein. For example, medications, fluid, or other substances can be given through a needle or soft tube inserted through the skin's surface directly into a vein.

Botulism (BOH-chu-lih-zum) is an uncommon, nerve-paralyzing illness caused by toxins* produced by Clostridium botulinum *(klos-TRIH-de-um boh-chu-LIE-num) bacteria.*

What Is Botulism?

There are seven types of botulinum toxin, each designated by a letter from A through G. Only four types (A, B, E, and F) make people sick. There are three forms of naturally occurring human botulism: infant botulism, food-borne botulism, and wound botulism. Inhalation (in-huh-LAY-shun) botulism is an additional form of the illness that could possibly be spread through the air intentionally by man. *Clostridium botulinum* is commonly found in soil and grows best in low-oxygen environments. The bacteria form spores* that remain dormant, or inactive, waiting for conditions that allow them to grow. The spores can exist everywhere, and people might eat food containing these spores without becoming sick. When conditions are right, however, the spores can activate and produce toxin.

Food contaminated with the toxin is the culprit in cases of food-borne botulism; most outbreaks stem from food that is improperly cooked or incorrectly canned or preserved. In food-borne botulism the toxin itself is swallowed, but in cases of infant botulism an infant swallows the spores and they then activate in the intestine and produce toxin. It is believed that the infant intestine lacks enough protective intestinal bacteria, stomach acid, and immune globulins* to prevent the spores from activating. Wound botulism is rare and develops when bacteria infect a wound and grow, producing the toxin. Bioterrorists have attempted to aerosolize* botulinum toxin without success, but the threat of inhalation botulism as a biological weapon has raised concerns.

How Common Is Botulism?

More than 100 cases of botulism are reported in the United States each year. Infant botulism accounts for about 72 percent of reported cases and food-borne botulism for about 25 percent. Wound botulism is the rarest form, but health officials have noted an increase in this type in California, a rise they attribute to the intravenous* use of illegal drugs from Mexico.

How Can a Person Contract Botulism?

Botulism is not contagious. Outbreaks of food-borne botulism usually can be traced to improperly home-canned foods, especially those with low amounts of acid, such as asparagus, green beans, beets, and corn, which allow the *Clostridium botulinum* bacteria to grow. Various frozen foods also have been implicated in outbreaks of the disease. Most infants contract botulism by inhaling or swallowing spores; honey is one source of these spores. Wound botulism sometimes is linked to crush injuries.

What Are the Signs and Symptoms of Botulism?

The classic symptoms of botulism include blurred or double vision*, droopy eyelids, slurred speech, difficulty in swallowing, dry mouth, and muscle weakness. These symptoms appear when the toxin interrupts nerve impulses to the muscles, which paralyzes the muscles. If untreated, paralysis may progress to involve the arms, legs, trunk, and muscles of the respiratory tract*. In food-borne botulism, symptoms generally begin 18 to 36 hours after eating the contaminated food, but they can occur after as little as 6 hours or as much as 10 days. Infants with botulism may appear drowsy or sluggish, not eat well, be constipated, and have a weak cry and muscle weakness. In infants, it can take 3 to 30 days for the symptoms to appear and progress.

How Do Doctors Make the Diagnosis?

Laboratory tests can detect the toxin in blood, stool (bowel movements), or wound samples. Because the symptoms of botulism are similar to those of stroke* and several other nerve diseases, doctors also may order a brain scan, spinal tap*, or other nerve- and muscle-function tests to check for other possible causes. The doctor may ask whether the patient has eaten any home-canned foods and, if so, order tests on the suspect food.

How Is Botulism Treated?

The U.S. Centers for Disease Control and Prevention (CDC) has a supply of antitoxin* against botulism. The antitoxin can slow or halt the damage caused by botulinum toxin. The sooner it is given, the more effective it is in easing the symptoms. To help rid the body of the toxin, doctors sometimes cause vomiting or use enemas*. In severe cases, patients who are unable to breathe well enough on their own might need a ventilator (VEN-tuh-lay-ter), a machine that can help a person breathe for several weeks. Wound botulism might require surgery to remove the source of the toxin-producing bacteria.

What Are the Complications and Duration of the Disease?

Most people with botulism require hospitalization, but they typically recover after weeks or perhaps months of care. Paralysis of the respiratory muscles can lead to pneumonia*. Even after recovery, some patients may be tired and feel short of breath.

How Can Botulism Be Prevented?

Although botulinum toxin is extremely potent, it can be destroyed easily. Heating food and drinks to an internal temperature of 185 degrees

* **double vision** is a vision problem in which a person sees two images of a single object.

* **respiratory tract** includes the nose, mouth, throat, and lungs. It is the pathway through which air and gases are transported down into the lungs and back out of the body.

* **stroke** is a brain-damaging event usually caused by interference with blood flow to the brain. A stroke may occur when a blood vessel supplying the brain becomes clogged or bursts, depriving brain tissue of oxygen. As a result, nerve cells in the affected area of the brain, and the specific body parts they control, do not properly function.

* **spinal tap,** also called a lumbar puncture, is a medical procedure in which a needle is used to withdraw a sample of the fluid surrounding the spinal cord and brain. The fluid is then tested, usually to detect signs of infection, such as meningitis, or other diseases.

* **antitoxin** (an-tih-TOK-sin) counteracts the effects of toxins, or poisons, on the body. It is produced to act against specific toxins, like those made by the bacteria that cause botulism or diphtheria.

* **enemas** (EH-nuh-muhz) are procedures in which liquid is injected through the anus into the intestine, usually to flush out the intestines.

* **pneumonia** (nu-MO-nyah) is inflammation of the lung, usually caused by infection.

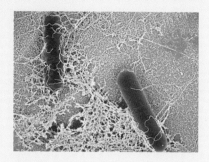

Clostridium botulinum bacteria as seen with an electron microscope. *Visuals Unlimited*

▶ See also
Intestinal Infections

Fahrenheit for at least 5 minutes will detoxify them. Boiling home-canned foods before eating them also lessens risk. Health officials advise using a pressure cooker and high temperatures—about 250 degrees Fahrenheit—to kill the spores when canning or preserving foods at home. It also is best to avoid eating commercially prepared foods from cans that are swollen, punctured, or leaking. Because honey can contain spores of *Clostridium botulinum,* doctors advise that infants younger than 1 year not be given this sweetener. Breast-feeding can help protect against infant botulism. Receiving prompt medical care for infected wounds and not injecting street drugs can help prevent wound botulism.

Resource

Website

KidsHealth.org. KidsHealth is a website created by the medical experts of the Nemours Foundation and is devoted to issues of children's health. It contains articles on a variety of health topics, including botulism. http://www.KidsHealth.org

FOR GOOD AND EVIL

Botulinum toxin is the first biological toxin licensed for treatment of human diseases. The U.S. government approves its use to relax painfully cramped or tight muscles and as an ingredient in medications for the treatment of migraine headache, chronic lower back pain, stroke, brain injury, and cerebral palsy. Botulinum toxin injections (called Botox) can paralyze muscles that cause the skin to wrinkle. Their use is popular among people looking to maintain a youthful appearance.

Ironically, the same substance has the potential to cause mass destruction if it is dispersed into the air or introduced into the food supply. The U.S. government developed botulinum toxin for potential use as a weapon during World War II. Japan, Iraq, and the Soviet Union have also experimented with botulinum toxin as a biological weapon, and Iran, North Korea, and Syria may have done so as well.

However, scientists have been perplexed and terrorists thwarted by how difficult it is to prepare botulism toxin for use as a weapon. Terrorists in Japan attempted to unleash it on at least three occasions between 1990 and 1995, but their plan for widespread destruction failed each time. In addition to tracking the efforts of bioterrorists, the U.S. government has developed elaborate methods to detect and respond to an attack with botulinum toxin. A national surveillance system involving doctors and hospitals has been designed to alert the U.S. Centers for Disease Control and Prevention to botulism outbreaks, and stores of antitoxin are on hand to treat victims.

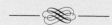

Bronchiolitis

Bronchiolitis (brong-kee-o-LYE-tis) is an infection that causes inflammation of the lung's smaller airways, also called the bronchioles (BRONG-kee-oles). It is common among very young children, particularly during the winter months.

What Is Bronchiolitis?

Bronchiolitis is caused by a virus that infects the bronchioles, the smallest airways that carry air through the lungs. The linings of these airways swell and become blocked with fluid and mucus*, making it difficult to breathe. The virus that most often causes bronchiolitis is called respiratory syncytial virus* (RSV). Other viruses, such as rhinovirus, parainfluenza* virus, influenza A*, and adenovirus*, also can cause bronchiolitis. Bronchiolitis is most common in late fall, winter, and early spring. It typically affects younger children, with most cases occurring in children 2 years old or younger. About 90,000 children are hospitalized for bronchiolitis each year in the United States.

How Does Bronchiolitis Spread?

The viruses that cause bronchiolitis are contagious. They usually are spread through the air when infected drops of fluid are released during a sneeze or cough. RSV stays alive on surfaces, such as countertops and toys, for long periods of time. When children touch these infected surfaces, they can easily pick up the virus. A child who is infected with RSV, however, may just get a bad cold and may not experience the symptoms of bronchiolitis.

Signs and Symptoms of Bronchiolitis

An infected child typically has a runny nose, mild cough, and low fever for a few days. Then the infection peaks; at this stage the cough may worsen, and breathing sometimes becomes difficult. The child may have rapid breathing and begin to wheeze. The child usually will not eat or sleep well because of these symptoms. The nostrils may flare (that is, they will open wide when the child breathes) and the upper belly and the skin covering the chest may retract (that is, it will look as though it is caving in) with each intake of breath. Sometimes the symptoms of bronchiolitis are so severe that the child needs extra oxygen and inhaled medications. If the child is not getting enough oxygen, cyanosis* may develop.

How Is Bronchiolitis Diagnosed and Treated?

It is important for children who have breathing problems to be examined by a doctor to make sure that they are getting enough oxygen. The

KEYWORDS
for searching the Internet
and other reference sources

Adenovirus

Influenza

Pneumonia

Respiratory syncytial virus (RSV)

Rhinovirus

* **mucus** (MYOO-kus) is a thick, slippery substance that lines the insides of many body parts.

* **respiratory syncytial** (RES-puh-ruh-tor-e sin-SIH-she-ul) **virus,** or RSV, is a virus that infects the respiratory tract and typically causes minor symptoms in adults but can lead to more serious respiratory illnesses in children.

* **parainfluenza** (pair-uh-in-floo-EN-zuh) is a family of viruses that cause respiratory infections.

* **influenza** (in-floo-EN-zuh) **A**, is one member of a family of viruses that attack the respiratory tract.

* **adenovirus** (ah-deh-no-VY-rus) is a type of virus that can produce a variety of symptoms, including upper respiratory disease, when it infects humans.

* **cyanosis** (sye-uh-NO-sis) is a bluish or purplish discoloration of the skin and mucous membranes due to a lack of oxygen in the blood.

75

* **dehydration** (dee-hi-DRAY-shun) is a condition in which the body is depleted of water, usually caused by excessive and unre-placed loss of body fluids, such as through sweating, vomiting, or diarrhea.

* **antigen** (AN-tih-jen) is a sub-stance that is recognized as a threat by the body's immune sys-tem, which triggers the formation of specific antibodies against the substance.

doctor also will check for signs of dehydration*. The child's nasal fluid can be examined for the presence of RSV in a laboratory with the rapid antigen* detection test. This test often is used to diagnose the infection in the emergency room during the winter months.

Most children can be treated at home. Doctors typically recommend that children with bronchiolitis drink lots of fluids and sleep with a cool-mist vaporizer or humidifier in the bedroom, to ease breathing. Over-the-counter medications for pain and fever, such as acetaminophen (uh-SEE-teh-MIH-noh-fen), also can help children feel better. Antibiotics do not help bronchiolitis, because a virus causes the illness and antibi-otics treat only infections caused by bacteria. Decongestants (medica-tions that decrease the amount of mucus) should not be used, because they often produce unwanted side effects in very young children. Instead, a child's nose can be cleared of mucus with suction from a rubber bulb and saltwater nose drops. Occasionally, a child with bronchiolitis, espe-cially one who was born prematurely or who has heart or lung problems, may have to be hospitalized so that extra oxygen and fluids can be given. Sometimes breathing treatments are required.

What to Expect

Most children with bronchiolitis do well with treatment at home guided by the child's doctor. A doctor should be called right away if the child has any signs of difficulty in breathing, such as breathing very fast or ex-periencing retractions or if the skin or lips turn pale or bluish. The doc-tor also should be called if the child is not able to take and hold down fluid by mouth. Most children get better after about a week, but the cough may last longer. In some cases the cough may not clear up for sev-eral weeks, even though the child is back to normal otherwise. Compli-cations of bronchiolitis include pneumonia*, apnea*, and respiratory fail-ure*. These are more common in children who are born prematurely or who have heart, lung, or other health problems. Children who have had bronchiolitis are more prone to asthma* later in childhood.

* **pneumonia** (nu-MO-nyah) is inflammation of the lung.

* **apnea** (AP-nee-uh) is a tempo-rary stopping of breathing.

* **respiratory failure** is a condition in which breathing and oxygen delivery to the body are danger-ously altered. This may result from infection, nerve or muscle damage, poisoning, or other causes.

* **asthma** (AZ-mah) is a condition in which the airways of the lungs repeatedly become narrowed and inflamed, causing breathing difficulty.

How Can Bronchiolitis Be Prevented?

The viruses that cause bronchiolitis, especially RSV, are spread easily. It is almost impossible to keep children away from others who are sick, but it is important to wash the hands often (children as well as the people caring for them, as in day care centers) to prevent the spread of RSV. Keeping sick children home from school and day care can help control the spread of infection to others. Children who are considered to be at high risk of becoming seriously ill from bronchiolitis, such as premature infants and those with chronic heart or lung disease, can be immunized against RSV to prevent infection.

Resource

Organization

American Academy of Family Physicians, 11400 Tomahawk Creek Parkway, Leawood, KS 66211-2672. The American Academy of Family Physicians posts information about bronchiolitis at its website. Telephone 800-274-2237
http://www.familydoctor.org

Bronchitis, Infectious

Bronchitis (brong-KYE-tis) is a disease that involves inflammation (irritation and swelling) of the larger airways in the respiratory tract, which can result from infection or other causes. These airways, called the bronchial (BRONG-kee-ul) tubes or bronchi (BRONG-kye), extend from the trachea* to the lungs.

What Is Bronchitis?

When a person has bronchitis, the tissue lining the airways swells, narrowing the air passages and making it difficult to breathe. The inflamed airways produce larger amounts of a thick, slippery substance called mucus (MYOO-kus), which can clog the air passages and complicate breathing even more. The excess mucus usually is coughed up. In addition, in bronchitis, the cilia (fine, hairlike structures on the surface of the cells lining the airways that help cleanse the airways of inhaled particles) become less able to clear impurities and bacteria from the airways, making it harder for the person to fight off lung infection. The disease can be brought on by a viral or bacterial infection, but it also can be the result of smoking or living or working in areas where there is heavy air pollution and dust.

Types of bronchitis There are three kinds of bronchitis. Acute bronchitis comes on quickly and is typically the result of a bad cold or flu. It generally lasts about 10 days. In severe cases, a bad cough can persist up to a month as the bronchi heal. The acute form also can be caused by an allergy or by inhaling irritating substances in the air, such as smoke from a fire. Chronic (KRAH-nik, persistent or recurring) bronchitis is caused by continuing or repeated inflammation of the lungs over a period of time, at least 2 to 3 months, and it can persist or come and go over years. Excess mucus is produced, and the lining of the bronchi thickens. This leads to a bad cough and restricted airflow. People who smoke heavily and those with chronic lung disease are most likely to experience chronic bronchitis. The third type, asthmatic bronchitis, is seen in people with persistent asthma.

 See also
Bronchitis, Infectious
Common Cold
Influenza
Pneumonia

KEYWORDS
for searching the Internet and other reference sources

Asthma

Chronic obstructive pulmonary disease (COPD)

Influenza

Lung disease

Pneumonia

* **trachea** (TRAY-kee-uh) is the windpipe—the firm, tubular structure that carries air from the throat to the lungs.

Kicking Butts

When a smoker quits smoking, it takes only 20 minutes to feel better. Statistics from the American Lung Association show that:

20 minutes after quitting

- blood pressure decreases
- pulse rate lowers

8 hours after quitting

- the carbon monoxide level in the blood returns to normal
- the oxygen level in the blood rises to normal

1 day after quitting

- the chance of a heart attack drops

2 days after quitting

- nerve endings begin to regrow, allowing the senses of taste and smell to return to normal

2 weeks to 3 months after quitting

- circulation of the blood improves
- walking becomes easier
- breathing becomes easier

1 to 9 months after quitting

- coughing, congestion, tiredness, and shortness of breath diminish

1 year after quitting

- the risk of heart disease becomes half that of a smoker

The long-term benefits are encouraging, too. After 5 years the risk of stroke drops to that of someone who has never smoked. At 10 years after quitting the risk of lung cancer is significantly lower, and at 15 years the likelihood of a person who has quit smoking having a heart attack is the same as that of someone who has never smoked at all.

Who Gets Bronchitis and How?

No matter who they are, what their job, or where they live, people who smoke cigarettes are more likely to experience chronic bronchitis. The American Lung Association reports that the disease develops in nearly nine million people in the United States every year. Bronchitis affects people of all ages, but those who are 45 years or older get it more often, and women are more susceptible than men. More than 10 million people have bouts of acute bronchitis every year; most are children less than 5 years of age, who typically get it in winter and early spring. The viruses that can cause acute bronchitis are contagious. People can get a viral infection from someone who is infected if they come into contact with that person's respiratory fluids. The virus also can spread from person to person through the air by way of the droplets from a sneeze or cough. Generally, chronic bronchitis is not contagious.

What Are the Signs and Symptoms of Bronchitis?

Bronchitis symptoms often mimic those of a cold. A cough that brings up mucus is common. Symptoms of acute bronchitis may include wheezing, tiredness, chest pain, and difficulty breathing. If the cause is a viral or bacterial infection, the patient may have a fever. Chronic bronchitis usually is marked by a cough that lasts 3 months or longer, tightness in the chest, and trouble breathing. Bronchitis often is confused or lumped together with other conditions. The doctor usually will rule out other causes for coughing and breathing problems to make the diagnosis. Besides listening to a person's breathing, the doctor may order a chest X ray to check for pneumonia or a lung function test to check for asthma.

How Is Bronchitis Treated?

Many doctors prescribe antibiotics for acute bronchitis, although these medicines often do not work because they cannot cure viral infections. Bronchodilator* drugs may be prescribed to help open the airways, either in pill form or as a spray inhaler. Over-the-counter medications can be used to minimize pain and lessen cough. Patients also are advised to get a lot of rest, eat a well-balanced diet, and drink lots of fluids. It is suggested that people who have chronic bronchitis stop smoking and avoid dust, fumes, and cold or dry air. Cough medicine and vaporizers may help. Antibiotics often are prescribed when symptoms flare up acutely in a person with chronic bronchitis.

How Long Does Bronchitis Last?

People with acute bronchitis usually begin to feel better within a few days, although they usually can expect to have a cough for 1 to 2 weeks or longer while the airways in the lungs heal. Chronic bronchitis symptoms last longer and may never resolve, because the damage to the lungs may be permanent. Because excess mucus is being produced, the body's natural reflex will be to cough it up, and this cough may come and go for a long time, flaring up, subsiding, and flaring up again. Occasionally, pneumonia may develop in people with acute bronchitis. If a person is already in poor health, bronchitis can worsen the condition. Chronic bronchitis can lead to heart failure, because it makes the heart work harder to compensate for the lack of oxygen. Severe respiratory problems can develop, and in some cases the disease can result in death.

How Can Bronchitis Be Prevented?

Since many cases are caused by a viral infection, washing the hands and not sharing drinks or eating utensils with someone who is infected can help to prevent acute bronchitis. Many cases of chronic bronchitis can be prevented or its symptoms made less severe by not smoking. In fact, if people did not smoke, most cases of chronic bronchitis would never develop. People with chronic bronchitis or other chronic lung diseases are usually advised to get a yearly influenza* vaccination to prevent symptoms from flaring up in response to infection with flu viruses.

Resource

Organization

American Lung Association, 61 Broadway, 6th Floor, New York, NY 10006. The American Lung Association posts information about chronic bronchitis and other lung conditions at its website. Telephone 212-315-8700
http://www.lungusa.org

** **bronchodilator** (brong-ko-DYE-lay-tor) is a medication that helps improve air flow through the lungs by widening narrowed airways.*

** **influenza** (in-floo-EN-zuh), also known as the flu, is a contagious viral infection that attacks the respiratory tract, including the nose, throat, and lungs.*

▶ *See also*
Bronchiolitis
Influenza
Pneumonia

C

Cat Scratch Disease

Cat scratch disease is an infectious illness that can cause flulike symptoms and swelling of lymph nodes*. It is caused by bacteria carried in cat saliva. The bacteria usually enter the body from a cat scratch or a bite that breaks the skin.

What Is Cat Scratch Disease?

Cat scratch disease (also called cat scratch fever) is caused by the bacterium *Bartonella henselae* (bar-tuh-NEH-luh HEN-suh-lay), which is found in the saliva of cats and kittens all over the world. About 3 to 10 days after a person is bitten or scratched by a cat, a blister or small bump may develop. This is called an inoculation (ih-nah-kyoo-LAY-shun) lesion, which means that it appears at the site where germs entered the body. Usually about 2 weeks later, there is inflammation of nearby lymph nodes. If the scratch or bite is on the arm, the lymph nodes on the arm or in the armpit will become swollen. Swelling also can develop in the lymph nodes in the neck or groin, depending on the site of the scratch or bite.

Who Gets Cat Scratch Disease?

People of any age can get the disease, but most cases occur in children and teens. It is estimated that there are about 24,000 cases of cat scratch disease each year in the United States. Members of the same household can become ill if they are scratched or bitten by the same infected cat. Cat scratch disease affects 9 of every 100,000 persons each year worldwide. People can get the disease only from infected cats and kittens. It cannot be transmitted from person to person, but it can spread among cats. It is thought that cats and kittens can become infected with *Bartonella henselae* from fleas.

What Are the Signs and Symptoms of the Disease?

The most common symptoms of cat scratch disease are a bite or scratch that does not heal normally; painful or swollen glands (lymph nodes), especially in the armpit or near the inside of the elbow; fever; headache; fatigue; joint pain; and sometimes a rash. Less common symptoms are weight loss, sore throat, and draining lymph nodes. If a person is suspected of

KEYWORDS
for searching the Internet and other reference sources

Bartonella henselae **bacteria**

Illnesses associated with cats

Parinaud oculoglandular syndrome

***lymph** (LIMF) **nodes** are small, bean-shaped masses of tissue that contain immune system cells that fight harmful microorganisms. Lymph nodes may swell during infections.

having cat scratch disease, the doctor will ask about any recent contact with a cat and will look for signs of a cat scratch or bite, swollen lymph nodes, or an inoculation lesion. In some cases, a person with cat scratch disease does not recall having had contact with a cat. Blood tests can rule out other causes of swollen nodes and check for the presence of antibodies* to the bacteria that cause the disease. In some cases, a doctor will use a needle to take a sample (a piece of tissue) from a swollen lymph node for examination under a microscope.

How Do Doctors Treat Cat Scratch Disease?

Antibiotics may be prescribed for cat scratch disease, but some doctors advise taking these medications only in severe cases. Most people eventually get well without treatment. If the patient is otherwise healthy, rest and over-the-counter medicines, such as acetaminophen (uh-see-teh-MIH-noh-fen), to relieve pain and fever are all that are needed while waiting for the disease to run its course. If a lymph node becomes very swollen and painful, the doctor may decide to drain it. Treatment with antibiotics often is recommended for patients who have weakened immune systems as the result of other illnesses. The symptoms in most patients usually resolve after several weeks of treatment with antibiotics and within 3 months without antibiotic treatment. Swollen lymph nodes may take several months to return to normal size. Most people recover completely from the illness. After an episode of cat scratch disease, people are usually immune to it, meaning that they cannot get the disease again.

Complications

Generally, cat scratch disease is not serious in people who are healthy. But people with weak immune systems, such as those with human immunodeficiency virus* (HIV) infection or poorly controlled diabetes* and those receiving chemotherapy for cancer, have a greater risk of complications and need to be watched closely by their health care providers. These complications include hepatitis*, osteomyelitis*, encephalitis*, and retinitis*. Sometimes cat scratch disease can appear in the form of Parinaud oculoglandular syndrome (PAH-rih-nod ok-yoo-lo-GLAN-dyoo-ler SIN-drome). In this condition, a small sore and inflammation develop in the membrane lining the inner eyelid, called the conjunctiva (kon-jung-TIE-vuh), accompanied by swollen lymph nodes around the ear. Rubbing one's eyes after handling an infected cat can transmit the infection to the conjunctiva, because the bacteria can be present on the cat's coat wherever it licks itself.

Prevention

About 30 percent of American households have pet cats. Keeping cats indoors and free of fleas may help prevent them from contracting the infection. It is a good idea to avoid stray or unfamiliar cats and not to pro-

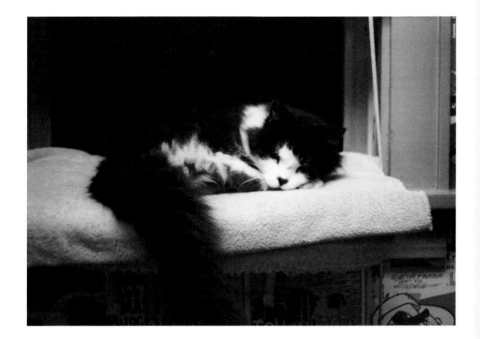

It was not until the 1980s that *Bartonella* bacteria were identified as the cause of cat scratch disease. Infection does not appear to make cats ill, making it easier for the disease to spread from cat to cat (through fleas) and then to people. *George Zebrowski*

voke any cat or kitten to the point that it scratches or bites. Thoroughly cleaning any wounds inflicted by a cat may help prevent infection.

Resources

Organizations

American Academy of Family Physicians, 11400 Tomahawk Creek Parkway, Leawood, KS 66211-2672. The American Academy of Family Physicians posts information about cat scratch disease at its website. Telephone 800-274-2237
http://www.familydoctor.org

U.S. National Library of Medicine, 8600 Rockville Pike, Bethesda, MD 20894. The National Library of Medicine has a website packed with information on diseases (including cat scratch disease) and drugs, consumer resources, dictionaries and encyclopedias of medical terms, and directories of doctors and helpful organizations. Telephone 888-346-3656
http://www.nlm.nih.gov

Website

KidsHealth.org. KidsHealth is a website created by the medical experts of the Nemours Foundation and is devoted to issues of children's health. It contains articles on a variety of health topics, including cat scratch disease.
http://www.KidsHealth.org

▶ *See also*
Encephalitis
Hepatitis, Infectious
The Nature of Germs and Infection
Osteomyelitis
Rabies
Toxoplasmosis

Chagas Disease *See* Trypanosomiasis

Chicken Pox *See* Varicella (Chicken Pox) and Herpes Zoster (Shingles)

Chlamydial Infections

Chlamydial (kla-MIH-dee-ul) infection can take various forms and can affect the urinary and genital systems of the body, as well as the eyes and lungs. One of its most common forms is a sexually transmitted disease (STD), which usually is passed from one person to another through unprotected sexual intercourse.

What Are Chlamydial Infections?

There are different types of chlamydia bacteria. *Chlamydia trachomatis* (kla-MIH-dee-uh truh-KO-mah-tis) is the bacterium that causes genital (and sometimes throat) infections. People with this form of chlamydial infection might not know they have the disease, because symptoms of infection often do not appear right away. In both men and women, long-term complications can result from an untreated infection. The penis, vagina, cervix*, anus, or urethra* can become infected. Babies born to mothers with chlamydial infection may develop a type of conjunctivitis* shortly after birth. A different type of *Chlamydia trachomatis* also causes the most common infection-related form of blindness in the world.

Infection with *Chlamydia pneumoniae* (kla-MIH-dee-uh nu-MO-nye) can lead to pneumonia in humans and may be linked to an increased risk of heart disease. Humans also can contract *Chlamydia psittaci* (kla-MIH-dee-uh sih-TAH-see) through contact with infected birds. This infection causes psittacosis (sih-tuh-KO-sis), or "parrot fever," a pneumonia-like illness. This form of chlamydial infection is the most rare, usually affecting only those people who work closely or live with birds.

Chlamydial infection is the most common STD in the United States. As many as 3 to 4 million new cases occur each year. Most people who contract chlamydia are younger than 25 years old. Of every 10 teenage girls tested for chlamydial infection, 1 girl has the infection.

How Do Chlamydial Infections Spread and What Are the Symptoms?

Spread by oral (by mouth), vaginal, and anal sexual intercourse, *Chlamydia trachomatis* is easily transmitted from person to person. Chlamydia

KEYWORDS
for searching the Internet and other reference sources

Chlamydia pneumoniae

Chlamydia psittaci

Chlamydia trachomatis

Conjunctivitis

Gonorrhea

Pelvic inflammatory disease (PID)

Psittacosis

Sexually transmitted disease

Venereal disease

* **cervix** (SIR-viks) is the lower, narrow end of the uterus that opens into the vagina.

* **urethra** (yoo-REE-thra) is the tube through which urine passes from the bladder to the outside of the body.

* **conjunctivitis** (kon-jung-tih-VY-tis), often called "pinkeye," is an inflammation of the thin membrane that lines the inside of the eyelids and covers the surface of the eyeball. Conjunctivitis can be caused by viruses, bacteria, allergies, or chemical irritation.

also can pass from a woman to her baby during birth; infants born to infected mothers have about a 25 percent chance of becoming infected with conjunctivitis or pneumonia.

The sexually-transmitted infection often is called "the silent epidemic," and up to half of men and three-fourths of women who have the disease do not know it, because symptoms can be mild or may not even be noticeable. Symptoms can take from 1 to 3 weeks to appear after a person becomes infected. Women may have a milky or yellowish discharge (mucus* or pus*) from the vagina and experience pain while urinating or having sex. Fever, bleeding between periods, abdominal* pain, and the urge to urinate frequently are also signs of infection. Men may have a burning sensation when they urinate or a thin yellowish or milky discharge from the penis and swollen or tender testicles. Some men may not experience any symptoms. Chlamydia spread through oral contact with the genitals can cause an infection in the throat.

How Are the Diseases Diagnosed?

Specific testing for chlamydia is usually included when a person is screened for STDs. Tests for chlamydial infection and gonorrhea usually are done together, because the symptoms of these two sexually transmitted infections are similar. A doctor will ask about sexual history, collect a sample of urine for examination in a laboratory, and take cotton-swab samples from the cervix or the tip of the penis. If swelling or discharge is present, swabs also will be taken from the throat or anus. The material picked up by the swab is tested for the bacteria. Testing can take up to 3 days. Sometimes a quicker test that diagnoses chlamydial infection from a urine sample is used. Results from a urine sample usually can be obtained from a laboratory within a few hours. It is necessary for all sexual partners of a person who is diagnosed with chlamydial infection to be tested for the disease, even if they do not have symptoms.

What Is the Treatment for Chlamydial Infection?

Once a person is diagnosed with chlamydial infection, treatment with antibiotics begins. It is important for an infected person to finish all prescribed medication, even if symptoms disappear. If symptoms persist after taking all the medication, a follow-up visit to the doctor is necessary. Babies who contract chlamydia from their mothers also are treated with antibiotics.

Complications

If chlamydial infection is left untreated in women, it can move through a woman's reproductive organs and spread to the cervix, uterus*, fallopian tubes*, or ovaries*, causing pelvic inflammatory disease (PID). PID is a serious condition that can result in infertility (the inability to become pregnant). Each year, PID develops in up to a million women in the United States; half of these cases are the result of chlamydial infection. PID can scar and block the fallopian tubes and cause a woman to be at increased

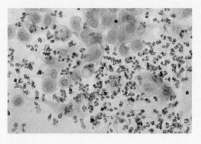

A microscopic image of a smear of material taken from the cervix of a woman infected with chlamydia shows the presence of the bacteria. *Custom Medical Stock Photo, Inc.*

* **mucus** (MYOO-kus) is a thick, slippery substance that lines the insides of many body parts.

* **pus** is a thick, creamy fluid, usually yellow or greenish in color, that forms at the site of an infection. Pus contains infection-fighting white cells and other substances.

* **abdominal** (ab-DAH-mih-nul) refers to the area of the body below the ribs and above the hips that contains the stomach, intestines, and other organs.

* **uterus** (YOO-teh-rus) is the muscular, pear-shaped internal organ in a woman where a baby develops until birth.

* **fallopian** (fah-LO-pee-uhn) **tubes** are the two slender tubes that connect the ovaries and the uterus in females. They carry the ova, or eggs, from the ovaries to the uterus.

* **ovaries** (O-vuh-reez) are the sexual glands from which ova, or eggs, are released in women.

* **HIV**, or human immunodeficiency virus (HYOO-mun ih-myoo-no-dih-FIH-shen-see), is the virus that causes AIDS (acquired immunodeficiency syndrome).

* **epididymitis** (eh-pih-dih-duh-MY-tis) is a painful inflammation of the epididymis, a structure attached to the testicles.

* **prostate** (PRAH-state) is a male reproductive gland located near where the bladder joins the urethra. The prostate produces the fluid part of semen.

* **arthritis** (ar-THRY-tis) refers to any of several disorders characterized by inflammation of the joints.

▶ *See also*

AIDS and HIV Infection

Congenital Infections

Conjunctivitis

Gonorrhea

Sexually Transmitted Diseases

risk for an ectopic (ek-TAH-pik) pregnancy, in which the fertilized egg develops outside the uterus, usually within one of the fallopian tubes. Ectopic pregnancies are removed by emergency surgery to prevent the fallopian tube from rupturing and causing internal bleeding. Without emergency medical treatment, a ruptured ectopic pregnancy can result in severe bleeding that can lead to death. Women with a history of PID are 10 times more likely to have ectopic pregnancies than are other women. Research has shown that women who have chlamydia are up to five times more likely to become infected with the human immunodeficiency virus (HIV)* if they have unprotected sex with someone who has HIV infection.

In men, chlamydia can spread from the urethra to the testicles and may result in a condition called epididymitis*, which can lead to sterility (the inability to impregnate a woman). Men also can develop prostatitis (pros-tah-TY-tis), an inflammation of the prostate*, or Reiter syndrome (RYE-ter SIN-drome), a condition associated with arthritis*.

Prevention

People who have chlamydial infection may pass the disease on to their sexual partners, even if they are not aware that they are infected. It is wise to approach any sexual relationship with a strong sense of responsibility. People who are sexually active are advised always to use a latex condom for all forms of sexual intercourse. Having several sexual partners puts a person at increased risk of all types of STDs. It is recommended that all men and women who are sexually active be screened regularly for STDs. The U.S. Centers for Disease Control and Prevention advises all sexually active women who have risk factors for chlamydial infection to be screened for STDs at least once a year, as part of a full gynecological exam. Women considered to be at risk are those who have new sex partners or who engage in sex with several partners and who do not use condoms during sex. Pregnant women are also screened, to prevent spreading the infection to their babies.

Resources

Organizations

Planned Parenthood Federation of America, 810 Seventh Avenue, New York, NY 10019. Planned Parenthood posts information about sexually transmitted infections at its website.
Telephone 212-541-7800
http://www.plannedparenthood.org

U.S. National Institute of Allergy and Infectious Diseases (NIAID), Building 31, Room 7A-50, 31 Center Drive MSC 2520, Bethesda, MD 20892-2520. NIAID, part of the National Institutes of Health, posts fact sheets about many STDs, including chlamydial infections, at its website.

Telephone 301-496-5717
http://www.niaid.nih.gov

Website

KidsHealth.org. KidsHealth is a website created by the medical experts
of the Nemours Foundation and is devoted to issues of children's
health. It contains articles on a variety of health topics, including
chlamydial infections and other STDs.
http://www.KidsHealth.org

Cholera

Cholera (KAH-luh-ruh) is an acute infection of the small intestine* that
can cause severe diarrhea (dye-uh-REE-uh).*

What Is Cholera?

Cholera is an illness caused by the bacterium *Vibrio cholerae*, which is
contracted by eating contaminated food or drinking contaminated water. The bacteria can cause serious diarrhea by producing a toxin that
makes the intestines release more water and minerals than usual. The
disease has a 1 to 5 day incubation period (the time between infection
and when symptoms appear) and progresses very quickly. Most cases of
cholera are mild, but in about 1 of 20 cases the disease is serious. If left
untreated, severe cholera can lead to death from dehydration within
hours. With treatment, the death rate is less than 1 percent.

Is Cholera Common?

Cholera has been rare in industrialized (or highly developed) countries
such as the United States since the turn of the twentieth century, thanks
to improved sanitation and water treatment. However, cholera is still
common in other parts of the world, including India and southern Asia,
parts of Africa, and Latin America.

In 1991, an epidemic* of cholera occurred in South America and
some cases appeared in the United States shortly thereafter. Most cases
of cholera reported in the United States can be traced to travel to an area
where cholera is endemic*.

How Do People Contract Cholera?

Cholera is spread when people eat food or drink water that has been
contaminated with feces (excreted waste) containing *Vibrio cholerae*.
Risk factors for epidemics of cholera include unsanitary and crowded
living conditions, war, famine (scarcity of food), and natural disaster.
For example, following a natural disaster such as a hurricane or flood,
supplies of drinking water can become contaminated. The disease is

KEYWORDS
*for searching the Internet
and other reference sources*

Dehydration

Diarrhea

Epidemics

Enteritis

Vibrio cholerae

* **acute** describes an infection or
other illness that comes on suddenly and usually does not last
very long.

* **small intestine** is the part of the
intestine—the system of muscular
tubes that food passes through
during digestion—that directly receives the food after it passes
through the stomach.

* **epidemic** (eh-pih-DEH-mik) is an
outbreak of disease, especially
infectious disease, in which the
number of cases suddenly becomes far greater than usual.
Usually epidemics are outbreaks
of diseases in specific regions,
whereas worldwide epidemics
are called pandemics.

* **endemic** (en-DEH-mik) describes
a disease or condition that is
present in a population or geographic area at all times.

most frequently spread in areas with poor sanitation and water treatment facilities.

During outbreaks of the disease, cholera may spread by contact with the feces of an infected person; *Vibrio cholerae* can live in feces for up to 2 weeks. It also spreads when people use contaminated water for cleaning or waste disposal. Eating raw or undercooked shellfish can be another source of the illness because the bacteria can survive in slow-moving rivers and coastal waters. The few cases in the United States are typically caused by contaminated seafood from the Gulf of Mexico or seafood brought home by people who have traveled to other countries.

What Happens to People Who Have Cholera?

Signs and symptoms   The major symptom of cholera is diarrhea, which can be severe and cause up to a quart of fluid loss per hour from the body. Diarrhea caused by cholera is painless, with stools that are fishy smelling and watery, often with flecks of mucus* in them (these are sometimes called "rice water" stools, because they look like rice floating in water).

Most cases of cholera are mild or moderate, and they can be difficult to distinguish from other causes of diarrhea. More serious cases can cause severe diarrhea, vomiting, and dehydration. Signs of dehydration include decreased urination, extreme tiredness, rapid heartbeat, dry skin, dry mouth and nose, thirstiness, and sunken eyes.

* **mucus** (MYOO-kus) is a thick, slippery substance that lines the insides of many body parts.

CONCERN OVER CHOLERA

Until the late 1800s, cholera was a very real threat in the United States, and the numbers of cases often reached epidemic proportions. In 1849, the immigrant boat *John Drew* brought cholera to the city of Chicago, where 678 people died of the disease that year.

By 1870, cholera was no longer a major threat in the United States because of improved sanitation and water treatment. However, the disease continues to be a significant concern in other parts of the world. In 1961, a pandemic (an epidemic that occurs over a large geographic area) that began in Indonesia spread to Bangladesh, India, Iran, and Iraq by 1965. In 1970, cholera appeared in West Africa, where it had not been seen in 100 years. It eventually became endemic to most of the continent.

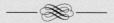

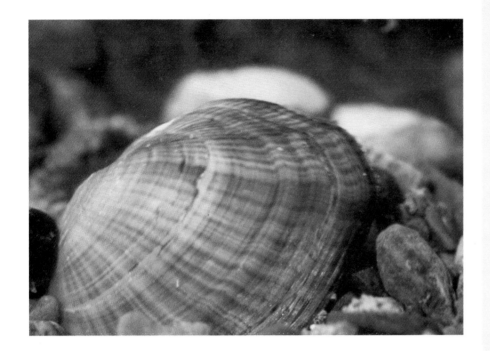

Diagnosis Because the symptoms of cholera are often identical to those of other illnesses that cause diarrhea, knowing that a person has traveled to a country where cholera is endemic is important in helping a doctor make the diagnosis. Blood and stool samples can be taken to look for signs of the bacteria.

Treatment Treatment of cholera can be very simple and effective, especially if it is given soon after symptoms appear. Rehydration, or replenishing the body with fluids, is the most important part of treatment. This can be accomplished most effectively by drinking a mixture of sugar, salts, and clean water, known as an oral rehydration solution. The World Health Organization has an oral rehydration solution that is distributed worldwide through the efforts of the United Nations. In the United States, solutions can be bought or mixed at home. Such solutions replenish the fluid and salts lost by the body due to diarrhea and vomiting.

More serious cases of cholera may require intravenous (in-tra-VEE-nus) fluids, or fluids injected directly into a vein. Antibiotics, which are given in severe cases, can shorten the time that the symptoms last and help prevent spread of the disease to others.

Complications from cholera are usually the result of severe dehydration. Seizures*, abnormal heart rhythms, shock*, damage to the kidneys*, coma*, and death can occur. Children, especially infants, are more likely to develop complications than adults because they are more prone to developing severe dehydration and body mineral imbalances.

* **seizures** (SEE-zhurs) are sudden bursts of disorganized electrical activity that interrupt the normal functioning of the brain, often leading to uncontrolled movements in the body and sometimes a temporary change in consciousness.

* **shock** is a serious condition in which blood pressure is very low and not enough blood flows to the body's organs and tissues. Untreated, shock may result in death.

* **kidneys** are the pair of organs that filter blood and remove waste products and excess water from the body in the form of urine.

* **coma** (KO-ma) is an unconscious state in which a person cannot be awakened and cannot move, see, speak, or hear.

How Can Cholera Be Prevented?

Steps people can take to prevent cholera when traveling or after a natural disaster include:

- drinking only bottled water, water that has been boiled or treated with chlorine or iodine, or bottled, carbonated beverages
- eating only food that has been thoroughly cooked and is still hot
- not eating raw fruit or vegetables unless they have been peeled
- avoiding food and drinks sold by street vendors
- avoiding raw or undercooked seafood
- not bringing seafood from abroad back to the United States.

Vaccines* for cholera exist, but their effectiveness is short lived and none are provided or recommended in the United States.

Resources

Organizations

U.S. Centers for Disease Control and Prevention (CDC), 1600 Clifton Road, Atlanta, GA 30333. The CDC is the U.S. government authority for information about infectious and other diseases. It has a fact sheet about cholera at its website.
Telephone 800-311-3435
http://www.cdc.gov

World Health Organization (WHO), Avenue Appia 20, 1211 Geneva 27, Switzerland. WHO's communicable disease surveillance and response division posts a global cholera update at its website to report numbers of cholera cases and deaths worldwide.
Telephone 011-41-22-791-2111
http://www.who.int

Chronic Fatigue Syndrome

Chronic fatigue syndrome (KRAH-nik fuh-TEEG SIN-drome), or CFS, is a condition that makes people feel extremely exhausted and affects their participation in normal activities, such as work or school. Although the cause of the syndrome is still not known, researchers are investigating the possibility that an infection might trigger the condition in some cases.

What Is Chronic Fatigue Syndrome?

Chronic fatigue syndrome is a condition that causes almost constant exhaustion. People with CFS cannot just get more sleep to feel better, be-

---

* **vaccines** (vak-SEENS) are preparations of killed or weakened germs, or a part of a germ or product it produces, given to prevent or lessen the severity of the disease that can result if a person is exposed to the germ itself. Use of vaccines for this purpose is called immunization.

▶ See also
Intestinal Infections

KEYWORDS
for searching the Internet and other reference sources

Exhaustion

Fatigue

Neurasthenia

cause their fatigue does not improve with rest. In addition, physical or mental work may make the fatigue worse. Doctors and scientists do not know what causes CFS. In the past, people with CFS often were told their symptoms were psychological, or "all in their heads." It was not until the 1980s that CFS began to be recognized as a medical condition associated with the physical symptoms of severe fatigue and weakness. CFS affects all racial groups, and the condition occurs in teens as well as adults. According to the National Institutes of Health, a woman is at least two to four times more likely than a man to develop CFS. Some studies have estimated that as many as 800,000 people in the United States have the syndrome.

What Are the Symptoms of CFS?

For a diagnosis of CFS, a person must have a sudden onset of exhaustion that continues for 6 months or recurs during that period of time. In addition, the person must have four of the following symptoms, and the symptoms must have started after the fatigue began:

- joint pain in several places in the body (without redness or swelling)
- muscle pain
- sore throat
- tender lymph nodes*
- difficulty in concentrating or short-term memory problems
- headaches different from those previously experienced
- general exhaustion that lasts for more than 24 hours after exercise or exertion
- a feeling of tiredness despite having slept

Some people with CFS also experience:

- dizziness
- abdominal* pain
- weight loss
- nausea
- night sweats
- chest pain
- continuing cough
- shortness of breath
- anxiety
- depression
- irregular heartbeat
- abnormal skin sensations

*** lymph** (LIMF) **nodes** are small, bean-shaped masses of tissue that contain immune system cells that fight harmful micro-organisms. Lymph nodes may swell during infections.

*** abdominal** (ab-DAH-mih-nul) refers to the area of the body below the ribs and above the hips that contains the stomach, intestines, and other organs.

People diagnosed with CFS are not just a little sleepy. The fatigue they experience is so great that it significantly interferes with work or school.

* **hypoglycemia** (hi-po-gly-SEE-mee-uh) is a condition that occurs when the amount of glucose, or sugar, in the blood becomes too low. Symptoms can include dizziness, trembling, sweating, and confusion.

* **candidiasis** (kan-dih-DYE-uh-sis) is an overgrowth of *Candida*, a type of yeast, in or on the body.

* **neurasthenia** (nur-us-THEE-nee-uh) is a disorder of the nervous system causing weakness and fatigue.

* **multiple sclerosis** (skluh-RO-sis) **(MS)** is an inflammatory disease of the nervous system that disrupts communication between the brain and other parts of the body. MS can result in paralysis, loss of vision, and other symptoms.

* **hypothyroidism** (hi-po-THY-royd-ih-zum) is an impairment of the functioning of the thyroid gland that causes too little thyroid hormone to be produced by the body. Symptoms of hypothyroidism can include tiredness, paleness, dry skin, and in children, delayed growth and mental and sexual development.

* **cognitive behavioral therapy** (KOG-nih-tiv be-HAY-vyuh-rul THAIR-uh-pee) is treatment that helps people identify negative ways of thinking and behaving and change them to more positive approaches.

* **rehabilitative therapy** helps people return to more normal physical, mental, or emotional function following an illness or injury. Rehabilitative therapy also helps people find ways to better cope with conditions that interfere with their lives.

What Causes CFS?

Doctors do not know what causes CFS. Because many people first experience the symptoms of CFS after an illness caused by a virus (such as mononucleosis or hepatitis), some scientists think that a viral illness can trigger the condition. Toxins, stress, and physical or emotional injury also have been suggested as possible causes of CFS. Some researchers think that CFS stems from a problem in the immune system, which helps the body fight disease. Because many people with CFS experience depression, other doctors believe that a psychological condition produces the physical symptoms of CFS. In the past, CFS has been blamed on many other conditions, such as allergies, hypoglycemia*, infection with Epstein-Barr virus (the virus that causes mononucleosis), candidiasis*, neurasthenia*, and Lyme disease.

Diagnosis and Treatment of CFS

CFS is diagnosed if a person has the symptoms listed earlier. There are no specific laboratory tests that can confirm the diagnosis of CFS, although a person may have to undergo blood tests and physical examinations to rule out other possible causes of symptoms, such as multiple sclerosis*, hypothyroidism*, or heart or kidney disease. A diagnosis of CFS often is made when nothing else is found to account for the symptoms.

Because the cause of CFS is unknown, treatment for CFS involves relieving the symptoms. Although there is no specific treatment for CFS, moderate exercise, such as yoga or tai chi; antidepressants (medications that can ease depression); and nonsteroidal anti-inflammatory drugs, such as ibuprofen, can help minimize the severity of many of the symptoms. It is also important for people with CFS to watch their stress levels, because mental, physical, or emotional overexertion can aggravate CFS symptoms. A few patients with CFS may respond to drinking extra fluids and eating extra salt. Some people also find cognitive behavioral therapy* and rehabilitative therapy* helpful in decreasing or coping with their symptoms. For most patients, the symptoms of CFS are most severe in the beginning, and later they may come and go. Some people recover completely from CFS, although it is not clear why this happens. Most CFS patients recover gradually within 5 years after symptoms begin.

Resources

Organizations

American Association for Chronic Fatigue Syndrome, 515 Minor Avenue, Suite 18, Seattle, WA 98104. People with CFS can find information about how to manage the symptoms of the disease at the American Association for Chronic Fatigue Syndrome website. Telephone 206-781-3544 http://www.aacfs.org

U.S. Centers for Disease Control and Prevention (CDC), 1600 Clifton Road, Atlanta, GA 30333. The CDC offers information about chronic fatigue syndrome and its diagnosis and treatment on its website.
Telephone 800-311-3435
http://www.cdc.gov

U.S. National Institute of Allergy and Infectious Diseases (NIAID), Building 31, Room 7A-50, 31 Center Drive MSC 2520, Bethesda, MD 20892-2520. NIAID, part of the National Institutes of Health, posts fact sheets about chronic fatigue syndrome on its website.
Telephone 301-496-5717
http://www.niaid.nih.gov

▶ *See also*
Lyme Disease
Mononucleosis, Infectious

Coccidioidomycosis (Valley Fever)

Coccidioidomycosis (kok-sih-dee-oyd-o-my-KO-sis), also know as valley fever, is a disease that can occur after breathing in the spores* of a fungus found naturally in the soil of dry regions, such as the southwestern United States.

What Is Coccidioidomycosis?

During World War II, American trainees sent to Arizona and parts of southern California for flight training took thousands of days of sick leave because of coccidioidomycosis, a disease caused by *Coccidioides immitis* (kok-sih-dee-OYD-eez IH-mih-tus), a fungus that hibernates a few inches beneath semi-dry soil. The disease's other name, valley fever, comes from the San Joaquin Valley region of California, where the fungus was first identified.

After regular rainfall, the *coccidioides* fungus blooms into tiny mold spores. If the soil is stirred by events such as dust storms, earthquakes, farming, excavation, or construction work, these microscopic spores spring into the air, where they are easily breathed into the lungs of people and animals.

Coccidioidomycosis cannot be passed from person to person. People must inhale the spores of the fungus in order to contract the disease. Most people who inhale the spores develop only a mild case of disease, in which the infection results in symptoms similar to those of a cold or the flu that go away on their own. Many people are not even aware that they are infected when the symptoms are mild. For those with weakened immune systems and for people of African or Filipino ancestry (who, for some unknown reason, get more severe forms of the disease), coccidioidomycosis can be much more serious, spreading from the lungs

KEYWORDS
for searching the Internet and other reference sources

Coccidioides immitis

Desert rheumatism

Fungal infection

San Joaquin Valley fever

* **spores** are a temporarily inactive form of a germ enclosed in a protective shell.

*meningitis (meh-nin-JY-tis) is an inflammation of the meninges, the membranes that surround the brain and the spinal cord. Meningitis is most often caused by infection with a virus or a bacterium.

*arthritis (ar-THRY-tis) refers to any of several disorders characterized by inflammation of the joints.

*endemic (en-DEH-mik) describes a disease or condition that is present in a population or geographic area at all times.

*antibodies (AN-tih-bah-deez) are protein molecules produced by the body's immune system to help fight specific infections caused by microorganisms, such as bacteria and viruses.

*culturing (KUL-chur-ing) means subjecting to a test in which a sample of fluid or tissue from the body is placed in a dish containing material that supports the growth of certain organisms. Typically, within days the organisms will grow and can be identified.

*sputum (SPYOO-tum) is a substance that contains mucus and other matter coughed out from the lungs, bronchi, and trachea.

*pneumonia (nu-MO-nyah) is inflammation of the lung.

to other parts of the body and even to the brain. Severe cases may result in meningitis*. *Coccidioides* infection that has spread throughout the body and occurs with arthritis* is sometimes called desert rheumatism (ROO-muh-tih-zum). In general, the more fungal spores inhaled by a person, the more serious the disease tends to be.

Is Coccidioidomycosis Common?

The fungus that causes coccidioidomycosis is found mainly in the desert climates of the southwestern United States, parts of Mexico, and Central and South America. The infection is considered endemic* in these regions. People who live in or visit "cocci country" and who often spend time outside for work or play are more likely to develop the disease, especially near areas of development and construction during the summer and fall. Up to 50 percent of people living in such areas have antibodies* against *Coccidioides immitis* in their blood, which indicates that they have been exposed to the fungus, although many of them never developed signs of the disease.

Signs and symptoms   About 60 percent of people infected by *Coccidioides immitis* develop no symptoms. When symptoms do occur, they are usually mild and include fever, aches, chills, headache, and tiredness. Those with weakened immune systems, such as people with AIDS, certain types of cancer, and diabetes, have a greater risk of developing a more severe form of the infection.

Diagnosis   A doctor diagnoses coccidioidomycosis by culturing* a patient's sputum* or by doing a skin test. If injecting the test material into the skin of the forearm causes a large circular welt to appear on the arm within 2 days, it is considered a positive test for the fungus. Blood tests may show antibodies to the fungus, which helps confirm the diagnosis. A chest X ray is sometimes taken to look for signs of infection or inflammation in the lungs.

Treatment   Most mild cases of the disease can be managed with bed rest, over-the-counter pain relievers such as acetaminophen (uh-see-teh-MIH-noh-fen), and sometimes oral (by mouth) anti-fungal medication. In more serious cases in which the fungus has spread throughout the body, intravenous (in-tra-VEE-nus, or given directly into a vein) anti-fungal medicines and hospitalization may be necessary. Mild cases of coccidioidomycosis last about 2 weeks, but recovery may take up to 6 months in more severe cases.

Complications   Pneumonia*, arthritis, meningitis, and other serious problems can result if the infection spreads throughout the lungs or to other parts of the body, such as the liver, heart, brain, bones, or joints.

Can Coccidioidomycosis Be Prevented?

No specific activities can prevent a person from becoming infected with the *coccidioides* fungus, other than avoiding the regions where it is found. Planting grass and paving roads may reduce dust in problem areas but will not kill the fungus.

Resources

Organizations

U.S. Centers for Disease Control and Prevention (CDC), 1600 Clifton Road, Atlanta, GA 30333. The CDC offers information about coccidioidomycosis at its website.
Telephone 800-311-3435
http://www.cdc.gov

U.S. National Library of Medicine, 8600 Rockville Pike, Bethesda, MD 20894. The National Library of Medicine has a website packed with information on diseases (including coccidioidomycosis) and drugs, consumer resources, dictionaries and encyclopedias of medical terms, and directories of doctors and helpful organizations.
Telephone 888-346-3656
http://www.nlm.nih.gov

▶ *See also*
Arthritis, Infectious
Fungal Infections
Meningitis
Pneumonia

Common Cold

The "common cold" is a nickname for the commonly occurring viral infections of the upper respiratory tract*.

What Is the Common Cold?

More than 200 different viruses can cause colds. Rhinoviruses are responsible for up to a third of all upper respiratory infections. Other common viruses that lead to stuffy heads and runny noses include adenoviruses (ah-deh-no-VY-rus-sez), coronaviruses (ko-ro-nuh-VY-rus-sez), parainfluenza (pair-uh-in-floo-EN-zuh) viruses, respiratory syncytial (RES-puh-ruh-tor-e sin-SIH-she-ul) virus, coxsackieviruses (kok-SAH-kee-vy-ruh-sez), echoviruses (EH-ko-vy-rus-sez), and influenza (in-floo-EN-zuh) viruses (although influenza may also trigger more serious complications). Children get colds most frequently, in part because of their close contact with so many other children in daycare or school. Younger children also tend to cough without covering their mouths and do not regularly wash their hands.

In North America, young children in daycare may catch several (sometimes as many as 10 or more) colds each year. People tend to get

KEYWORDS
for searching the Internet and other reference sources

Adenovirus

Coronavirus

Coxsackievirus

Echovirus

Influenza virus

Parainfluenza virus

Respiratory infection

Respiratory syncytial virus (RSV)

Rhinovirus

* **respiratory tract** includes the nose, mouth, throat, and lungs. It is the pathway through which air and gases are transported down into the lungs and back out of the body.

Common Cold Myths

Colds are so common that everyone seems to have a theory on what brings them on and how to cure them. Just consider these common cold myths (and some myth-busting explanations):

MYTH: Running around in the cold and having a wet head or wet feet can bring on a cold.

REALITY: These two beliefs probably stem from the accurate observation that more colds seem to occur in the cold, wet weather that often accompanies winter months in the United States. In reality, though, it is not the cold or wet that brings on the illness. Colder weather drives people indoors, which means increased and closer contact with others and a higher risk for colds.

MYTH: "Feed a cold (and starve a fever)."

REALITY: A recent study found that eating might actually boost the power of the immune system against certain illnesses, such as long-lasting colds, whereas decreased food intake may stimulate immune system chemicals that keep fever away. Until more studies are done, many doctors continue to urge patients with colds to down warm soup and other light fare.

MYTH: Taking large doses of vitamin C prevents colds.

REALITY: Vitamin C may have other body-boosting benefits, but there is no scientific proof that it prevents the common cold. Although garlic (which may have antiviral properties) and chicken soup appear to have some beneficial effects, studies of other widely touted cold remedies such as echinacea (eh-kih-NAY-see-uh), a plant product, and zinc supplements have mostly yielded negative, inconsistent, or unconvincing results.

fewer colds as they grow older because they develop immunity* to some of these viruses after being infected with them. For this reason, healthy adults average 2 to 4 colds a year, and those over age 60 tend to get even fewer (maybe 1 cold a year, or less).

Cold season in the United States generally occurs during the fall and winter months, although people can get sick from viral respiratory infections year round. Many people believe the cold air is responsible for catching a cold, but there is no evidence that viruses spread more easily or that our immune system is weaker in the cold. However, winter is the time of year when more people stay inside, bringing them into closer contact with others and their germs.

How Common Is the Common Cold?

As many as a billion colds occur each year in the United States. The U.S. Centers for Disease Control and Prevention's National Center for Health Statistics notes that on a yearly basis close to 22 million school days are lost due to illness from colds, and 45 million days are spent resting while recovering from colds.

Is the Common Cold Contagious?

Colds are very contagious. In general, they are most contagious during the first few days of illness, when symptoms like congestion (stuffy nose) and sneezing are starting. Cold viruses often spread through direct contact. Shaking the unwashed hand of someone with a cold (who has just touched his or her face) can easily spread the virus. When an infected person laughs, sneezes, or coughs, virus-packed droplets of moisture from the person's mouth and nose can become suspended in the air, where they can be inhaled by others. Sometimes these drops of respiratory secretions land on a surface such as a kitchen or bathroom counter, where they can infect the next person who comes along and touches the surface.

What Happens to Someone Who Has a Cold?

Signs and symptoms Cold symptoms usually appear within 2 to 3 days after the person becomes infected. They often include a runny or stuffy nose, watery eyes, coughing, mild muscle aches, tiredness, headache, low fever, and a scratchy, sore throat. Sneezing and coughing up mucus* are also common.

Diagnosis Doctors diagnose colds based on a history of symptoms and findings from a physical examination. Cultures* and other tests for the viruses are available but are not done in most situations. However, the doctor will want to distinguish a cold, caused by a virus, from bacterial infections of the sinuses or throat, such as strep throat.

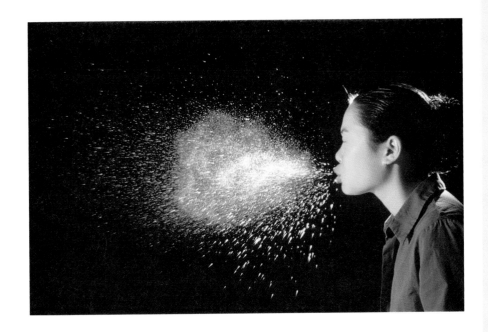

This high-speed photograph captures a sneeze in action. Virus-packed droplets are expelled from the respiratory system and can spread widely to contaminate surfaces. *Custom Medical Stock Photo, Inc.*

Treatment At the present time, there remains no true medical "cure" for the common cold. People who come down with colds can help themselves feel better by taking care of themselves at home until the infection goes away on its own. Bed rest helps tiredness, and inhaling mist in a steamy bathroom or running a humidifier in the bedroom to moisten dry air can relieve congestion and make it easier to breathe. Drinking plenty of clear or warm fluids may also reduce congestion, and tea with honey can soothe a scratchy throat. Over-the-counter medicines such as acetaminophen (uh-see-teh-MIH-noh-fen) can ease headaches and body aches and lower fever. Over-the-counter cold medicines may also help relieve symptoms. Symptoms of a cold can last up to a couple of weeks, but most people recover within a few days.

Because viruses cause colds, antibiotics are not useful in fighting these infections. Scientists are studying newer antiviral drugs that may be effective in fighting some cold-causing viruses (such as rhinoviruses). These medicines might change the treatment of colds in the future.

Complications Sometimes colds can cause swelling and irritation in the nasal passages, eustachian tubes*, and airways leading to the lungs. Bacteria that invade the body can flourish in these areas, causing additional infections. This is why it is not uncommon for someone to develop sinusitis*, an ear infection (otitis, o-TIE-tis), or bronchitis at the end of a bad cold. For those with weaker immune systems, such as the very young, the elderly, or those with chronic illnesses, these secondary infections can lead to breathing problems from severe bronchitis or pneumonia, which may sometimes be life threatening. Colds also can trigger flare-ups or worsening of respiratory symptoms in people who have asthma.

* **immunity** (ih-MYOON-uh-tee) is the condition of being protected against an infectious disease. Immunity often develops after a germ is introduced to the body. One type of immunity occurs when the body makes special protein molecules called antibodies to fight the disease-causing germ. The next time that germ enters the body, the antibodies quickly attack it, usually preventing the germ from causing disease.

* **mucus** (MYOO-kus) is a thick, slippery substance that lines the insides of many body parts.

* **culture** (KUL-chur) is a test in which a sample of fluid or tissue from the body is placed in a dish containing material that supports the growth of certain organisms. Typically, within days the organisms will grow and can be identified.

* **eustachian** (yoo-STAY-she-un) **tubes** are the tiny channels that connect and allow air to flow between the middle ears and the throat.

* **sinusitis** (sy-nyoo-SY-tis) is an infection in the sinuses, which are hollow cavities in the facial bones near the nose.

Can Colds Be Prevented?

To lower the risk of catching (or spreading) a cold, experts advise that people wash their hands frequently and cover the mouth with a tissue when coughing or sneezing. Avoiding touching the eyes or nose as much as possible, regularly cleaning bathroom and kitchen surfaces to get rid of germs, and avoiding close, extended contact with anyone who has a cold are also helpful.

Researchers have explored the idea of a cold vaccine, but many different viruses can cause colds, making the development of a single, effective vaccine a great challenge.

Resources

Organization

U.S. National Institute of Allergy and Infectious Diseases (NIAID), Building 31, Room 7A-50, 31 Center Drive MSC 2520, Bethesda, MD 20892. The NIAID, part of the National Institutes of Health, posts information about viral infections that cause colds at its website. http://www.niaid.nih.gov

Website

KidsHealth.org. KidsHealth is a website created by the medical experts of the Nemours Foundation and is devoted to issues of children's health. It contains articles on a variety of health topics, including the common cold. http://www.KidsHealth.org

Congenital Infections

Congenital infections affect babies as the result of infection of the mother during pregnancy. Infection of the infant can occur before the infant is born or during the birth process.

What Are Congenital Infections?

Bacteria, parasites, or viruses can cause congenital infections, which are infections that are present at birth. These infections can be passed to the fetus or newborn in two ways. Some infections, such as rubella or cytomegalovirus, are passed from the mother to the baby through the placenta (pluh-SEN-ta), the organ that nourishes the baby in the uterus, or womb. A baby can also become infected during the passage through the birth canal, as happens with group B streptococcus.

▶ *See also*

Bronchiolitis

Bronchitis, Infectious

Coxsackievirus and Other Enteroviruses

Croup

Influenza

Laryngitis

Otitis (Ear Infection)

Pneumonia

Sinusitis

KEYWORDS
for searching the Internet and other reference sources

Chlamydia

Cytomegalovirus

Gonorrhea

Group B streptococcus

Hepatitis

Herpes

Newborn infections

Parvovirus

Pregnancy infections

Rubella

Syphilis

Toxoplasmosis

Varicella

Some infections that can seriously endanger the health of a developing fetus or newborn cause few or no symptoms in a pregnant woman. The mother's health and immunity to disease play a role in whether or not she contracts an illness. In addition, the stage during the pregnancy when a woman becomes infected can also affect the severity of the infant's illness. For example, being exposed to an infection in early pregnancy is often more dangerous for the fetus, placing the baby at higher risk for miscarriage*, birth defects, or other problems.

What Are Some Common Congenital Infections?

There are many infections that can be passed from mother to child during pregnancy or childbirth.

Chlamydial Infection   Chlamydial (kla-MIH-dee-ul) infection is a sexually transmitted disease (STD) caused by the bacterium *Chlamydia trachomatis* (kla-MIH-dee-uh truh-KO-mah-tis). Many women who are infected do not even realize it because they often have no symptoms. However, when untreated, chlamydia can cause a scarring infection of the woman's internal reproductive organs, increasing her risk of a potentially fatal tubal pregnancy*. If passed to the baby during the passage through the birth canal, chlamydia can cause conjunctivitis* and pneumonia*. These infections usually respond well to antibiotic treatment.

Cytomegalovirus   Cytomegalovirus (sye-tuh-meh-guh-lo-VY-rus) infection (CMV) is caused by the cytomegalovirus, a member of the herpesvirus family*. It is transmitted through infected blood, saliva, urine, or other body fluids. CMV is a common infection, affecting about 1 in 100 newborns. Many people who have CMV do not realize it because it often produces no symptoms in healthy adults, but mothers who are infected with the virus during pregnancy can pass the virus to the baby in the uterus. A woman can also pass the virus to her infant during delivery or through breast milk, however, infection by these routes is less likely to cause severe problems for the baby. Newborns who have contracted CMV in the womb may have no initial symptoms, but over the first few years of life the infection has been associated with problems with growth and development, as well as trouble with vision and hearing. About 10 percent of infants with congenital CMV infection will have signs or symptoms at birth that may include jaundice*, retinitis*, microcephaly*, or signs of brain damage. Antiviral medications may help in some cases of congenital CMV infection.

Gonococcal infection   Gonorrhea (gah-nuh-REE-uh) is an STD caused by the bacterium *Neisseria gonorrhoeae* (nye-SEER-e-uh gah-no-REE-eye). Women often do not know that they are infected because the infection may not cause noticeable symptoms. Newborns can be infected

* **miscarriage** is the ending of a pregnancy through the death of the embryo or fetus before birth.

* **tubal** (TOO-bal) **pregnancy** is a condition in which a fertilized egg implants in the fallopian tube instead of the wall of the uterus.

* **conjunctivitis** (kon-jung-tih-VY-tis), often called "pinkeye," is an inflammation of the thin membrane that lines the inside of the eyelids and covers the surface of the eyeball. Conjunctivitis can be caused by viruses, bacteria, allergies, chemical irritation, and other conditions or diseases that cause inflammation.

* **pneumonia** (nu-MO-nyah) is inflammation of the lung.

* **herpesvirus** (her-peez-VY-rus) **family** is a group of viruses that can store themselves permanently in the body. The family includes varicella virus, Epstein-Barr virus, and herpes simplex virus.

* **jaundice** (JON-dis) is a yellowing of the skin, and sometimes the whites of the eyes, caused by a buildup in the body of bilirubin, a chemical produced in and released by the liver. An increase in bilirubin may indicate disease of the liver or certain blood disorders.

* **retinitis** (reh-tin-EYE-tis) is an inflammation of the retina, the nerve-rich membrane at the back of the eye on which visual images form.

* **microcephaly** (my-kro-SEH-fah-lee) is the condition of having an abnormally small head, which typically results from an underdeveloped or malformed brain.

during birth and develop an eye infection called gonococcal ophthalmia (gah-nuh-KOH-kul opf-THAL-me-uh). In rare cases, babies will develop gonorrhea that causes blindness or meningitis*. In the United States, newborns routinely receive eye medication at birth to prevent gonococcal eye infection. Antibiotics are given by injection to newborns if gonococcal infection is suspected.

Group B streptococcal infection

Group B streptococcal, or GBS, infection is caused by a bacterium that can be passed from mother to child shortly before or during birth. In newborns it can cause sepsis*, pneumonia, and meningitis. Although most pregnant women with GBS infection have no symptoms, it can cause bladder infections, infections in the womb (known as amnionitis, am-nee-o-NYE-tiss), and stillbirth. GBS disease is the most frequent cause of life-threatening infection in newborns, and according to the U.S. Centers for Disease Control and Prevention (CDC), the rate of infection in newborns is 0.5 per 1,000 live births. Since the beginning of preventive screening and treatment in pregnant women, the number of babies affected by GBS infection has declined by 70 percent. Newborns with GBS infection are treated with intravenous* antibiotics and require hospitalization.

Hepatitis

Hepatitis (heh-puh-TIE-tis) is an inflammation of the liver*. Viruses, bacteria, and a number of other noninfectious medical conditions can cause hepatitis. Hepatitis that is of concern with regard to congenital infection usually is caused by the hepatitis B or C viruses. Both can be transmitted from mother to newborn during birth. If not vaccinated, about 90 percent of newborns infected with hepatitis B at birth will develop chronic* hepatitis, although newborns may not have symptoms of hepatitis at first. In the United States, newborns now routinely receive vaccinations* against hepatitis B infection.

Herpes

Herpes (HER-peez) refers to the infections caused by the two types of herpes simplex virus: HSV-1 and HSV-2. HSV-1 causes cold sores; HSV-2 is sexually transmitted and in women can cause lesions (LEE-zhunz), or sores, on the vagina, cervix*, or skin around the birth canal. The virus can be passed to babies who have contact with these lesions during birth. Herpesvirus infection in newborns can be limited to the skin or it can involve the lungs, brain, and other organs. More widespread infection in the infant can result in permanent brain damage, mental retardation, or death. Newborns with herpes are given intravenous antiviral medication.

Parvovirus

Parvovirus infection is caused by parvovirus B19, which causes fifth disease in children. Fifth disease usually results in a distinctive red rash on the face, body, arms, and legs. Women who are infected during pregnancy typically experience only mild illness, with symptoms such as a rash or joint pain or swelling. However, in some cases the infection can cause severe anemia* in the unborn baby and miscarriage.

Rubella   Rubella (roo-BEH-luh) infection (German measles) is caused by the rubella virus, which is transmitted by contact with fluid from the mouth or nose (usually from coughs or sneezes) of someone who is infected. If a woman contracts the disease early in her pregnancy, she can pass it to her unborn baby. It can lead to congenital rubella syndrome (CRS), which is associated with fetal death, miscarriage, premature delivery, and various birth defects, including deafness, cataracts*, mental retardation, microcephaly, enlarged liver and spleen*, bone marrow* problems, and heart defects. CRS occurs in about 25 percent of infants born to women who had rubella infection during the first 3 months of pregnancy. Babies born with CRS are treated for specific defects.

Syphilis   Syphilis (SIH-fih-lis) is an STD caused by the bacterium *Treponema pallidum.* If a pregnant woman has syphilis, she can pass it to the fetus. If not treated early, syphilis can lead to serious complications in infants, including blindness, deafness, central nervous system* problems, and death. Nearly half of all infants infected with syphilis during pregnancy die before or shortly after birth, unless the mother has received treatment with antibiotics (usually penicillin) early in the pregnancy. Penicillin is given to infants whose mothers were infected but inadequately treated. Babies who show evidence of possible congenital syphilis, based on either physical signs or the results of a routine newborn blood test that screens infants for exposure to syphilis, also are treated with penicillin.

Toxoplasmosis   Toxoplasmosis (tox-o-plaz-MO-sis) is caused by the parasite *Toxoplasma gondii,* which is commonly found in cats and can be passed to humans in cat feces*. The March of Dimes estimates that a pregnant woman who contracts toxoplasmosis has a 40 percent chance of passing it to her baby. Handling soiled cat litter is the typical way that the disease is transmitted to humans, but the parasite also may be present in raw or undercooked meat. Women who are first infected with the parasite shortly before they become pregnant or when they are pregnant can pass the organism to the fetus, leading to congenital toxoplasmosis; the symptoms of this condition include jaundice, rash, fever, anemia, inflammation of the retina of the eye, and an enlarged spleen and liver. A baby with congenital toxoplasmosis may be blind or have learning and motor (movement) disabilities and other central nervous system problems. The problems associated with congenital toxoplasmosis may be present at birth or appear as the child develops.

Varicella   Infection with the varicella zoster (var-uh-SEH-luh ZOS-ter) virus can cause chicken pox and shingles (an infection that can

* **anemia** (uh-NEE-me-uh) is a blood condition in which there is a decreased amount of oxygen-carrying hemoglobin in the blood and, usually, fewer than normal numbers of red blood cells.

* **cataracts** (KAH-tuh-rakts) are areas of cloudiness of the lens of the eye that can interfere with vision.

* **spleen** is an organ in the upper left part of the abdomen that stores and filters blood. As part of the immune system, the spleen also plays a role in fighting infection.

* **bone marrow** is the soft tissue inside bones where blood cells are made.

* **central nervous system** (SEN-trul NER-vus SIS-tem) is the part of the nervous system that includes the brain and spinal cord.

* **feces** (FEE-seez) is the excreted waste from the gastrointestinal tract.

Should Pregnant Women Receive Vaccinations?

One way for a woman to prevent pregnancy- and newborn-related infections is to make sure her vaccinations are updated before becoming pregnant. Vaccinations can prevent some diseases, such as rubella and varicella, but if a pregnant woman does not have immunity to these diseases, she should not be vaccinated while pregnant because of potential risk to the fetus (these vaccines contain live viruses). Instead, vaccinating those around her can help protect her from infection. Other vaccines, such as the flu vaccine (not a live virus vaccine), are recommended during pregnancy.

* **antibodies** (AN-tih-bah-deez) are protein molecules produced by the body's immune system to help fight specific infections caused by microorganisms, such as bacteria and viruses.

* **immune globulin** (ih-MYOON GLAH-byoo-lin), also called gamma globulin, is the protein material that contains antibodies.

cause a painful rash with blisters), and it can be spread through contact with the sneezes or coughs of an infected person. Because most adults had chicken pox as children, it is uncommon for a pregnant woman to become infected with the varicella virus. The American College of Obstetricians and Gynecologists estimates that a woman's risk of contracting varicella during pregnancy is less than 1 in 1,000. However, becoming infected during pregnancy can cause serious complications. If a woman is infected with varicella early in the pregnancy, the baby can have multiple birth defects. Features of congenital varicella syndrome may include scarring, malformed limbs, and damage to the eyes and brain. Up to 2 percent of women who become infected with varicella during the first 20 weeks of pregnancy have babies with congenital varicella syndrome. If a mother contracts chicken pox immediately before or after delivery, the baby may develop severe or even fatal chicken pox.

Can Congenital Infections Be Prevented?

There are many preventive steps pregnant women can take to avoid becoming infected with diseases that could harm their infants. Practicing abstinence (not having sex) or safe sex by using a latex condom can reduce the risk of contracting STDs such as syphilis, chlamydia, gonorrhea, and herpes. Experts recommend that every pregnant woman be screened for these infections and, if needed, treated with antibiotics or other medications to reduce the risk of passing them to her baby.

Because between 20 and 30 percent of pregnant women carry GBS bacteria, pregnant women often are tested for the bacteria between the thirty-fifth and thirty-seventh weeks of pregnancy. The woman's doctor takes samples from the vagina and rectum, and the samples are examined under a microscope. If a woman is infected with GBS, intravenous antibiotics given during delivery can help reduce the risk of transmitting the bacteria to her baby.

Avoiding contact with cat feces and not eating or handling raw meat can reduce the risk of contracting toxoplasmosis. Wearing gloves when handling soil, especially outside, and cooking all meat thoroughly before eating can also help prevent infection. Women who are considering becoming pregnant can be screened for antibodies* to CMV and toxoplasmosis. If tests show that they already have antibodies, there is no risk of acquiring the disease during pregnancy and therefore no risk to the baby. If they do not have antibodies, they should practice particularly good hygiene while pregnant, including frequent hand washing, especially after contact with diapers or someone's bodily fluids. Good hygiene can also help prevent infection with parvovirus.

Women with herpes lesions will likely have their babies delivered via cesarean section to reduce the risk of passing the virus to the baby during delivery. Administering hepatitis B immune globulin* and hepatitis B vaccine to the infant within 12 hours of birth can prevent hepatitis B infection in the newborn. Experts recommend that rubella and varicella vaccines be given before pregnancy to women who have not already had these diseases or received the vaccines.

Resources

Organizations

March of Dimes, 1275 Mamaroneck Avenue, White Plains, NY 10605. The March of Dimes provides information about how to prevent birth defects, such as those caused by CMV and rubella infection. Telephone 888-MODIMES
http://www.modimes.org

U.S. Centers for Disease Control and Prevention (CDC), 1600 Clifton Road, Atlanta, GA 30333. The CDC is the U.S. government authority for information about infectious and other diseases. The organization offers fact sheets about pregnancy- and newborn-related infections at its website. Telephone 800-311-3435
http://www.cdc.gov

Conjunctivitis

Conjunctivitis (kon-jung-tih-VY-tis), often called pinkeye, is an inflammation of the conjunctiva (kon-jung-TIE-vuh), the thin membrane that lines the inside of the eyelids and covers the surface of the eyeball. Conjunctivitis can be caused by viruses, bacteria, allergies, or chemical irritation.

What Is Conjunctivitis?

Conjunctivitis, is an inflammation of the thin membrane that lines the inside of the eyelids and covers the white surface of the eye. The inflammation can produce redness, burning, or itching of the eyes and sometimes a discharge. Bacterial or viral infections most often cause conjunctivitis. Many different bacteria can be the culprit, most commonly *Streptococcus pneumoniae* (strep-tuh-KAH-kus nu-MO-nye), *Haemophilus influenzae* (he-MOH-fih-lus in-floo-EN-zuh), and *Staphylococcus aureus* (stah-fih-lo-KAH-kus ARE-ree-us). Infections with adenoviruses* and influenza viruses are common causes of conjunctivitis. About 80 percent of all cases of conjunctivitis result from viral or bacterial infection.

Rarely, parasites* and fungal infections can cause conjunctivitis. The condition also can stem from various allergies, irritants, chemicals, and

▶ *See also*

Chlamydial Infections

Cytomegalovirus (CMV) Infection

Fifth Disease

Gonorrhea

Hepatitis, Infectious

Herpes Simplex Virus Infections

Rubella (German Measles)

Sexually Transmitted Diseases

Streptococcal Infections

Syphilis

Toxoplasmosis

Varicella (Chicken Pox) and Herpes Zoster (Shingles)

KEYWORDS
for searching the Internet and other reference sources

Chlamydia

Eye infections

Gonorrhea

Herpesvirus

Pinkeye

* **adenoviruses** (ah-deh-no-VY-ruh-sez) can produce a variety of symptoms, including upper respiratory disease, when they infect humans.

* **parasites** (PAIR-uh-sites) are organisms such as protozoa (one-celled animals), worms, or insects that must live on or inside a human or other organism to survive. An animal or plant harboring a parasite is called its host. Parasites live at the expense of the host and may cause illness.

103

* **chlamydia** (kla-MIH-dee-uh) are microorganisms that can infect the urinary tract, genitals, eye, and respiratory tract, including the lungs.

* **gonorrhea** (gah-nuh-REE-uh) is a sexually transmitted disease (STD) spread through all forms of sexual intercourse. The bacteria can also be passed from an infected mother to her baby during childbirth. Gonorrhea can affect the genitals, urethra, rectum, eyes, throat, joints, and other tissues of the body.

pollutants. Reactions to smoke, dust, makeup, contact lenses, and pollen all can produce symptoms in some people. The sexually transmitted diseases chlamydia* and gonorrhea*, which can be passed from infected mothers to their babies during birth, are the most common causes of conjunctivitis in newborns. These two diseases can lead to conjunctivitis in adults as well. Conjunctivitis usually does not cause problems with vision.

How Does Conjunctivitis Spread and Who Gets It?

Conjunctivitis, especially of viral origin, typically is seen in children and adults who are caregivers of children, such as parents or day-care workers. Bacterial conjunctivitis is less common in healthy older children and adults. Both the bacterial and viral forms of the condition are contagious. The germs that cause conjunctivitis may be present in nasal secretions and in the discharge from the eyes. People can become infected simply by touching the face of someone with the disease and then rubbing their own eyes without first washing their hands. Sharing contaminated towels or eye makeup also can spread the infection. Infectious conjunctivitis can spread quickly through child-care and school settings and among members of the same family. Bacterial conjunctivitis can remain contagious until treatment with antibiotics is started. The viral form is usually contagious before the symptoms appear and for as long as symptoms, including any discharge from the eye, last.

What Are the Signs and Symptoms of Conjunctivitis?

The first symptoms typically appear within a few days or up to a week after infection. A person may feel discomfort, a gritty sensation under the eyelids, or a feeling that there is something in the eye. Redness develops in the eye, and the eyelids may swell. Bacterial infections usually produce a thick yellowish or greenish discharge. When the person wakes up in the morning, the eyelids might stick together as the result of dried discharge. In viral conjunctivitis, the discharge is often thin, watery, and clear. Viral infections are more likely to affect both eyes and can be accompanied by other symptoms of viral infection, such as cold or flu symptoms.

How Is Conjunctivitis Diagnosed?

Eye discharge and inflammation (redness) of the conjunctiva are the hallmarks of conjunctivitis. The doctor also will ask whether the person has had any recent contact with someone with conjunctivitis and will examine the eyes, making sure the person's vision is normal. Sometimes the doctor will swab the inside of the eyelids to obtain fluid for laboratory testing, to determine the type of infection. This is more likely to be done in newborn babies or someone at risk of a sexually transmitted disease, such as chlamydial infection or gonorrhea.

How Do Doctors Treat Conjunctivitis?

Treatment depends on the cause of conjunctivitis. If bacterial conjunctivitis has been diagnosed, antibiotic eyedrops usually are prescribed for about a week. An antibiotic ointment is used for babies. Viral conjunctivitis disappears by itself and does not typically require treatment. (One exception is conjunctivitis caused by herpesvirus* infection, which is treated with antiviral eyedrops.) Over-the-counter pain relievers, such as acetaminophen (uh-see-teh-MIH-noh-fen), and warm compresses placed over the eyelids several times a day may ease the discomfort. Conjunctivitis usually clears up within a week. Cases of viral conjunctivitis can take longer to resolve than bacterial conjunctivitis.

Are There Complications?

Complications of conjunctivitis are rare. In newborns, untreated gonorrheal infection of the conjunctiva can cause a spreading infection of the eye that can lead to blindness. A few viruses cause conjunctivitis that affects deeper parts of the eye, resulting in keratitis (kare-uh-TY-tis), an inflammation of the cornea* that causes changes in vision and sometimes permanent scarring of the cornea. Trachoma (truh-KO-mah), a type of chlamydial conjunctivitis seen in developing countries, also can lead to blindness.

Can Conjunctivitis Be Prevented?

The best way to prevent infectious conjunctivitis is to wash hands frequently, especially after touching the face of someone who has the infection. It is a good idea for people with infectious conjunctivitis to wash their hands often to avoid spreading the infection. It is also wise not to share makeup; disposable items, such as paper towels and cotton balls; or towels. Washing towels and clothing in hot water can disinfect them.

Resource

Website

KidsHealth.org. KidsHealth is a website created by the medical experts of the Nemours Foundation and is devoted to issues of children's health. It contains articles on a variety of health topics, including conjunctivitis.
http://www.KidsHealth.org

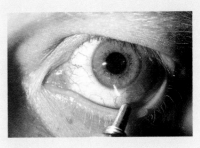

Antibiotic eyedrops or ointments are applied to the eye to treat bacterial conjunctivitis. *Custom Medical Stock Photo, Inc.*

* **herpesvirus** (her-peez-VY-rus) is a member of a family of viruses that can store themselves permanently in the body. The family includes varicella virus, Epstein-Barr virus, and herpes simplex virus.

* **cornea** (KOR-nee-uh) is the transparent circular layer of cells over the central colored part of the eyeball (the iris) through which light enters the eye.

▶ *See also*
Chlamydial Infections
Congenital Infections
Gonorrhea
Influenza

Coxsackieviruses and Other Enteroviruses

The enteroviruses (en-tuh-ro-VY-rus-sez) are a family of viruses that usually enter the body by infecting the gastrointestinal* tract. They cause several types of infection, mostly in children. Coxsackieviruses (kok-SAH-kee-vy-ruh-sez) are some of the most well known enteroviruses.

What Are Enteroviruses?

There are many different kinds of viruses in the enterovirus family, which cause infections with different symptoms, mostly in children. These viruses make their home in the digestive tract and are related to the viruses that cause poliomyelitis* and hepatitis A*. The largest subgroups of the enterovirus family are coxsackieviruses and echoviruses. In most cases, coxsackievirus infection causes fever and sometimes a mild rash in children, but a variety of other symptoms can occur. Coxsackievirus is well known for its link to hand, foot, and mouth disease, which causes red bumps and blisters to appear inside the mouth and on the hands and feet.

Are Enteroviruses Contagious?

Everyone is at risk of contracting enteroviral infections. They most commonly infect infants and children younger than 5 years old and spread easily among children in group settings, such as day-care centers or schools. These viruses are most likely to cause infections during late summer and early fall and are very contagious. People with coxsackievirus are most contagious during the first week that they are sick.

How Are Enteroviruses Spread?

Enteroviruses are usually spread through contact with feces*, especially on unwashed hands and on surfaces that an infected person has touched, such as a countertop, phone, or toy. The viruses can stay alive for days on these surfaces, waiting to be touched by the next person. Parents, babysitters, and day-care workers who change diapers typically have a higher risk of becoming infected with enteroviruses and passing them on to others, especially if they do not wash their hands often. Like many other viruses, enteroviruses also can spread through tiny droplets of fluid that are sprayed into the air when someone sneezes, coughs, or stands close to another person while talking. A person can become infected by breathing in these droplets or by touching something that the infected person has handled, sneezed at, or coughed on.

What Are the Signs and Symptoms?

Many people who become infected with enteroviruses have no symptoms or experience only mild symptoms that do not require medical at-

KEYWORDS
for searching the Internet and other reference sources

Coxsackievirus

Echovirus

Enterovirus

Hand, foot, and mouth disease

Herpangina

Pleurodynia

Poliomyelitis

* **gastrointestinal** (gas-tro-in-TES-tih-nuhl) means having to do with the organs of the digestive system, the system that processes food. It includes the mouth, esophagus, stomach, intestines, colon, and rectum and other organs involved in digestion, including the liver and pancreas.

* **poliomyelitis** (po-lee-o-my-uh-LYE-tis) is a condition caused by the polio virus that involves damage of nerve cells. It may lead to weakness and deterioration of the muscles and sometimes paralysis.

* **hepatitis A** (heh-puh-TIE-tis) is an inflammation of the liver that is caused by an infection with the hepatitis A virus.

* **feces** (FEE-seez) is the excreted waste from the gastrointestinal tract.

tention. Some have a fever and a rash, while others may get a sore throat, headache, mild abdominal* pain, or nausea. Fever can be as high as 104 degrees Fahrenheit and may come and go over the course of several days. Some enteroviruses can cause conditions characterized by groups of specific symptoms:

- Hand, foot, and mouth disease: red, painful blisters on the tongue and gums, inside the cheeks, on the palms of hands and the soles of feet, and sometimes on the buttocks.
- Herpangina (her-pan-JY-na): sore throat with blisters that appear on the tonsils and palate*.
- Pleurodynia (ploor-o-DIN-e-uh), also known as Bornholm disease: stabbing pain in the chest or upper abdomen.
- Hemorrhagic conjunctivitis (heh-muh-RAH-jik kon-jung-tih-VY-tis): sudden and severe eye pain with red and watery eyes, eye swelling, and sometimes blurred vision.

Rarely, enteroviruses can cause myositis*, meningitis*, or encephalitis*. Myocarditis* or pericarditis* also can occur. In some cases, these infections can be serious or even lead to death.

How Do Doctors Diagnose and Treat Enteroviruses?

Usually a doctor will diagnose an enterovirus infection by getting a history of the patient's symptoms and performing a physical, paying particular attention to any rash or blisters. Sometimes doctors use cotton swabs to take a fluid sample from the back of the mouth or throat, which is tested to find out if an enterovirus is present. Samples of bowel movements also might be tested. Like other viral infections, enteroviral infections do not respond to antibiotics, which treat only bacterial infections. New antiviral medications can be used to treat some severe cases of enterovirus infection. Usually, treatment is aimed at relieving discomfort. Doctors recommend that people with these viruses get plenty of rest, drink cool fluids, and take over-the-counter, non-aspirin pain relievers such as acetaminophen (uh-see-teh-MIH-noh-fen) to ease fever, headache, muscle aches, and painful mouth blisters. Doctors may prescribe a medicated cream or gel to numb sores inside the mouth or on the gums or tongue. Rarely, hospitalization is necessary for infants and children who experience complications.

How Long Do Enterovirus Symptoms Last and What Are the Complications?

Enteroviruses can cause illness that lasts from 3 days to 2 weeks, depending on the type of infection. Fevers usually last a few days, whereas rash and blisters take longer to disappear. Dehydration* can become a problem, especially in infants and young children, because mouth sores can make eating and drinking painful. In such cases, intravenous* fluids

* **abdominal** (ab-DAH-mih-nul) refers to the area of the body below the ribs and above the hips that contains the stomach, intestines, and other organs.

* **palate** (PAL-it) is the structure at the roof of the mouth. Damage or poor functioning of the palate can affect swallowing, the voice, and breathing.

* **myositis** (my-oh-SY-tis) is an inflammation of the muscles.

* **meningitis** (meh-nin-JY-tis) is an inflammation of the meninges, the membranes that surround the brain and the spinal cord. Meningitis is most often caused by infection with a virus or a bacterium.

* **encephalitis** (en-seh-fuh-LYE-tis) is an inflammation of the brain, usually caused by a viral infection.

* **myocarditis** (my-oh-kar-DYE-tis) is an inflammation of the muscular walls of the heart.

* **pericarditis** (per-ih-kar-DYE-tis) is an inflammation of the sac surrounding the heart.

* **dehydration** (dee-hi-DRAY-shun) is a condition in which the body is depleted of water, usually caused by excessive and unreplaced loss of body fluids, such as through sweating, vomiting, or diarrhea.

* **intravenous** (in-tra-VEE-nus) means within or through a vein. For example, medications, fluid, or other substances can be given through a needle or soft tube inserted through the skin's surface directly into a vein.

DID YOU KNOW?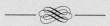

Coxsackievirus got its name from the town of Coxsackie, New York, the site of the first recognized outbreak of the virus infection in 1948.

may be required. It is recommended that people with enterovirus infections seek medical attention if they start to experience pain in the chest or abdomen, a sore throat that does not improve, difficulty in breathing, severe headaches, neck stiffness, or vomiting.

How Are Enterovirus Infections Prevented?

There is no vaccine to prevent enterovirus infections. As with most contagious infections, washing hands with soap and water after going to the bathroom, changing diapers, shaking hands with other people, and touching surfaces, especially those in public places, may help prevent the spread of infection. It is a good idea to cover the mouth and nose when coughing and sneezing and to avoid contact with other people who are coughing and sneezing. It is recommended that toys shared by infants and toddlers, especially in day-care settings, be cleaned with a disinfectant daily, because enteroviruses and other viruses can survive on them for days. Doctors usually advise that an infected child be kept out of day care or school for a few days to avoid spreading the virus to others.

Resources

Organization

U.S. Centers for Disease Control and Prevention (CDC), 1600 Clifton Road, Atlanta, GA 30333. The CDC offers information about coxsackievirus and other enterovirus infections at its website. Telephone 800-311-3435
http://www.cdc.gov

Website

KidsHealth.org. KidsHealth is a website created by the medical experts of the Nemours Foundation and is devoted to issues of children's health. It contains articles on a variety of health topics, including coxsackievirus.
http://www.KidsHealth.org

▶ *See also*

Conjunctivitis

Encephalitis

Hepatitis, Infectious

Meningitis

Myocarditis/Pericarditis

Polio

Creutzfeldt-Jakob Disease

Creutzfeldt-Jakob (KROYTZ-felt YAH-kub) disease is a disorder of the brain that is ultimately fatal.

What Is Creutzfeldt-Jakob Disease?

Creutzfeldt-Jakob disease (CJD) is a very rare disorder that damages the tissues of the brain, causing a rapid decline in mental function and muscle coordination, eventually leading to death. It is believed that a tiny transmissible* protein particle called a prion triggers the disease, which is divided into three categories:

- Familial CJD accounts for up to about 10 percent of cases. In these instances, there exists a family history of the disease, suggesting that certain genes* shared by family members make them more susceptible to CJD.

- Sporadic cases, in which people have no known risk factors for the disease, make up about 85 percent of occurrences.

- Acquired CJD is the rarest form. Less than 5 percent of all cases result from exposure to infected brain or spinal tissue, usually during a medical procedure.

CJD belongs to a family of illnesses known as transmissible spongiform (SPUN-jih-form) encephalopathies (en-seh-fuh-LAH-puh-theez). Spongiform refers to the appearance of brain tissue affected by the disease—the damaged tissue is full of holes, much like a sponge. Other diseases in the CJD family include kuru*; bovine spongiform encephalopathy (BSE), which infects cattle and is known as mad cow disease; and scrapie*, which affects sheep. The disease generally affects people age 60 or older, but in 1996 scientists described a new form of CJD, called variant CJD or new variant CJD (vCJD). Variant CJD differs from classic CJD in that it typically affects people under the age of 30 and causes different symptoms. So far, cases of vCJD have been limited mostly to the United Kingdom and France, and all the people in whom vCJD has developed have been exposed to areas where BSE has been found.

How Common Is CJD?

Creutzfeldt-Jakob disease remains extremely rare, occurring in about one in 1 million people each year.

Is the Disease Contagious?

Although CJD may be transmissible, it does not appear to spread through usual types of direct person-to-person contact. CJD can be transmitted through contact with infected brain or central nervous system* tissue or

KEYWORDS
for searching the Internet and other reference sources

Bovine spongiform encephalopathy (BSE)

Kuru

Mad cow disease

Prions

Scrapie

Transmissible spongiform encephalopathies

* **transmissible** (trans-MIH-sih-bul) means able to be transferred or spread.

* **genes** (JEENS) are chemical structures composed of deoxyribonucleic acid (DNA) that help determine a person's body structure and physical characteristics. Inherited from a person's parents, genes are contained in the chromosomes found in the body's cells.

* **kuru** (KUR-ew) is a progressive, fatal brain disease characterized by tremors and loss of muscle coordination that is caused by eating contaminated brain tissue from other humans who had the disease.

* **scrapie** (SKRAY-pee) is a fatal brain disorder of sheep that is characterized by itching of the skin and difficulty walking.

* **central nervous system** (SEN-trul NER-vus SIS-tem) is the part of the nervous system that includes the brain and spinal cord.

Mad Cow Disease and the Human Connection

A disease called bovine spongiform encephalopathy (BSE or mad cow disease), which is similar to CJD but is found in cattle, has been linked to variant CJD. Cattle had long been fed ground-up carcasses from sheep and other livestock as a nutritional supplement. This practice may have caused an epidemic of BSE among cows in the United Kingdom that began in 1986. It is thought that the carcasses fed to the cows could have been those of animals infected with various forms of transmissible spongiform disease. In 1988 this feeding practice was banned in the United Kingdom. Millions of cows have since been slaughtered to protect the food supply, and the number of new BSE cases has dropped sharply.

* **cornea** (KOR-nee-uh) is the transparent circular layer of cells over the central colored part of the eyeball (the iris) through which light enters the eye.

* **dura mater** (DUR-uh MAY-ter) is the outermost of three membranes covering the brain and spinal cord.

* **grafts** are tissue or organ transplants.

* **microorganisms** are tiny organisms that can be seen only using a microscope. Types of microorganisms include fungi, bacteria, and viruses.

* **mutation** (myoo-TAY-shun) is a change in an organism's gene or genes.

fluid, usually during a medical procedure. For example, the disease has been reported after cornea* transplants and dura mater* grafts*, following injection of human pituitary*–derived growth hormone*, and after contact with medical instruments used during brain surgery on a person with the disease. Cerebrospinal fluid can spread CJD, but there is no evidence of transmission through other body fluids, including saliva, blood, or urine. Variant CJD has occurred only where cases of BSE also have been found, leading researchers to theorize that eating beef from cattle with BSE could spread the agent and lead to CJD in humans. Although this explanation is widely accepted, it has not been proved.

What Are the Signs and Symptoms of CJD?

The most characteristic symptom of CJD is quickly worsening dementia*, including memory loss and impaired thinking. Patients often have problems with vision and muscle coordination. The inability to sleep, unusual sensations, and depression are also common. Many patients experience muscle jerking known as myoclonus (my-AH-kloh-nus), which consists of brief, rapid muscle contractions. If the disease is contracted from human tissue (such as from a transplanted cornea), symptoms may not appear for decades after exposure to the contaminated tissue. Vari-

PRIONS: ARE THEY "INFECTIOUS"?

Like bacteria, viruses, and parasites, prions, which are abnormal protein particles, have been linked to certain transmissible diseases. Yet prions are different from other infectious agents. While microorganisms* contain genetic material, prions do not, which means that they are not alive. According to the prion theory, the protein at first cannot transmit disease. Instead, it undergoes a change that allows it to fold into a different shape, its "infectious" form. When a prion enters a brain cell in the course of CJD, it binds to normal proteins, causing them to change shape. This sets off a chain reaction leading to cell death and the release of more prions to enter and affect more cells. As cells die, holes form in brain tissue giving it the characteristic "spongelike" appearance. Prions can be acquired during a medical procedure or from some other exposure to brain tissue or fluids containing brain tissue. In the inherited form of CJD, it is believed that a gene mutation* allows some normal proteins to change into prions under certain conditions.

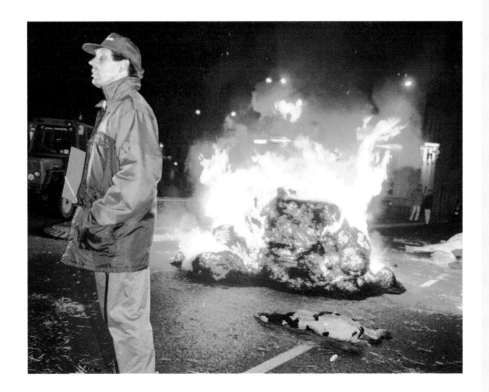

Variant Creutzfeld-Jakob disease has occurred only where cases of bovine spongiform encephalopathy also have been found, leading researchers to theorize that eating beef from cattle with BSE could spread the agent. In France and England whole herds of cattle have been put to death in an effort to prevent the spread of disease. *AP/Wide World Photos*

ant CJD at first causes psychiatric (sy-kee-AH-trik) symptoms, such as depression, anxiety (ang-ZY-uh-tee), or personality changes; dementia and myoclonus typically occur later than in classic CJD.

How Do Doctors Make the Diagnosis?

CJD can be diagnosed by a brain biopsy (BI-op-see), which requires removing a small piece of brain tissue during surgery to examine for signs of the disease, or by an autopsy*. Other, less invasive tests may point to a diagnosis of CJD or help identify another cause of the patient's symptoms, such as meningitis or encephalitis. During a physical examination, the doctor checks for muscle twitching and spasms. An eye exam may show areas of blindness that the patient may not have noticed, and a spinal tap* and blood tests may identify certain proteins associated with CJD. An electroencephalogram (EEG) test records electrical activity in the brain and may show a pattern of brain waves seen in many patients with CJD, although the typical EEG findings are not present in vCJD. Some people with CJD have negative test results, making a diagnosis difficult without a brain biopsy.

What Is the Treatment and Course of the Disease?

Because CJD cannot be cured, the goal of treatment is to make the patient as comfortable as possible. Medications can help control aggressive behavior, lessen pain, and ease muscle jerks. Dementia can progress to

* **pituitary** (pih-TOO-ih-tare-e) is a small oval-shaped gland at the base of the skull that produces several hormones—substances that affect various body functions, including growth.

* **growth hormone** is a chemical substance produced by the pituitary gland that regulates growth and other body functions.

* **dementia** (dih-MEN-sha) is a loss of mental abilities including memory, understanding, and judgment.

* **autopsy** (AW-top-see) is an examination of a body after death to look for the cause of death or the effects of a disease.

* **spinal tap**, also called a lumbar puncture, is a medical procedure in which a needle is used to withdraw a sample of the fluid surrounding the spinal cord and brain. The fluid is then tested, usually to detect signs of infection, such as meningitis, or other diseases.

Genetically Engineered Bacteria to the Rescue

Growth hormone once was obtained from the pituitary glands of cadavers—that is, the bodies of people who have died—and patients who needed injections of growth hormone were at risk of getting CJD. Now growth hormone can be produced in laboratories by inserting the genes controlling the production of growth hormone into bacteria, thus avoiding the need to extract the hormone from human tissue and eliminating the risk of transmitting CJD.

▶ *See also*
Encephalitis
Meningitis

KEYWORDS
*for searching the Internet
and other reference sources*

Adenovirus

Parainfluenza virus

Respiratory infections

Respiratory syncytial virus (RSV)

Stridor

*trachea (TRAY-kee-uh) is the windpipe, the firm, tubular structure that carries air from the throat to the lungs.

loss of speech, the inability to take care of oneself, blindness, and even coma. As patients become bedridden, they are vulnerable to infections, such as pneumonia, and most eventually need to be hospitalized. Many patients die within a year after symptoms appear.

How Can CJD Be Prevented?

No known measures can prevent the onset of CJD in a person whose brain tissue contains the prion. Because the ways by which the disease can be transmitted are still not well understood, blood banks forbid people with confirmed or suspected CJD or those who may be at high risk, such as persons with a family history of the disease, to donate blood, and doctors advise that they not be organ or tissue donors. Family members of a person with CJD may wish to have genetic counseling to learn more about any family risk. Special handling of surgical instruments can limit the chance of transmission during certain medical procedures, particularly those involving the brain.

Resource

Organization

Creutzfeldt-Jakob Disease Foundation, Inc., P.O. Box 5312, Akron, OH 44334. The foundation gives an overview of CJD and lists CJD-related websites, along with the latest news and research. Telephone 800-659-1991
http://cjdfoundation.org

Croup

Croup (KROOP) is an infection involving the trachea (windpipe) and larynx (voice box) that typically occurs in childhood. It causes inflammation and narrowing of the upper airway, sometimes making it difficult to breathe. The characteristic symptom is a barking cough.

What Is Croup?

Croup is an infection of the throat typically occurring in childhood that causes the lining of the trachea* and larynx* to swell, narrowing the upper airway and sometimes making it difficult to breathe. The characteristic symptom is a barking cough. In more severe cases of croup, a high-pitched or squeaking noise called stridor* can be heard when the child takes a breath. The symptoms of the infection can appear suddenly, or develop over a few days. Common cold symptoms, such as a runny nose, usually precede the onset of the barking cough. An allergy or a bacterial infection can produce symptoms of croup, but the most common culprit is a virus, usually parainfluenza* virus. Influenza viruses, adenovirus*, respiratory syncytial virus*, and measles virus also can cause croup.

Who Gets Croup?

Croup is most common during the winter months and in the early spring. The condition tends to develop in children who are between the ages of 3 months and 5 years. In the same way that an adult with a cold might have laryngitis*, a child with a cold might get croup. In fact, many of the viruses that cause croup in children can lead to laryngitis in adults. Some children are more prone to croup, such as those who are born prematurely or who have narrowed upper airways. These children may get symptoms of croup every time they have a respiratory illness. Although the viruses that cause croup can pass easily between children through respiratory secretions, most children who come into contact with those viruses will not get croup.

What Are the Symptoms and Complications of Croup?

A low fever is common, and children with croup usually have a barking cough. In severe cases, when their airways become more swollen and narrowed, children might experience difficulty breathing. Fast breathing and stridor may develop. If the body is not getting enough oxygen, the lips, tongue, and skin around the mouth can start to appear bluish. Crying can make the breathing symptoms worse. The symptoms also tend to worsen at night, when children are tired, and a child with croup often will have trouble sleeping or even resting. Croup symptoms typically peak 2 to 3 days after they start, and the illness generally lasts less than a week. In a small number of cases, children may have such complications as an ear infection or pneumonia.

How Is Croup Diagnosed?

A barking cough and stridor are telltale signs of croup. Other clues to the diagnosis are low fever, common cold symptoms, previous bouts of croup, or a history of intubation* or other upper-airway problems. If the symptoms are severe, or if the child does not respond quickly to treatment, a neck X ray may be taken to check for other reasons for the breathing difficulty. The X ray might show a foreign object lodged in the throat or, possibly, epiglottitis*. If the air passage at the top of the trachea is narrowed almost to a point (called a "steeple sign"), it helps confirm the diagnosis of croup.

Can Croup Be Treated and Prevented?

Mild cases of croup can be treated safely at home. Moist air is especially helpful, and mist from a steam-filled bathroom or cool-mist humidifier will moisten the child's airway, help open the air passage, and relieve

*larynx (LAIR-inks) is the voice box (which contains the vocal cords) and is located between the base of the tongue and the top of the windpipe.

*stridor (STRY-dor) is a high-pitched, squeaking noise that occurs while breathing in, present usually only if there is narrowing or blockage of the upper airway.

*parainfluenza (pair-uh-in-floo-EN-zuh) is a family of viruses that cause respiratory infections.

*adenovirus (ah-deh-no-VY-rus) is a type of virus that can produce a variety of symptoms, including upper respiratory disease, when it infects humans.

*respiratory syncytial (RES-puh-ruh-tor-e sin-SIH-she-ul) virus, or RSV, is a virus that infects the respiratory tract and typically causes minor symptoms in adults but can lead to more serious respiratory illnesses in children.

*laryngitis (lair-in-JY-tis) is an inflammation of the vocal cords that causes hoarseness or a temporary loss of voice.

*intubation (in-too-BAY-shun) is the insertion of a tube into the windpipe to allow air and gases to flow into and out of the lungs in a person who needs help breathing.

*epiglottitis (eh-pih-glah-TIE-tis) is a condition involving life-threatening swelling of the epiglottis (a soft flap of tissue that covers the opening of the trachea when a person swallows), which is usually caused by a bacterial infection of the epiglottis. The condition can result in a blockage of the trachea and severe breathing difficulty.

epinephrine (eh-pih-NEH-frin) is a chemical substance produced by the body that can also be given as a medication to constrict, or narrow, small blood vessels, stimulate the heart, and cause other effects, such as helping to open narrowed airways in conditions like asthma and croup.

corticosteroids (kor-tih-ko-STIR-oyds) are chemical substances made by the adrenal glands that have several functions in the body, including maintaining blood pressure during stress and controlling inflammation. They can also be given to people as medication to treat certain illnesses.

▶ See also

Common Cold

Epiglottitis

Influenza

Laryngitis

Measles (Rubeola)

Pneumonia

KEYWORDS
for searching the Internet
and other reference sources

Epstein-Barr virus

Herpes simplex virus

Herpesvirus

Immune deficiencies

Mononucleosis

Varicella zoster virus

coughing. Taking the child outdoors for a few minutes, even in the winter, can ease a coughing attack quickly, because the cool air can shrink the swollen tissues lining the airway. As with most illnesses, drinking fluids and getting plenty of rest help the body heal. Cigarette smoke near a child with croup or any other respiratory illness can make symptoms worse. Doctors advise prompt medical treatment for serious croup infections. Inhaled medications, including epinephrine*, can minimize swelling in the upper airways. Doctors often will administer corticosteroid* medicines to ease airway swelling for a few days while the child recovers from the virus infection that causes croup. There is no way to prevent croup, but frequent hand washing and avoiding contact with people who have respiratory infections can lessen the chance of spreading the viruses that cause croup.

Resources

Organization

U.S. Centers for Disease Control and Prevention (CDC), 1600 Clifton Road, Atlanta, GA 30333. The CDC offers information about croup at its website.
Telephone 800-311-3435
http://www.cdc.gov

Website

KidsHealth.org. KidsHealth is a website created by the medical experts of the Nemours Foundation and is devoted to issues of children's health. It contains articles on a variety of health topics, including croup.
http://www.KidsHealth.org

Cytomegalovirus (CMV) Infection

Cytomegalovirus (sye-tuh-MEH-guh-lo-vy-rus), or CMV infection is very common and usually causes no symptoms. It poses little risk for healthy people, but it can lead to serious illness in people with weak immune systems.

What Is CMV?

CMV is part of the herpesvirus (her-peez-VY-rus) family, which also includes the viruses that cause herpes*, chicken pox, and mononucleosis*. As with other members of the herpesvirus family, once CMV enters a person's body, it remains there for life. CMV infection can bring about flulike symptoms when a person is first infected, but many people have no symptoms at all. The virus usually becomes dormant after it enters the body, meaning that it remains "hidden" and does not cause symptoms of illness. The virus can emerge at a later time, however, and produce illness in people with weakened immune systems, such as people who have cancer or AIDS or those who have received organ or bone marrow* transplants. CMV is a risk for pregnant women because of the danger that it can be transmitted to their babies. The disease is the leading cause of mental retardation and hearing defects in newborns in the United States as a result of congenital (kon-JEH-nih-tul) infection, that is, infection that is present at birth.

How Is CMV Spread?

CMV is contagious and can spread through bodily fluids, including blood, saliva, semen, breast milk, tears, and urine. The virus can be transmitted by sexual contact, by close person-to-person contact, or from mother to baby during pregnancy or birth or while breast-feeding. It often spreads among children in day care or preschool or among family members. In the United States, as many as three of every five adults have been infected with CMV by the time they reach age 40. CMV infects people all over the world and is even more widespread in developing countries and those with poor living conditions.

What Are the Symptoms of CMV?

Most people who have been infected with CMV never show symptoms. In some people, the virus causes mild symptoms that mimic the flu or infectious mononucleosis, such as fever, chills, body aches, headache, swollen lymph nodes*, sore throat, and fatigue. Newborns who contract CMV infection in the womb may be born with jaundice*, microcephaly*, signs of brain damage, and a serious inflammation of the eyes known as retinitis*. Others seem healthy when they are born but later have growth problems and signs of hearing loss or mental retardation.

How Are CMV Infections Diagnosed and Treated?

Most cases of CMV infection are never diagnosed because they produce few or no symptoms. When doctors do suspect CMV, they often base the diagnosis on symptoms, physical examination, and blood tests for antibodies* to the virus. They also will rule out other diseases that cause similar symptoms, such as infectious mononucleosis caused by the Epstein-Barr virus. Sometimes blood tests show evidence of past infection with CMV but do not indicate active infection. A test known as the polymerase (pah-LIM-er-ace) chain reaction, or PCR, can test specifically for active CMV infection by finding traces of DNA* from the virus in body fluids. People with healthy immune systems who contract CMV infection usually do not require medical treatment. When people with weakened immune systems develop CMV infection, doctors often prescribe medication made to fight viruses. These antiviral medicines may

* **herpes** (HER-peez) is a viral infection that can produce painful, recurring skin blisters around the mouth or the genitals, and sometimes symptoms of infection elsewhere in the body.

* **mononucleosis** (mah-no-nu-klee-O-sis) is an infectious illness caused by a virus that often leads to fever, sore throat, swollen glands, and tiredness.

* **bone marrow** is the soft tissue inside bones where blood cells are made.

* **lymph** (LIMF) **nodes** are small, bean-shaped masses of tissue that contain immune system cells that fight harmful microorganisms. Lymph nodes may swell during infections.

* **jaundice** (JON-dis) is a yellowing of the skin, and sometimes the whites of the eyes, caused by a buildup in the body of bilirubin, a chemical produced by the liver. An increase in bilirubin may indicate disease of the liver.

* **microcephaly** (my-kro-SEH-fah-lee) is the condition of having an abnormally small head, which typically results from having an underdeveloped or malformed brain.

* **retinitis** (reh-tin-EYE-tis) is inflammation of the retina, the nerve-rich membrane at the back of the eye on which visual images form.

* **antibodies** (AN-tih-bah-deez) are protein molecules produced by the body's immune system to help fight specific infections caused by microorganisms, such as bacteria and viruses.

* **DNA**, or deoxyribonucleic acid (dee-OX-see-ry-bo-nyoo-klay-ik AH-sid), is the specialized chemical substance that contains the genetic code necessary to build and maintain the structures and functions of living organisms.

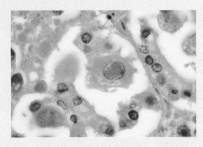

▲

Once inside the human body, the cytomegalovirus can invade many organs and systems. In this microscopic image, viral components are visible in the lining of the stomach. If the virus becomes active in the stomach, it can produce ulcers. *Visuals Unlimited*

* **pneumonia** (nu-MO-nyah) is inflammation of the lung.

▶ *See also*

AIDS and HIV Infection

Congenital Infections

Herpes Simplex Virus Infections

Immune Deficiencies

Laboratory Tests

Mononucleosis, Infectious

Pneumonia

need to be given by injection, and patients sometimes have to take them for months or even years. Symptoms of initial CMV infection usually last 2 to 3 weeks in healthy people. After that, the virus remains in the body for life. Flare-ups of illness from CMV in healthy people are rare and typically occur when the immune system has been stressed by fighting another illness.

What Are the Complications of CMV Infection?

CMV infection can cause more severe illness in people with weakened immune systems, such as pneumonia* and retinitis. If it is untreated, retinitis can lead to blindness. CMV also can cause severe inflammation of the esophagus and colon, leading to difficulty in swallowing, long-lasting diarrhea, and weight loss. It also can affect the brain or nerves. Infants born with CMV infection may have jaundice, poor growth, problems with vision and hearing, and other disabilities, including slow development and mental retardation.

How Is CMV Infection Prevented?

The best way to help prevent the spread of CMV is to wash the hands regularly, especially after changing diapers or touching bodily fluids. Doctors advise women who are pregnant and people who work in child care to be particularly careful. Patients scheduled to have organ or bone marrow transplants typically receive medication before the operation to prevent CMV disease from developing, as the transplant process weakens their immune systems.

Resources

Organizations

U.S. Centers for Disease Control and Prevention (CDC), 1600 Clifton Road, Atlanta, GA 30333. The CDC offers information about cytomegalovirus infection at its website.
Telephone 800-311-3435
http://www.cdc.gov

U.S. National Institute of Allergy and Infectious Diseases (NIAID), Building 31, Room 7A-50, 31 Center Drive MSC 2520, Bethesda, MD 20892-2520. The NIAID, part of the National Institutes of Health, posts fact sheets on cytomegalovirus at its website.
Telephone 301-496-5717
http://www.niaid.nih.gov

D

Dengue Fever

Dengue (DENG-gay) fever is a serious illness commonly occurring in tropical and subtropical regions of the world. It is caused by a virus that passes from person to person through the bite of mosquitoes, and causes high fever and pain in the muscles, joints, and bones.

KEYWORDS
for searching the Internet and other reference sources

Aedes mosquito

Arbovirus

Flavivirus

Hemorrhagic fever

What Is Dengue Fever?

Dengue fever is characterized by a sudden high fever and severe pain in the muscles, joints, and bones. (It originally was named "break-bone fever.") The disease is more likely to cause serious illness in children, and some cases are fatal. Dengue fever is caused by four varieties of flaviviruses*, which are part of the arbovirus* family of viruses. Each virus can cause illness, but being infected by one type does not make a person immune* to the other three.

Who Gets Dengue Fever and How?

Dengue fever is widespread in Asia, Africa, South America, and Central America. About 20 million cases develop annually worldwide, and the number of cases is on the rise. It occurs most frequently in highly populated areas, often in cities. Although the number of places where dengue fever is found continues to grow, the disease remains rare in the United States, with most cases appearing in travelers arriving from other countries.

The virus does not spread directly from person to person. Instead, the bite of a mosquito, usually the female *Aedes* mosquito, transmits the disease. The insect takes in the virus with its meal of blood when it bites an infected person. Because the virus remains in the mosquito for the rest of its life, the mosquito can pass the infection to many people. In areas with large populations of mosquitoes, dengue fever epidemics* can occur.

What Are the Symptoms of Dengue Fever?

A sudden high fever, sometimes reaching 104 or 105 degrees Fahrenheit, often is the first symptom. The affected person also may have a flushed (reddish) face. As other symptoms develop, a person might experience muscle, joint, or bone pain; a severe headache; a rash; pain behind the eyes; and signs of small hemorrhages*, such as bleeding gums,

** **flaviviruses** (FLAY-vih-vy-ruh-sez) are a group of viruses that includes those that cause dengue fever and yellow fever.*

** **arbovirus** (ar-buh-VY-rus) is a member of a family of viruses that multiply in blood-sucking organisms, such as mosquitoes and ticks, and spread through their bites.*

** **immune** (ih-MYOON) means resistant to or not susceptible to a disease.*

** **epidemics** (eh-pih-DEH-miks) are outbreaks of diseases, especially infectious diseases, in which the number of cases suddenly becomes far greater than usual. Usually, epidemics that involve worldwide outbreaks are called pandemics.*

** **hemorrhages** (HEH-muh-rih-jes) are areas of uncontrolled or abnormal bleeding.*

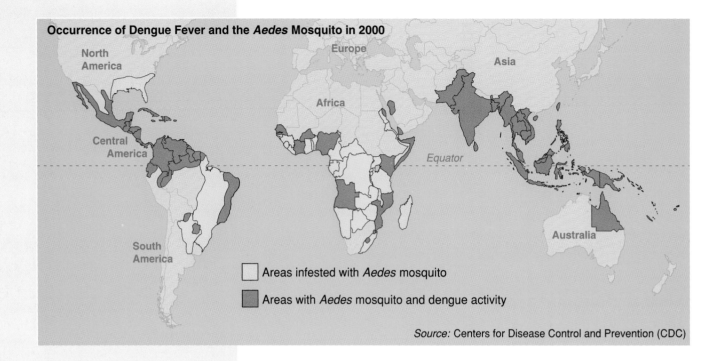

Occurrence of Dengue Fever and the *Aedes* Mosquito in 2000

☐ Areas infested with *Aedes* mosquito

■ Areas with *Aedes* mosquito and dengue activity

Source: Centers for Disease Control and Prevention (CDC)

This map shows the occurrence of Dengue fever and its relationship to the regions where the *Aedes* mosquito lives. The disease is widespread close to the equator, in the tropical areas of Asia, Africa, South America, and Central America, the mosquito's preferred habitat.

* **petechiae** (puh-TEE-kee-eye) are tiny dots of blood beneath the skin that indicate bleeding from small vessels.

* **antibodies** (AN-tih-bah-deez) are protein molecules produced by the body's immune system to help fight specific infections caused by microorganisms, such as bacteria and viruses.

* **dehydration** (dee-hi-DRAY-shun) is a condition in which the body is depleted of water, usually caused by excessive and unreplaced loss of body fluids, such as through sweating, vomiting, or diarrhea.

petechiae*, or a nosebleed. Fever typically lasts 2 to 7 days. Once the fever goes away, the other signs and symptoms usually fade as well. Some symptoms may linger for a few weeks.

How Is Dengue Fever Diagnosed and Treated?

Doctors typically diagnose dengue fever from a patient's history of symptoms and risk factors, including whether that person has been anywhere where dengue fever is found. The doctor looks for three signs: high fever, pain, and rash. These symptoms are known as the dengue triad. To help confirm the diagnosis, doctors may order blood tests or tests on spinal fluid to look for antibodies* to the virus.

No specific treatment exists for dengue fever, but the disease usually clears up on its own. In serious cases, supportive care in a hospital can make recovery easier or even save a person's life. It is important to drink plenty of fluids to avoid dehydration*. Over-the-counter medicine, such as acetaminophen (uh-see-teh-MIH-noh-fen), can relieve pain and fever while the disease runs its course.

What Are the Complications of Dengue Fever?

The most serious form of the disease is called dengue hemorrhagic (heh-muh-RAH-jik) fever, which is characterized by high fever, serious hemorrhage, pneumonia, and sometimes failure of the circulatory system* (heart failure) or shock*. People who develop dengue hemorrhagic fever usually require hospitalization, where they receive fluids. It is possible to die from this form of the disease, though most people recover.

118

How Is Dengue Fever Prevented?

Scientists are working on a vaccine for dengue fever, but one is not yet available. The only way to control the spread of the disease is to reduce mosquito populations. Using pesticides, stocking lakes and ponds with special fish that eat mosquito larvae*, and covering or eliminating small pools of standing water in which the insects breed can help keep mosquito levels in check. People can protect themselves from bites by using insect repellent and wearing clothing that covers much of the body.

* **circulatory** (SIR-kyoo-luh-tor-e) **system** is the system composed of the heart and blood vessels that moves blood throughout the body.

* **shock** is a serious condition in which blood pressure is very low and not enough blood flows to the body's organs and tissues. Untreated, shock may result in death.

* **larvae** (LAR-vee) are the immature forms of an insect or worm that hatches from an egg.

WHAT'S IN A NAME?

The history of medicine is replete with fanciful names derived from the symptoms or causes of various medical conditions, like "break-bone fever." Here are just a few:

- **Alice in Wonderland syndrome**
  a condition in which a person has delusions or hallucinations

- **cri-du-chat, or cat-cry, syndrome**
  a genetic disease with many symptoms, including mental retardation and a high-pitched, catlike mewing cry

- **cauliflower ear**
  thickening of the ear with distortion of the contours, also known as boxer's ear

- **happy puppet syndrome**
  a genetic disorder marked by a jutting out of the jaw, seizures, and prolonged spasms of laughter

- **jumping disease**
  an exaggerated response to being startled, causing a person to jump, fling the arms around, and yell; sometimes called jumping Frenchmen of Maine disease after the French loggers it was first found to affect

- **kissing disease**
  infectious mononucleosis, an acute illness that can spread through saliva

- **mitten hand**
  a birth defect involving the fusion of several fingers, with a single fingernail

- **vagabond's disease**
  discoloration of the skin in people who are exposed to lice bites over a long period of time.

Resources

Organizations

U.S. Centers for Disease Control and Prevention (CDC), 1600 Clifton Road, Atlanta, GA 30333. The CDC offers information about dengue fever at its website.
Telephone 800-311-3435
http://www.cdc.gov

World Health Organization (WHO), Avenue Appia 20, 1211 Geneva 27, Switzerland. WHO posts fact sheets on dengue fever and information about outbreaks in different regions of the world on its website.
Telephone 011-41-22-791-2111
http://www.who.int

▶ *See also*
Ebola Virus Infection
Travel-related Infections
Yellow Fever

KEYWORDS
for searching the Internet and other reference sources

Antitoxin

Corynebacterium diphtheriae

Epidemic

Respiratory infection

Vaccination

* **exotoxin** (ek-so-TOK-sin) is a substance produced by bacteria that has harmful effects on the infected person.

* **shock** is a serious condition in which blood pressure is very low and not enough blood flows to the body's organs and tissues. Untreated, shock may result in death.

* **epidemic** (eh-pih-DEH-mik) is an outbreak of disease, especially infectious disease, in which the number of cases suddenly becomes far greater than usual. Usually epidemics are outbreaks of diseases in specific regions, whereas worldwide epidemics are called pandemics.

Diphtheria

Diphtheria (dif-THEER-e-uh) is an infection of the lining of the upper respiratory tract (the nose and throat). It is a serious disease that can cause breathing difficulty and other complications, including death. Routine vaccination against diphtheria has made it rare in the United States.

What Is Diphtheria?

Diphtheria is an infection caused by a bacterium called *Corynebacterium diphtheriae* (kor-ih-nee-bak-TEER-e-um dif-THEER-e-eye) that infects the upper respiratory tract. As the bacteria infect the nose, throat, or larynx (LAIR-inks, the voicebox), a distinctive thick membrane forms over the site of infection. The membrane can become large enough to interfere with a person's breathing and swallowing. Some strains of *Corynebacterium diphtheriae* also produce an exotoxin* that can cause arthritis and damage to the nerves and heart. Sepsis, a potentially serious spreading of infection (usually bacterial) through the bloodstream and body, can result from diphtheria, causing shock*, heart failure, and even death.

How Common Is Diphtheria?

Diphtheria infection occurs throughout the world and is common in developing regions of Africa, Asia, and South America where children often do not receive the diphtheria vaccine. Cases usually occur in winter and the cooler months of autumn and spring.

Diphtheria infection is extremely rare in the United States because of the widespread use of routine diphtheria vaccination during childhood. From 1980 through 2000, 51 cases of diphtheria were reported in the United States. However, a diphtheria epidemic* has affected the countries that make up the former Soviet Union; since 1990 more than 150,000 cases have been reported.

Is Diphtheria Contagious?

Diphtheria is highly contagious. An untreated person who has diphtheria can spread the infection for up to a month. Within 48 hours of receiving antibiotics, however, people infected with diphtheria are usually no longer contagious.

The bacteria that cause diphtheria are spread through the air in drops of moisture from the respiratory tract, often from coughing or sneezing. Sharing drinking glasses or eating utensils or handling soiled tissues or handkerchiefs that have been used by a person with the disease can also transmit the bacteria. A person can get diphtheria from someone who has symptoms of the disease or from someone who is just a carrier* of the bacteria.

What Are the Signs and Symptoms of Diphtheria?

Within 5 days after becoming infected, a person typically begins to have symptoms of diphtheria. Early symptoms often include a severe sore throat, runny nose, mild fever, and swollen glands in the neck. People infected with diphtheria in the nose, throat, or larynx usually develop a thick membrane at the site of the infection. Membranes in the nose are often white, whereas those at the back of the throat are gray-green.

As diphtheria progresses, respiratory symptoms can become more severe and include difficulty breathing or swallowing and a bark-like cough. Sometimes inflammation and swelling in the throat and the diphtheria membrane itself can cause blockage of the upper airways, making emergency treatment necessary.

How Is Diphtheria Diagnosed and Treated?

Diphtheria is diagnosed when the membrane that signals the disease is seen in the nose or throat during an examination of someone with symptoms of the disease. The diagnosis is confirmed by taking a swab of the coating from underneath the membrane and performing a laboratory test that identifies diphtheria bacteria.

Hospitalized people who are known to have diphtheria are kept isolated to prevent the disease from spreading to others. Patients are treated in the hospital with antibiotics and diphtheria antitoxin*. The antitoxin, which is produced in horses, is given intravenously (directly into a vein).

In severe cases of diphtheria, patients may need a ventilator (VEN-tuh-lay-ter) to help with breathing or medication to treat complications of the disease, such as septic shock*, heart inflammation, or heart failure. After they leave the hospital, bed rest at home for several weeks is generally recommended. Members of the same household are usually given a diphtheria booster vaccine to protect against possible infection. Recovery from diphtheria often takes 4 to 6 weeks or more.

A Canine Hero

In the winter of 1925, a diphtheria epidemic swept through Nome, Alaska. Antitoxin was located almost 1,000 miles away in the city of Anchorage. The only way to transport the medicine was by dog sled. A relay of sled-dog teams, with the last leg led by a dog named Balto, successfully carried the medicine through frigid Alaskan temperatures in time to save many lives. In honor of that achievement, a statue of Balto was erected in Central Park in New York City.

* **carrier** is a person who has in his body a bacterium or virus that he can transmit to other people without getting sick himself.

* **antitoxin** (an-tih-TOK-sin) counteracts the effects of a toxin, or poison, in the body. Antitoxins are produced to act against specific toxin, like those made by the bacteria that cause botulism or diphtheria.

* **septic shock** is shock due to overwhelming infection, and is characterized by decreased blood pressure, internal bleeding, heart failure, and, in some cases, death.

121

* **neuritis** (nuh-RYE-tis) is an inflammation of the nerves that disrupts their function.

* **tetanus** (TET-nus) is a serious bacterial infection that affects the body's central nervous system.

* **pertussis** (per-TUH-sis) is a bacterial infection of the respiratory tract that causes severe coughing.

* **seizures** (SEE-zhurs) are sudden bursts of disorganized electrical activity that interrupt the normal functioning of the brain, often leading to uncontrolled movements in the body and sometimes a temporary change in consciousness.

 See also

Arthritis, Infectious

Public Health

Sepsis

Vaccination (Immunization)

Complications of diphtheria include abnormal heart rhythms, arthritis, and neuritis*. Diphtheria is most dangerous for children under 5 and adults over 40. Death occurs in up to 10 percent of people with diphtheria who receive medical treatment; death rates are higher in some parts of the world where treatment is not readily available.

Can Diphtheria Be Prevented?

In the United States, immunization programs have been very effective in preventing diphtheria. The diphtheria vaccine is given in combination with vaccines for tetanus* and pertussis* (this is called the DTaP vaccine) as part of a child's routine immunizations. Four doses of the vaccine are given before 2 years of age. A first booster dose is given at 4 to 6 years of age when a child enters school. Additional booster doses are recommended every 10 years, in combination with a tetanus booster.

Sometimes people have mild reactions to the vaccine, including a low-grade fever, tenderness at the injection site, and irritability. Very rarely, stronger reactions such as seizures* or allergic reactions can occur.

Resources

Organizations

Immunization Action Coalition, 573 Selby Avenue, Suite 234, St. Paul, MN 55104. The Immunization Action Coalition provides information about infectious diseases and immunization.
Telephone 651-647-9009
http://www.immunize.org

U.S. Centers for Disease Control and Prevention (CDC), 1600 Clifton Road Atlanta, GA 30333. The CDC provides information about infectious and other diseases, including diphtheria, at its website.
Telephone 800-311-3435
http://www.cdc.gov

E

Ear Infections *See* Otitis (Ear Infections)

Ebola Virus Infection

Ebola hemorrhagic (e-BO-luh heh-muh-RAH-jik) fever is a rare viral disease that causes severe bleeding and results in death in up to 90 percent of those infected.

KEYWORDS
for searching the Internet and other reference sources

Filovirus

Marburg virus

Viral hemorrhagic fever

Ebola appeared without warning in late 2000 in the northern district of Gulu in Uganda, Africa. Health workers responded quickly, caring for people infected with the disease and isolating them so that they would not spread the devastating virus to others. Despite the workers' efforts, more than 40 people died in the first wave of the epidemic*, and the disease spread throughout the district and beyond.

By February 2001, the epidemic had killed 224 people. Then, suddenly, it was over. The Ebola virus seemed to disappear back into the jungle.

* **epidemic** (eh-pih-DEH-mik) is an outbreak of disease, especially infectious disease, in which the number of cases suddenly becomes far greater than usual. Usually epidemics are outbreaks of diseases in specific regions, whereas worldwide epidemics are called pandemics.

What Is Ebola?

Although much remains unknown about Ebola, scientists have begun to piece together some of the puzzle. Ebola was first identified in 1976 in the Democratic Republic of Congo (formerly Zaire) and named for a river that flows through that African nation. Part of the filovirus family, Ebola virus has four subtypes, each named for the location in which it was discovered: Ebola-Zaire, Ebola-Sudan, Ebola-Ivory Coast, and Ebola-Reston. The Ebola-Reston virus, first detected in the United States in 1989, was discovered in sick monkeys imported from the Philippines to a research laboratory in Reston, Virginia. Although a few laboratory workers later showed signs of the virus in the blood, none of them became ill.

Decades after its identification, researchers continue to search for the natural reservoir, or origin, of the Ebola virus. The virus probably resides in the rain forests of Africa and Asia. Scientists think that the Ebola virus is animal-borne (or zoonotic) and that it is passed to primates (monkeys and apes) and humans by another animal.

How Common Is Ebola?

Although outbreaks of Ebola have been widely publicized because of the horrifying symptoms of the disease and the suddenness with which it

Ebola Virus Infection

In October 2000 an epidemic of Ebola broke out in Gulu, Uganda, and in 4 months it killed 224 people. Some doctors believe that eating ape meat contaminated with the virus may be one source of infection. It is hoped that research to determine the natural source of the virus and the ways in which it is transmitted to primates and humans will provide information about how to prevent future outbreaks. ▶

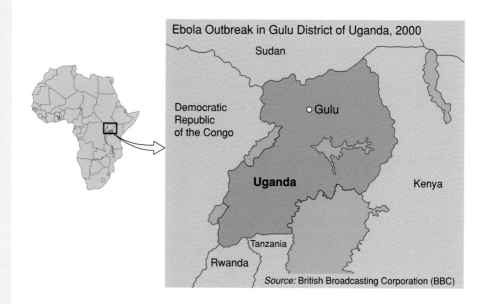

Ebola Outbreak in Gulu District of Uganda, 2000

Source: British Broadcasting Corporation (BBC)

* **contagious** (kon-TAY-jus) means transmittable from one person to another, usually referring to an infection.

* **biohazard** is a biological agent or condition that causes a threat to humans.

* **shock** is a serious condition in which blood pressure is very low and not enough blood flows to the body's organs and tissues. Untreated, shock may result in death.

kills, the disease is actually quite rare. Since the virus was discovered, about 1,500 cases of Ebola virus infection have been reported in humans, and over 1,000 of those infected died.

Is Ebola Contagious?

Ebola virus is extremely contagious*, but scientists do not know exactly how it spreads. They do know that it can spread through direct contact with infected blood, especially on contaminated needles, and possibly through the nasal or respiratory secretions of someone who is infected. Health care workers and family members tending to the people who have the virus risk becoming infected. The needles used to take blood samples are an extreme biohazard* because accidental needle pricks to health care workers can transmit the infection to them. Traditions in some African cultures may contribute to the spread of Ebola virus. For example, some funeral rites require a ritual cleansing of the corpse, which can bring a loved one into contact with the blood or other body fluids of the deceased. Also, ape meat is considered a delicacy in parts of Africa. Some scientists recommend that people not eat it because it might contain the Ebola virus, which can infect non-human primates such as monkeys and chimpanzees.

What Are the Signs and Symptoms of Ebola Virus Infection?

In the first few days after infection with Ebola virus, symptoms resemble those of other diseases: fever, headache, and muscle aches. The disease rapidly progresses to more serious symptoms such as rash, chest pain, severe bloody vomiting and diarrhea, uncontrolled internal bleeding, kidney and liver failure, and shock*.

124

Doctors can diagnose Ebola fever based on symptoms seen in patients as they quickly become ill during outbreaks. Blood tests can sometimes identify the virus directly, or antibodies* to Ebola produced by the body during infection can be detected in the blood. Doctors have to be careful when performing tests because simply injecting a needle into a patient who is prone to hemorrhage* can trigger uncontrolled bleeding.

How Is Ebola Treated?

There is no medication to treat or cure Ebola infection. Patients with Ebola fever are hospitalized and receive supportive care to treat symptoms. They may receive intravenous* (IV) fluids to protect against dehydration*; monitoring of blood pressure, heart rate, and breathing; and treatment for bleeding or other infections that may develop during the illness. During past outbreaks, 50 to 90 percent of people who developed symptoms of the disease died. Those who survive usually recover in several weeks.

Researchers have recently discovered a protein on the surface of the Ebola virus that is involved in attacking blood vessels, and this finding may help to explain the massive bleeding that leads to most Ebola deaths. Researchers are attempting to develop new drugs or a vaccine directed against this protein, which might prevent the disease or at least reduce the severity of the symptoms and the number of deaths caused by the virus.

Can Ebola Be Prevented?

Because there is no vaccine to prevent Ebola virus infection and no medication to halt it, the first line of defense for health officials is to isolate infected patients in a hospital. Health care workers use gloves and masks when coming into contact with patients to try to prevent the virus from

* **antibodies** (AN-tih-bah-deez) are protein molecules produced by the body's immune system to help fight specific infections caused by microorganisms, such as bacteria and viruses.

* **hemorrhage** (HEH-muh-rij) is uncontrolled or abnormal bleeding.

* **intravenous** (in-tra-VEE-nus) means within or through a vein. For example, medications, fluid, or other substances can be given through a needle or soft tube inserted through the skin's surface directly into a vein.

* **dehydration** (dee-hi-DRAY-shun) is a condition in which the body is depleted of water, usually caused by excessive and unreplaced loss of body fluids, such as through sweating, vomiting, or diarrhea.

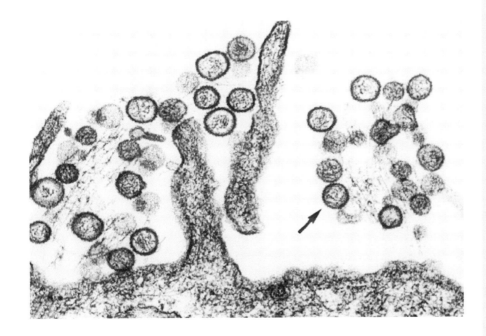

An electron micrograph shows Ebola virus particles. *Delmar Publishers, Inc.*

STRANGER THAN FICTION

The tale read like something from a Stephen King novel. Ebola virus had infected and killed monkeys in a laboratory in Reston, Virginia. A biohazard SWAT team descended on the Reston Primate Quarantine Unit and, working in secret just miles from the nation's capital, struggled to decontaminate the monkey house.

In his tense and terrifying book, *The Hot Zone*, Richard Preston recounts in detail how the U.S. Veterinary Corps at Frederick, Maryland, spotted Ebola at Reston in 1989 and recruited the secret SWAT team to contain the deadly virus.

Scientists later named the virus subtype Ebola-Reston and determined that, although it is deadly to monkeys, it does not cause Ebola fever in humans. The following year, the same virus was found in monkeys in labs in Texas and Pennsylvania.

Researchers were able to trace the infected monkeys back to a single exporter in the Philippines. In the United States, several of the monkeys died and four people were infected with the virus, although none of them became ill.

spreading. However, as the epidemic in Gulu showed, even those precautions sometimes fail.

Research efforts to determine the natural source of the virus and how it is carried to primates and humans will likely provide information about how to prevent future outbreaks.

Resources

Book

Preston, Richard. *The Hot Zone*. New York: Random House, 1994. A dramatic account of Ebola's destructive effects, including the story of Ebola-Reston, the virus that infected monkeys in a suburban Washington, D.C., laboratory.

Website

All the Virology on the WWW maintains *The Big Picture Book of Viruses*, which includes a catalog of virus pictures and a section on emerging viruses such as Ebola.
http://www.virology.net

▶ *See also*
Public Health
Zoonoses

Ehrlichiosis

Ehrlichiosis (air-lik-e-O-sis) is an infectious disease caused by various strains of Ehrlichia (air-LIH-kee-uh) bacteria, transmitted to humans by ticks.

Caused by an organism once thought to infect only dogs, sheep, cattle, goats, and horses, ehrlichiosis was first discovered in humans in 1953 when researchers in Japan found that Sennetsu fever, an illness that resembles mononucleosis*, was caused by *Ehrlichia sennetsu* bacteria. Since the 1980s, scientists have identified three additional strains* of *Ehrlichia* bacteria that cause forms of human ehrlichiosis in the United States: *E. chaffeensis*, which causes human monocytic ehrlichiosis (HME); bacteria similar or identical to *E. phagocytophila* or *E. equi* (known to cause ehrlichiosis in animals), which cause human granulocytic ehrlichiosis (HGE); and *E. ewingii*, which has only been seen in a few patients in the midwestern United States and Tennessee.

What Is Ehrlichiosis?

Ehrlichiosis interferes with the body's immune system by attacking white blood cells, a vital part of the body's defense against invading bacteria, viruses, and other microbes* or harmful substances. Untreated, the disease can leave people vulnerable to other infections.

Ehrlichiosis does not spread from person to person. The *Ehrlichia* bacteria that cause the disease are spread through tick bites. The species that most commonly spread the disease are the lone star tick, the black-legged tick, and the western black-legged tick.

Between 1986 and 1997, 1,223 cases of human ehrlichiosis were reported in the United States. Most occurred along the Atlantic Coast and in southern and central states, although cases were reported in almost every region of the country. The number of cases peaks during tick season, which runs from April to October.

What Happens When People Get Ehrlichiosis?

Most cases of ehrlichiosis are associated with mild flulike symptoms, such as fever, chills, headaches, muscle or joint pain, nausea and vomiting, cough, stomach pain, and sore throat. Some people with the infection show no symptoms at all. Symptoms usually start within 2 weeks of a tick bite but can take up to a month to appear.

Because ehrlichiosis shares many symptoms with Lyme disease* and other infections transmitted by ticks, diagnosis based on symptoms alone can be difficult. Blood tests are done to look for evidence of *Ehrlichia* infection, such as antibodies* to the bacteria or the presence of the germ itself in the blood.

KEYWORDS
for searching the Internet and other reference sources

Arthropod-borne infections

Ehrlichia sennetsu

Lyme disease

Rickettsial infections

Sennetsu fever

Tick-borne infections

* **mononucleosis** (mah-no-nu-klee-O-sis) is an infectious illness caused by a virus that often leads to fever, sore throat, swollen glands, and tiredness.

* **strains** are subtypes of particular species of organisms, such as viruses or bacteria.

* **microbes** (MY-krobes) are microscopic living organisms, especially bacteria and viruses.

* **Lyme** (LIME) **disease** is a bacterial infection that is spread to humans by the bite of an infected tick. It begins with a distinctive rash and/or flulike symptoms and, in some cases, can progress to a more serious disease with complications affecting other body organs.

* **antibodies** (AN-tih-bah-deez) are protein molecules produced by the body's immune system to help fight specific infections caused by microorganisms, such as bacteria and viruses.

*anemia (uh-NEE-me-uh) is a blood condition in which there is a decreased amount of oxygen-carrying hemoglobin in the blood and, usually, fewer than normal numbers of red blood cells.

*seizures (SEE-zhurs) are sudden bursts of disorganized electrical activity that interrupt the normal functioning of the brain, often leading to uncontrolled movements in the body and sometimes a temporary change in consciousness.

*human immunodeficiency (HYOO-mun ih-myoo-no-dih-FIH-shen-see) virus, or HIV, is the virus that causes AIDS (acquired immunodeficiency syndrome), an infection that severely weakens the immune system.

► See also

Lyme Disease

Mononucleosis, Infectious

Rickettsial Infections

Rocky Mountain Spotted Fever

Tick-borne Infections

If treated early, ehrlichiosis responds very well to certain antibiotics. Over-the-counter medicine such as acetaminophen (uh-see-teh-MIH-noh-fen) can help lower fever and relieve pain. Usually, people recover from mild cases of ehrlichiosis soon after finishing a week of antibiotic treatment. In severe cases, patients may need treatment in the hospital.

Although many cases of ehrlichiosis are mild, the infection can become serious if it is not treated. Some people who get ehrlichiosis develop anemia* and inflammation of the liver and kidneys. Breathing problems, internal bleeding, brain inflammation (encephalitis, en-seh-fuh-LYE-tis), and seizures* can also develop. People with weakened immune systems, such as those with HIV (human immunodeficiency virus*) infection, certain types of cancer, or the elderly, tend to develop more severe symptoms and complications. For these people, ehrlichiosis can be fatal.

Can Ehrlichiosis Be Prevented?

Avoiding direct contact with ticks is the best way to prevent ehrlichiosis. Experts recommend that people use tick repellent and wear light-colored, long-sleeved shirts (to help find ticks more easily) and long pants tucked into socks when entering potentially tick-infested areas such as woods or campgrounds. After visiting such areas, it is wise to carefully check the body, clothes, and hair for ticks. Pets need to be checked as well.

Resources

Organizations

Lyme Disease Foundation, Inc., One Financial Plaza, 18th Floor, Hartford, CT 06103. The Lyme Disease Foundation offers information on tick-borne illnesses and avoiding tick bites on its website. Telephone 860-525-2000
http://www.lyme.org

National Center for Infectious Diseases, U.S. Centers for Disease Control and Prevention, Mailstop C-14, 1600 Clifton Road, Atlanta, GA 30333. The website for this government agency provides information about ehrlichiosis.
Telephone 800-311-3435
http://www.cdc.gov/ncidod

Encephalitis

Encephalitis (en-seh-fuh-LYE-tis) is inflammation of the brain.

What Is Encephalitis?

There are several different causes of encephalitis. The most common is infection, usually by a virus. The condition can range from mild to severe, depending on the type of germ producing the infection. Encephalitis can occur with certain childhood viral illnesses, such as mumps, measles, varicella (chicken pox), rubella (German measles), or mononucleosis.

A much more serious type of encephalitis is caused by the herpes simplex virus* (HSV). HSV rarely infects the brain, but when it does, it can be life threatening. West Nile virus, which first arrived in the United States from other parts of the world in the late 1990s, can cause encephalitis as well. Infected birds carry this virus, but mosquitoes can pick up the virus when they bite infected birds and then spread the virus to humans through a bite.

Encephalitis may develop in a person who has meningitis (meh-nin-JY-tis), an inflammation of the membranes surrounding the brain and spinal cord, called the meninges (meh-NIN-jeez). It also can be a complication of other infectious diseases, such as rabies, cytomegalovirus* infection, listeriosis*, syphilis*, or Lyme disease. In people with a weakened immune system, for instance, those with HIV/AIDS, infection by parasites can lead to encephalitis, especially the parasite that causes toxoplasmosis*.

How Common Is Encephalitis?

Each year, several thousand cases of encephalitis are reported to the U.S. Centers for Disease Control and Prevention. Health officials believe that many more cases go unreported when the symptoms are mild.

Is the Disease Contagious?

Although the brain inflammation itself is not contagious, viruses that cause encephalitis may be contagious. When someone contracts the same virus that a person with encephalitis has, however, it does not mean that he or she also will develop encephalitis.

How Is Encephalitis Spread?

Because several different germs can cause encephalitis, spread of the infection may take place in different ways. For example, mosquitoes transmit viruses that cause West Nile encephalitis, St. Louis encephalitis, and western equine encephalitis. Other viruses (such as herpes simplex virus or varicella-zoster, var-uh-SEH-luh ZOS-ter, virus, which causes chicken pox) are spread in fluids from the mouth, throat, or nose; tiny drops of these fluids, such as saliva and nasal mucus*, may be sprayed into the air

KEYWORDS
for searching the Internet
and other reference sources

Arboviruses

Herpes simplex virus

Immunizations

La Crosse encephalitis

Meningitis

Mosquito-borne illnesses

St. Louis encephalitis

Tick-borne illnesses

West Nile virus

* **herpes simplex** (HER-peez SIM-plex) **virus** is a virus that can cause infections of the skin, mouth, genitals, and other parts of the body.

* **cytomegalovirus** (sy-tuh-MEH-guh-lo-vy-rus), or CMV, infection is very common and usually causes no symptoms. It poses little risk for healthy people, but it can lead to serious illness in people with weak immune systems.

* **listeriosis** (lis-teer-e-O-sis) is a bacterial infection that can cause a form of meningitis in infants and other symptoms in children and adults.

* **syphilis** (SIH-fih-lis) is a sexually transmitted disease that, if untreated, can lead to serious lifelong problems throughout the body, including blindness and paralysis.

* **toxoplasmosis** (tox-o-plaz-MO-sis) is a parasitic infection that usually causes no symptoms in healthy people, but it can cause serious problems in unborn babies and people with weak immune systems.

* **mucus** (MYOO-kus) is a thick, slippery substance that lines the insides of many body parts.

129

Causes of Encephalitis	How Spread
Enteroviruses	Contact with body fluids
Herpes simplex virus	Person to person contact
HIV (human immunodeficiency virus)	When an infected person's blood or body fluids are introduced into the bloodstream of a healthy person
Arboviruses	Bites from mosquitoes that pick up the virus from infected birds, chipmunks, squirrels, or other animals
Animal-borne illnesses	Bites from infected animals such as cats, dogs, and bats

by a cough or sneeze from someone who is infected. Ticks spread Lyme disease, and humans can contract rabies from the bite of infected animals, such as raccoons and bats.

What Are the Signs and Symptoms?

Many people who are infected with a virus that can cause encephalitis have only mild symptoms. Symptoms in people who develop encephalitis may appear suddenly and include headache, fever, sensitivity to light, loss of appetite, and a stiff neck and back. In more serious cases there may be high fever, nausea (NAW-zee-uh), vomiting, confusion, double vision*, personality changes, problems with hearing and speech, hallucinations*, sleepiness, clumsiness, muscle weakness, loss of sensation, and irritability. In the most severe cases, seizures* and loss of consciousness may occur. A person who has any of these symptoms requires immediate medical attention.

How Do Doctors Make the Diagnosis?

Doctors use several tests to diagnose encephalitis. Imaging tests, such as computerized tomography* scans or magnetic resonance imaging*, provide special views of the brain that allow doctors to check for swelling,

* **double vision** is a vision problem in which a person sees two images of a single object.

* **hallucinations** (ha-loo-sin-AY-shuns) occur when a person sees or hears things that are not really there. Hallucinations can result from nervous system abnormalities, mental disorders, or the use of certain drugs.

* **seizures** (SEE-zhurs) are sudden bursts of disorganized electrical activity that interrupt the normal functioning of the brain, often leading to uncontrolled movements in the body and sometimes a temporary change in consciousness.

bleeding, or other abnormalities. An electroencephalogram (e-lek-tro-en-SEF-a-loh-gram), which measures brain electrical activity, will show abnormal patterns in a person with encephalitis. Doctors also might order blood tests to look for the microorganism in the blood and tests that can tell whether the person's body is producing antibodies* in response to a specific virus or bacterium. A spinal tap, also called a lumbar puncture, often is performed. In this procedure a needle is inserted into the lower end of the spine and a small sample of cerebrospinal (seh-ree-bro-SPY-nuhl) fluid, which surrounds the brain and spinal cord, is removed. This fluid is examined under a microscope and tested for signs of infection. In addition, cotton swabs can be used to take fluid samples from the nose, throat, and rectum* to test for certain viruses that might be causing the infection.

How Do Doctors Treat Encephalitis?

Encephalitis is a very serious disease that can be life threatening. Although very mild cases can be treated at home, it is often necessary for patients to be hospitalized. Patients usually are admitted to an intensive care unit, where doctors carefully monitor blood pressure, heart rate, and ability to breathe. Such patients may require a ventilator (VEN-tuh-lay-ter), a machine that does the breathing for very ill people until they can breathe on their own again. Doctors also monitor the body fluids to help prevent or control swelling of the brain, which can lead to a dangerous increase in the pressure within the skull.

Several medications may be given to people with encephalitis. Over-the-counter medicines such as acetaminophen (uh-SEE-teh-MIH-noh-fen) may be used to treat minor symptoms such as fever and headache. Antiviral medications sometimes can help prevent the spread of the virus and are very important in the treatment of encephalitis caused by herpes simplex virus. If a patient is having seizures, anticonvulsants* may help control them. Anti-inflammatory medications called corticosteroids (kor-tih-ko-STIR-oyds) may lessen swelling in the brain.

How Long Does the Illness Last?

The acute phase of the disease, the time when symptoms are most severe, usually lasts up to a week. Full recovery can take much longer, often several weeks or months.

What Are the Complications?

Most people recover from encephalitis completely. For some people, however, swelling of the brain may lead to permanent brain damage. These patients may face long-term complications, such as learning disabilities, seizures, speech problems, memory loss, lack of muscle control, paralysis*, or coma*. In the rare cases where brain damage is severe, death can result. Infants younger than 1 year and adults older than 55 have the greatest risk of permanent brain damage and death from encephalitis.

* **computerized tomography** (kom-PYOO-ter-ized toe-MAH-gruh-fee), or CT, also called computerized axial tomography (CAT), is a technique in which a machine takes many X rays of the body to create a three-dimensional picture.

* **magnetic resonance imaging (MRI)** uses magnetic waves, instead of X rays, to scan the body and produce detailed pictures of the body's structures.

* **antibodies** (AN-tih-bah-deez) are protein molecules produced by the body's immune system to help fight specific infections caused by microorganisms, such as bacteria and viruses.

* **rectum** is the final portion of the large intestine, connecting the colon to the anus.

* **anticonvulsants** (an-tie-kon-VUL-sents) are medications that affect the electrical activity in the brain and are given to prevent or stop seizures.

* **paralysis** (pah-RAH-luh-sis) is the loss or impairment of the ability to move some part of the body.

* **coma** (KO-ma) is an unconscious state in which a person cannot be awakened and cannot move, see, speak, or hear.

How Is Encephalitis Prevented?

Some of the viral infections that can cause encephalitis, including measles, mumps, and chicken pox, can be prevented with vaccines given in childhood. To prevent encephalitis caused by West Nile virus or other viruses transmitted by mosquitoes, people are encouraged to avoid being outside at dawn and dusk, when mosquitoes are most active. If they do go out, they are advised to wear light-colored, long-sleeved shirts and long pants and to use insect repellent. Mosquitoes breed in places where there is standing water, such as in buckets, birdbaths, and flower pots, so draining these containers frequently can help control the mosquito population and decrease the risk of infection.

CAUSES OF ENCEPHALITIS

Encephalitis may be caused by a variety of viruses, bacteria, and other organisms. These agents include:

- Measles, chicken pox, rubella (German measles), mumps, polio, and other viral illnesses, which generally lead to a mild form of encephalitis known as postinfectious or para-infectious encephalitis.

- Enteroviruses (en-tuh-ro-VY-ruh-sez), viruses that typically infect the intestines and then may spread to other parts of the body, including the brain.

- Herpes simplex virus, a virus that can infect the mouth, skin, and other parts of the body.

- HIV (human immunodeficiency virus), the virus that causes AIDS (acquired immunodeficiency syndrome) and is transmitted when an infected person's blood or body fluids are introduced into the bloodstream of a healthy person.

- Arboviruses (ar-buh-VY-ruh-sez), which multiply in and are transmitted by blood-sucking insects (such as ticks and mosquitoes) when they bite infected birds, rodents (chipmunks and squirrels, for example), and other small animals and then bite humans.

- Animal-borne illnesses, such as rabies, toxoplasmosis, cat scratch disease, and Lyme disease, that are transmitted to humans by contact with an infected animal's saliva (through a bite or lick, for example), contact with an infected animal's feces (FEE-seez, or bowel movements), or an insect that bites an infected animal and then bites a person.

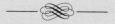

Resources

Organization

U.S. Centers for Disease Control and Prevention (CDC), 1600
Clifton Road, Atlanta, GA 30333. The CDC provides fact sheets and
other information on encephalitis at its website.
Telephone 800-311-3435
http://www.cdc.gov

Website

KidsHealth.org. KidsHealth is a website created by the medical experts
of the Nemours Foundation and is devoted to issues of children's
health. It contains articles on a variety of health topics, including
encephalitis.
http://www.KidsHealth.org

Endocarditis, Infectious

Infectious endocarditis (in-FEK-shus en-do-kar-DYE-tis) is an inflam-
mation of the valves and internal lining of the chambers of the heart,
known as the endocardium (en-doh-KAR-dee-um), caused by an infection.

What Is Endocarditis?

The heart has four chambers and four valves that regulate the flow of
blood through the heart. Each valve is made up of two or three smaller
parts, known as leaflets, that swing open and shut. As the heart beats, it
pumps blood through the chambers and out of the heart to the lungs and
the rest of the body. The valves open to allow blood to pass through and
out of the heart and then close to keep the blood from flowing backward.

In a normal heart, the swift, smooth movement of blood sweeps foreign material such as bacteria away from the heart. However, some people have defects in the heart's valves, the endocardium, or other parts of
the heart's structure that disrupt the flow of blood. This disruption can
allow bacteria or other germs that reach the heart through the bloodstream to lodge there and multiply, which results in an infection that inflames the heart's valves, muscles, and endocardium, producing endocarditis. The inflammation (in-flah-MAY-shun), which is the body's
response to injury or infection, can be serious, and sometimes it damages or destroys heart valves.

What Causes Endocarditis?

Viruses, fungi, or other microscopic organisms can all cause infectious
endocarditis, but the disease usually arises from a bacterial infection.

▶ *See also*

AIDS and HIV Infection

**Cytomegalovirus (CMV)
Infection**

**Herpes Simplex Virus
Infections**

Immune Deficiencies

Lyme Disease

Measles (Rubeola)

Meningitis

Mononucleosis, Infectious

Mumps

Rabies

Rubella (German Measles)

Syphilis

**Varicella (Chicken Pox)
and Herpes Zoster
(Shingles)**

West Nile Fever

KEYWORDS
*for searching the Internet
and other reference sources*

Bacteremia

Cardiovascular system

Endocardium

Heart valve

A common bacterium that lives in the mouth, *Streptococcus viridans* (strep-tuh-KAH-kus VEER-ih-danz), is responsible for up to half of all cases of bacterial endocarditis. Other bacterial culprits include bacteria from the staphylococcus, streptococcus, and enterococcus families and, less commonly, other types.

In most cases of endocarditis, bacteria that normally live harmlessly on the body, such as in the mouth, on the skin, in the intestines*, or in the urinary tract* (YOOR-ih-nair-e TRAKT), enter the blood (a condition known as bacteremia, bak-tuh-REE-me-uh). The bacteria can enter through a cut or a tear, frequently caused by a dental or medical procedure, or they may come from an infection somewhere else in the body. Once in the bloodstream, the bacteria travel to the heart and become stuck to the endocardium or heart valves. As they grow and multiply, the bacteria may form vegetations, which are composed of clumps of bacteria, red and white blood cells, and fibrin, a protein that helps blood clot*.

Who Gets Endocarditis?

Endocarditis is not contagious, so there is no reason to avoid contact with someone who has it. The disease is not very common in people with normal hearts, but some people are more susceptible to it. Because bacteria can easily attach to a malformed part of the heart, people with an artificial or damaged heart valve or a heart defect are more likely to get endocarditis. Anyone who has had it before or who has a catheter* in a blood vessel also has a greater chance of becoming infected. Although many people with heart defects are born with them, other people develop defects during their lifetime, such as from intravenous* drug use or rheumatic fever*, which puts them at increased risk for endocarditis as well. Overall, between 1 and 4 cases per 100,000 people occur each year in the United States.

What Are the Signs and Symptoms of Endocarditis?

Flulike symptoms, such as fever and chills, are the most common symptoms of endocarditis. Some people experience weight loss, weakness, headache, tiredness, shortness of breath, joint and muscle pain, and excessive sweating at night (night sweats). A heart murmur* usually develops, and the person may look pale, have red spots on their skin, and see blood in their urine. An enlarged spleen*, small hemorrhages* on the nails and on the whites of the eyes, and swelling of the feet, legs, and abdomen also can occur with endocarditis.

How Do Doctors Diagnose and Treat Endocarditis?

Doctors may suspect endocarditis if someone with a known heart abnormality develops an unexplained long-lasting fever, an abnormal heart sound (a murmur), or symptoms of heart failure such as shortness of breath or swelling of the legs.

* **intestines** are the muscular tubes that food passes through during digestion after it exits the stomach.

* **urinary tract** is the system of organs and channels that makes urine and removes it from the body. It consists of the urethra, bladder, ureters, and kidneys.

* **clot** is the process by which the body forms a thickened mass of blood cells and protein to stop bleeding.

* **catheter** (KAH-thuh-ter) is a small plastic tube placed through a body opening into an organ (such as the bladder) or through the skin directly into a blood vessel. It is used to give fluids to or drain fluids from a person.

* **intravenous** (in-tra-VEE-nus) means within or through a vein. For example, medications, fluid, or other substances can be given through a needle or soft tube inserted through the skin's surface directly into a vein.

* **rheumatic** (roo-MAH-tik) **fever** is a condition associated with fever, joint pain, and inflammation affecting many parts of the body, including the heart. It occurs following infection with certain types of strep bacteria.

* **heart murmur** is an abnormal sound from the heart, heard with a stethoscope, that is usually related to the flow of blood through the heart. Some murmurs indicate a problem with a heart valve or other part of the heart's structures, but many murmurs do not indicate any problem.

* **spleen** is an organ in the upper left part of the abdomen that stores and filters blood. As part of the immune system, the spleen also plays a role in fighting infection.

Certain tests can help doctors diagnose endocarditis, including blood cultures to detect bacteria in the bloodstream, a complete blood count, and laboratory tests that look for inflammation. For example, checking a patient's erythrocyte sedimentation rate (ESR) shows how quickly the person's red blood cells, or erythrocytes (eh-RITH-ruh-sites), settle to the bottom of a test tube, which is a measure of inflammation in the body. Another blood test identifies levels of C-reactive protein, which is increased in the blood when there is significant inflammation in the body. Doctors may also use an echocardiogram to look for signs of infection on the heart valves or in the heart. An echocardiogram (eh-ko-KAR-dee-uh-gram) is a diagnostic test that uses sound waves to produce images of the heart's chambers and valves and observe blood flow through the heart.

Doctors treat infectious endocarditis with antibiotics. The medication is given intravenously in the hospital at first, but sometimes patients finish treatment at home. Several weeks of antibiotic treatment may be necessary to eliminate the infection. In more serious cases, patients may need oxygen and medications to support heart function while hospitalized, and some people require surgery to repair damage to the heart caused by inflammation.

Do People Recover from Endocarditis?

The infection can start suddenly or come on gradually over weeks to months. Left untreated, endocarditis is often fatal. However, when treated successfully with antibiotics and when there has been little damage done to the heart valves, patients usually begin to feel better within a few days. If the infection does not improve with antibiotics, or if there is evidence that the heart valves have been damaged significantly, surgery may be required to replace the valve to clear the infection from the body and restore heart function.

Endocarditis can cause other complications. In some people with the disease, pieces of the infected material (vegetations) in the heart may break off and travel through the blood to other organs. If these pieces travel to the brain and block a blood vessel there, for example, the person may develop a stroke*. If they reach other organs, they may cause serious infections there. Endocarditis can also cause an irregular heartbeat, jaundice*, and kidney failure, as well as heart failure.

How Is Endocarditis Prevented?

Doctors give antibiotics to people who are at risk for infectious endocarditis before they undergo procedures that could introduce bacteria into the bloodstream. For example, simple dental work, removal of the tonsils, or medical procedures involving parts of the upper respiratory tract* (such as the mouth and throat), urinary tract (such as the urethra*), or lower gastrointestinal* tract can all provide an avenue for bacteria to enter the bloodstream and travel to the heart.

* **hemorrhages** (HEH-muh-rih-jes) are areas of uncontrolled or abnormal bleeding.

* **stroke** is a brain-damaging event usually caused by interference with blood flow to the brain. A stroke may occur when a blood vessel supplying the brain becomes clogged or bursts, depriving brain tissue of oxygen. As a result, nerve cells in the affected area of the brain, and the specific body parts they control, do not properly function.

* **jaundice** (JON-dis) is a yellowing of the skin, and sometimes the whites of the eyes, caused by a buildup in the body of bilirubin, a chemical produced in and released by the liver. An increase in bilirubin may indicate disease of the liver or certain blood disorders.

* **respiratory tract** includes the nose, mouth, throat, and lungs. It is the pathway through which air and gases are transported down into the lungs and back out of the body.

* **urethra** (yoo-REE-thra) is the tube through which urine passes from the bladder to the outside of the body.

* **gastrointestinal** (gas-tro-in-TES-tih-nuhl) means having to do with the organs of the digestive system, the system that processes food. It includes the mouth, esophagus, stomach, intestines, colon, and rectum and other organs involved in digestion, including the liver and pancreas.

▶ See also
Staphylococcal Infections
Streptococcal Infections

** epiglottis (eh-pih-GLAH-tis) is a
soft flap of tissue that covers the
opening of the trachea (windpipe) when a person swallows to
prevent food or fluid from entering the airway and lungs.*

Resources

Organizations

American Heart Association, National Center, 7272 Greenville Avenue, Dallas, TX 75231. The American Heart Association posts a fact sheet about bacterial endocarditis at its website.
Telephone 800-242-8721
http://americanheart.org

U.S. National Library of Medicine, 8600 Rockville Pike, Bethesda, MD 20894. The National Library of Medicine has a website packed with information on diseases (including endocarditis) and drugs, consumer resources, dictionaries and encyclopedias of medical terms, and directories of doctors and helpful organizations.
Telephone 888-346-3656
http://www.nlm.nih.gov

Epiglottitis

Epiglottitis (eh-pih-glah-TIE-tis) is a condition involving life-threatening swelling of the epiglottis*. It is usually caused by a bacterial infection of the epiglottis and can result in a blockage of the trachea (windpipe) and severe breathing difficulty.

What Is Epiglottitis?

Epiglottitis, also known as supraglottitis (su-pra-glah-TIE-tis), is characterized by inflammation and swelling of the epiglottis and other upper airway structures. The epiglottis can become dangerously swollen within just a few hours, leading to narrowing of the airway and severe breathing difficulty.

Epiglottitis is usually caused by bacterial infection. *Haemophilus influenzae* type B (Hib) bacteria accounted for the majority of epiglottitis cases before the widespread use of the Hib vaccine. *Staphylococcus aureus*; *Streptococcus pneumoniae* and group A, B, and C streptococci bacteria; certain viruses; traumatic injuries; scalding; and severe smoke inhalation (causing burns in the upper airway) can also lead to epiglottitis.

Who Gets Epiglottitis?

Epiglottitis is most common in children under 7 years of age. In the United States, cases of epiglottitis have declined greatly since the Hib vaccine was introduced in 1985.

Epiglottitis itself is not contagious, but the bacterial infections that can lead to the condition are. This means the bacteria can spread through

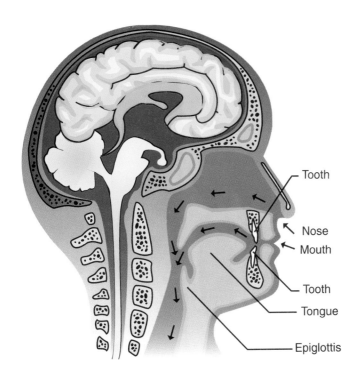

Tooth

Nose

Mouth

Tooth

Tongue

Epiglottis

Bacterial infection may cause inflammation and swelling of the epiglottis, which can quickly bring about narrowing or even closing of the airway and severe breathing problems.

person-to-person contact, often in drops of moisture from the respiratory tract when someone sneezes, coughs, or breathes.

What Are the Signs and Symptoms of Epiglottitis?

Epiglottitis often begins with a sore throat. Symptoms may come on suddenly and include:

- high fever
- inability to swallow and drooling
- difficulty breathing
- muffled voice
- stridor (STRY-dor, a high-pitched, squeaking noise that occurs while breathing in; it is present usually only if there is narrowing or blockage of the upper airway)
- a "sniffing" posture (when a young child leans forward, with chin extended, to make it easier to breathe)

Because their airways are smaller than those of adults, children with epiglottitis are at higher risk for developing severe breathing problems.

How Do Doctors Diagnose and Treat Epiglottitis?

Epiglottitis is a medical emergency that must be treated in a hospital. Ensuring that the person is able to breathe is the first and most important concern. Often a procedure called intubation (in-too-BAY-shun) is

Normal airways allow the free flow of air through the nose and mouth past the epiglottis, and then into the lungs. ▶

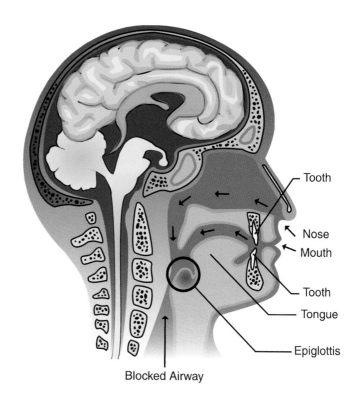

Tooth

Nose

Mouth

Tooth

Tongue

Epiglottis

Blocked Airway

* **tracheostomy** (tray-kee-AHS-tuh-me) refers to a small opening through the neck into the trachea, or windpipe, which has been made to allow air to enter the lungs more directly. The surgical procedure to create a tracheostomy is usually performed when a person's upper airway is narrowed or blocked or when there are other problems causing breathing difficulty.

* **intravenous** (in-tra-VEE-nus) (IV) means within or through a vein. For example, medications, fluid, or other substances can be given through a needle or soft tube inserted through the skin's surface directly into a vein.

performed, in which a tube is inserted into the windpipe through the mouth or nose to ensure that air can continue to flow into the lungs. In some cases, an emergency tracheostomy* must be performed to bypass the blocked part of the person's airway.

Doctors usually diagnose epiglottitis based on a physical examination and the patient's medical history. If the diagnosis is not clear, a doctor may order an X ray of the neck that will show if the epiglottis is swollen. Blood cultures or other blood tests may be used to confirm that the person has a bacterial or viral infection.

Intravenous* (IV) antibiotics are usually given to combat the infection that led to epiglottitis. Corticosteroid* medication is sometimes given to further reduce the swelling of the upper airway so the person can breathe more easily.

How Long Does It Take to Recover from Epiglottitis?

People with epiglottitis are hospitalized, usually in intensive care, for several days to a week or more to manage the infection that led to epiglottitis. The time it takes to fully recover varies depending on the particular infection.

Possible complications of epiglottitis include pneumonia*, ear infection and, rarely, meningitis* or bacteremia* caused by the same microorganism that caused the epiglottitis.

If not treated quickly, epiglottitis can result in complete airway obstruction (air can no longer flow into the lungs) and death.

Can Epiglottitis Be Prevented?

The best way to prevent epiglottitis is to avoid infection by the bacteria that most commonly cause it. The Hib vaccine, which is part of the routine childhood immunization schedule in the United States, has been extremely successful in decreasing the number of cases of epiglottitis resulting from *H. influenzae* infection. The Hib vaccine is given as four separate injections (shots) before 2 years of age.

Resources

Organization

The U.S. National Library of Medicine, 8600 Rockville Pike, Bethesda, MD 20894. A search of the National Library of Medicine website provides information about epiglottitis and the Hib vaccine. Telephone 888-346-3656
http://www.nlm.nih.gov

Website

KidsHealth.org. KidsHealth is a website created by the medical experts of the Nemours Foundation and is devoted to issues of children's health. It contains articles on a variety of health topics, including Hib immunization information.
http://www.KidsHealth.org

* **corticosteroids** (kor-tih-ko-STIR-oyds) are chemical substances made by the adrenal glands that have several functions in the body, including maintaining blood pressure during stress and controlling inflammation. They can also be given to people as medication to treat certain illnesses.

* **pneumonia** (nu-MO-nyah) is inflammation of the lung.

* **meningitis** (meh-nin-JY-tis) is an inflammation of the meninges, the membranes that surround the brain and the spinal cord. Meningitis is most often caused by infection with a virus or a bacterium.

* **bacteremia** (bak-tuh-REE-me-uh) is the presence of bacteria in the blood.

 See also
Staphylococcal Infections
Streptococcal Infections
Vaccination (Immunization)

F

Fifth Disease

Fifth disease, also known as erythema infectiosum (air-uh-THEE-muh in-fek-she-O-sum), is a common viral infection of infants and young children that causes a characteristic "slapped cheek" rash.

What Is Fifth Disease?

Fifth disease, sometimes called slapped-cheek disease, is an infection caused by a virus called human parvovirus B19. Its most characteristic feature is a bright red rash that begins on the face, making the cheeks look as if they have been slapped. After a few days, the rash may spread down the body and onto the arms and legs. As it spreads, the rash takes on a pink, lacy appearance.

Most people with fifth disease have mild symptoms and do not become seriously ill; some may not have any symptoms at all. However, the disease can be serious for people with certain blood disorders, such as sickle-cell disease*, because parvovirus B19 can temporarily cause or worsen existing anemia*. For most people, temporary anemia is not a problem, but for those who already have anemia, the condition can become severe, causing paleness, fatigue, and a fast pulse. People with weakened immune systems, such as those who have AIDS*, cancer, or who have had an organ transplant, can also develop severe anemia as a result of fifth disease.

Parvoviruses can infect animals, but these are not the same strains* that affect humans. Therefore, a person cannot catch fifth disease from a dog or cat, and a pet cannot catch it from an infected person.

How Common Is Fifth Disease?

Fifth disease occurs most commonly in children between the ages of 5 and 15 years, but adults can get it too. It often occurs in outbreaks (for example, among classmates at school or children in a child-care center) in the winter and spring, but people can get it throughout the year.

Fifth disease spreads quickly. At home, up to half of family members exposed to someone with fifth disease will become infected. If an outbreak occurs in school, up to 60 percent of students may get the virus.

A person with fifth disease can spread the infection in the early part of the illness, before the rash develops. By the time the rash appears (about a week after being exposed to the virus), a person likely is no longer

KEYWORDS
for searching the Internet and other reference sources

Erythema infectiosum

Parvovirus

Slapped-cheek rash

Viral infections

* **sickle-cell disease** is a hereditary condition in which the red blood cells, which are usually round, take on an abnormal crescent shape and have a decreased ability to carry oxygen throughout the body.

* **anemia** (uh-NEE-me-uh) is a blood condition in which there is a decreased amount of oxygen-carrying hemoglobin in the blood and, usually, fewer than normal numbers of red blood cells.

* **AIDS**, or acquired immunodeficiency (ih-myoo-no-dih-FIH-shen-see) syndrome, is an infection that severely weakens the immune system; it is caused by the human immunodeficiency virus (HIV).

* **strains** are various subtypes of organisms, such as viruses or bacteria.

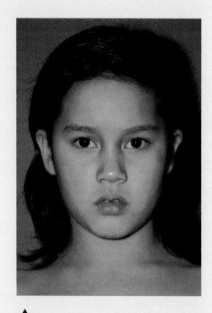

▲

A few days after infection with the virus that causes fifth disease, the telltale "slapped cheek" rash appears on the face. *Custom Medical Stock Photo, Inc.*

*immunity (ih-MYOON-uh-tee) is the condition of being protected against an infectious disease. Immunity often develops after a germ has entered the body. One type of immunity occurs when the body makes special protein molecules called antibodies to fight the disease-causing germ. The next time that germ enters the body, the antibodies quickly attack it, usually preventing the germ from causing disease.

*miscarriage is the ending of a pregnancy through the death of the embryo or fetus before birth.

contagious. Once someone is infected with parvovirus B19, that person develops immunity* to it and will not usually become infected again.

Parvovirus B19 passes from one person to another through nose and mouth fluids, such as saliva and mucus. Any direct contact with the fluids of an infected person, whether through a cough or sneeze or by sharing drinking glasses or utensils, can spread the infection.

Fifth disease can also be passed from pregnant women to their unborn babies. Most of the time, the baby is not harmed. Occasionally the infection can cause severe anemia in the baby and lead to miscarriage*, especially if the baby was infected in the first half of pregnancy.

What Happens When People Get Fifth Disease?

Signs and symptoms The first symptoms of fifth disease are similar to those of a common cold and include low fever, a runny or stuffy nose, sore throat, cough, headache, diarrhea, and fatigue. It is during this early period that fifth disease is most contagious. After a few days, especially in children, the slapped-cheek rash usually first appears on the face, and it soon begins to involve the rest of the body in a pink, lacy-looking pattern. Not everyone with fifth disease develops this rash; it is much more likely to appear in children under 10 years of age. For some people it will fade and reappear if triggered by heat, exercise, stress, or exposure to the sun. Sometimes the rash may itch, and adults in particular may experience pain and swelling of the joints in the hands, or the wrists, knees, or ankles.

Diagnosis In children, doctors can usually diagnose fifth disease simply by looking for the telltale rash on the face and body. In cases where there is no rash, blood tests can confirm the presence of parvovirus B19.

Treatment Most people with fifth disease do not require treatment. Antibiotics will not help because the illness is caused by a virus. Symp-

NAMING A DISEASE

Fifth disease was named in the late 1800s. It was the fifth classic childhood rash-associated disease to be named, following measles (first disease), scarlet fever (second disease), rubella or German measles (third disease), and a fourth condition with a rash that is unknown to doctors today (fourth disease). The name fifth disease probably stuck because it is a lot easier to say than erythema infectiosum.

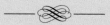

toms such as fever or joint pain may be treated with acetaminophen (uh-see-teh-MIH-noh-fen), a medication commonly used to reduce fever and relieve pain.

The rash clears up on its own, often within 1 to 3 weeks. Joint pain and swelling can take longer to go away, sometimes up to several months. People with joint pain may need to rest and restrict their activities until they feel better.

People with blood disorders or immune deficiencies who develop severe anemia as a result of fifth disease may require blood transfusions* and other specialized medical care.

Complications The vast majority of people who are infected with parvovirus B19 recover completely without any complications. Severe anemia, the complication most often associated with fifth disease, usually affects people with weakened immune systems or blood disorders and, rarely, unborn babies that were infected during the first half of pregnancy.

In healthy people, parvovirus B19 infection can sometimes affect the ability of the bone marrow (the soft tissue inside bones where blood cells are made) to make new red blood cells, but this effect is usually temporary and does not cause significant anemia or other problems.

* **blood transfusions** (trans-FYOO-zhunz) are procedures in which blood or certain parts of blood (such as specific cells) are given to a person who needs them because of illness or blood loss.

Can Fifth Disease Be Prevented?

There is no vaccine to prevent fifth disease. The best way to prevent the spread of infection is to practice good hygiene, including frequent hand washing and not sharing drinking glasses and eating utensils. Because the disease is most contagious before the telltale rash appears, it is difficult to keep the infection from spreading among family members or young children in school or day care. By the time the rash appears and the illness is diagnosed, the person is usually no longer contagious.

Resources

Organization

U.S. Centers for Disease Control and Prevention (CDC), 1600 Clifton Road, Atlanta, GA 30333. The CDC provides fact sheets about fifth disease at its website.
Telephone 800-311-3435
http://www.cdc.gov

Website

KidsHealth.org. KidsHealth is a website created by the medical experts of the Nemours Foundation and is devoted to issues of children's health. It contains articles on a variety of health topics, including fifth disease.
http://www.KidsHealth.org

▶ *See also*
Measles (Rubeola)
Rubella (German Measles)

Filariasis

Filariasis (fih-luh-RYE-uh-sis) is a tropical disease caused by tiny worms.

What Is Filariasis?

Filariasis is caused by different species of microscopic parasitic* round-worms that are passed to people through the bites of insects, most commonly mosquitoes. Several strains* of these worms, known as filariae (fih-LAIR-e-e), can infect humans, including *Wuchereria bancrofti* (voo-ker-E-re-ah ban-CROFT-e). There are also different types of filariasis itself, including cutaneous (kyoo-TAY-nee-us) or skin-related, body cavity, and lymphatic* infections. In the cutaneous disease, the worms live in the layers of the skin; in body cavity filariasis, they inhabit certain body openings and surrounding tissue; and in the lymphatic form of infection, they invade the vessels of the lymphatic system and the lymph nodes*.

Lymphatic filariasis, which can progress to a condition called elephantiasis*, is the most serious form of the disease. It begins when an infected female mosquito injects worm larvae* into a person's blood while feeding. The larvae travel to the lymphatic vessels, where they grow into adult worms. As adults, the worms can survive and reproduce for up to 7 years. The gradual buildup of worms in the vessels hinders the lymphatic system's ability to fight infection, and causes lymph fluid to collect—typically in the arms, legs, breasts, and male genitals—leading to swelling and disfigurement.

How Common Is the Infection?

Filariasis is most common in tropical and subtropical regions, including parts of Africa, the western Pacific, Asia (especially India), and Central and South America. In these areas, the number of cases of filariasis continues to rise. It is estimated that more than 120 million people worldwide have the lymphatic form of illness today, and approximately 40 million of them have been disabled or disfigured by the disease. Although contracting filariasis is not a risk in the United States, some recent immigrants may have it, and people who have traveled to other countries can contract the disease as well. Missionaries and Peace Corps volunteers are considered to be most at risk.

Is Filariasis Contagious?

The disease does not spread from direct person-to-person contact. Instead, it is transmitted by the bite of a mosquito. When one of these insects bites someone who is infected, it takes in the parasites along with its meal of blood. The mosquito then can pass those parasites on to the next person it bites. Usually, someone must be bitten many times, typically over a long period, to develop symptoms of filariasis.

KEYWORDS
for searching the Internet
and other reference sources

Brugia malayi

Brugia timori

Elephantiasis

Filariae

Lymphatic system

Mosquito-borne illnesses

Nematodes

Parasites

Roundworms

Travel-related illnesses

Wuchereria bancrofti

*parasitic (pair-uh-SIH-tik) refers to organisms such as protozoa (one-celled animals), worms, or insects that can invade and live on or inside human beings and may cause illness. An animal or plant harboring a parasite is called its host.

*strains are various subtypes of organisms, such as viruses or bacteria.

*lymphatic (lim-FAH-tik) means relating to the system of vessels and other structures that carry lymph, a colorless fluid, throughout the body's tissues; the lymphatic system plays an important role in protecting the body from infections.

*lymph (LIMF) nodes are small, bean-shaped masses of tissue that contain immune system cells that fight harmful microorganisms. Lymph nodes may swell during infections.

*elephantiasis (eh-luh-fan-TIE-uh-sis) is the significant enlargement and thickening of body tissues caused by an infestation of parasites known as filaria.

What Are the Signs and Symptoms of the Disease?

The lymphatic form of filariasis usually produces fever, swollen or painful lymph nodes in the neck and groin, pain in the testicles*, and swelling in the limbs or genitals. Males and the male urinary and genital systems are particularly likely to be affected. In elephantiasis, a severe form of chronic* lymphatic filariasis, the blocked flow of lymph causes one or both legs to swell significantly. Over time, the skin on the leg also can change, taking on a rough texture so that it resembles the skin of an elephant. Although elephantiasis is unusual, up to half of all men with lymphatic filariasis may show serious symptoms, such as swelling of the scrotum*. In some cases people may have no obvious symptoms, but they still may have serious damage to the kidneys and lymphatic system.

Making the Diagnosis

Knowing that the person lives in or has spent time in a country where filariasis poses a risk can help a doctor diagnose the disease. The doctor may also take skin and blood samples from the patient to look for signs of the parasite.

What Is the Treatment for Filariasis?

Ideally, treatment begins as soon as possible after the patient becomes infected. Prompt treatment may not be possible, however, because the disease can be difficult to detect in its early stages. When the diagnosis is made, treatment may include:

- medication to kill the young worms in the bloodstream and stop the parasite's life cycle (although the medicine cannot kill adult worms)
- exercising and moving swollen limbs to improve lymph flow
- bed rest and compression bandages to treat swelling
- medications to lessen swelling and discomfort
- hospitalization and intravenous* (IV) antibiotics for secondary infections that might appear because the damaged lymphatic system is less able to assist in defending the body against infectious agents
- surgical treatment for deformities, such as enlarged limbs and scrotum, sometimes with several procedures and skin grafts* to correct cases of disfigurement

How Long Does the Disease Last and What Are the Complications?

Filariasis can last a lifetime, and without treatment it can worsen. The disease can lead to permanent disfigurement and damage to the lymphatic system and kidneys, secondary infections, hardening and thickening of the skin, and sexual and psychological problems. In countries where the disease is common, a serious social stigma* often accompanies it.

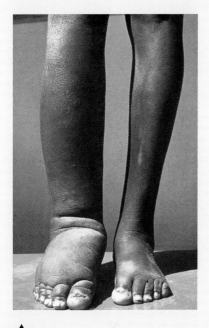

Lymphatic filariasis can progress to elephantiasis, a swelling and thickening of body tissues from accumulation of fluid. The skin may look thick, pebbly, and dark. *Phototake*

* **larvae** (LAR-vee) are the immature forms of an insect or worm that hatch from an egg.

* **testicles** (TES-tih-kuls) are the paired male reproductive glands that produce sperm.

* **chronic** (KRAH-nik) means continuing for a long period of time.

* **scrotum** is the sac of skin that contains the testicles.

* **intravenous** (in-tra-VEE-nus) means within or through a vein. For example, medications, fluid, or other substances can be given through a needle or soft tube inserted through the skin's surface directly into a vein.

* **grafts** are tissue or organ transplants.

* **stigma** is a mark of shame.

145

Can Filariasis Be Prevented?

There is no vaccine to prevent filariasis, but controlling the populations of blood-sucking insects, especially mosquitoes, can limit the spread of the disease. In some areas where filariasis is common, people are treated yearly with preventive medicine to kill any immature worms in their blood. To protect themselves, people can also:

- Stay inside as much as possible from dusk to dawn, when mosquitoes are most active.
- Sleep under mosquito netting.
- Place screens in all windows.
- Use insecticides around living areas.
- Apply insect repellent to exposed skin.

Resources

Organizations

U.S. Centers for Disease Control and Prevention (CDC), 1600 Clifton Road, Atlanta, GA 30333. The CDC provides a fact sheet and other information on filariasis at its website.
Telephone 800-311-3435
http://www.cdc.gov

World Health Organization (WHO), Avenue Appia 20, 1211 Geneva 27, Switzerland. The WHO tracks disease outbreaks around the world and offers information about filariasis at its website.
Telephone 011-41-22-791-2111
http://www.who.int

▶ See also

Skin Parasites

Travel-related Infections

West Nile Fever

Food Poisoning *See* Intestinal Infections

Fungal Infections

Fungal (FUNG-gul) infections are caused by fungi (FUNG-eye) that can grow on the skin, nails, and hair and within internal organs.

What Are Fungal Infections?

Fungal infections are caused by fungi, tiny microbes* found in soil, air, and water, as well as on plants, animals, and people. There are at least 100,000 species of fungi. The most familiar types are the mushrooms

** **microbes** (MY-krobes) are microscopic living organisms, such as bacteria, viruses and fungi.*

that some people like to eat on pizza, the fuzzy white or blue-green mold that grows on forgotten foods in the back of the refrigerator, and the mildew on the shower curtain. Fungi grow best in warm, moist areas, like a steamy bathroom or the spaces between the toes.

Relatively few species of fungi cause fungal infections, also called mycoses (my-KO-seez). Those that produce infection can cause two basic types: superficial and systemic infections. Superficial infections are found on the skin, nails, or hair and usually are not serious. Systemic infections take hold inside the body, in individual organs or throughout the body, and can be severe. Systemic infections are more likely to appear in people who have weak immune systems, such as those who have cancer or AIDS*. In these people, the infections can cause chronic* disease and, in some cases, death.

What Are the Common Signs and Symptoms of Fungal Infections?

Superficial fungal infections, such as jock itch, vaginal yeast infection, athlete's foot, and ringworm, typically are annoying but not very serious. Their symptoms generally include itchy, dry, red, scaly, or irritated skin. Systemic fungal infections often begin in the lungs and take time to develop. Severe infections occur in people whose immune systems have been weakened, allowing the infection to spread beyond the lungs to other organs. Symptoms of systemic fungal infections depend on which organs become infected and may include respiratory problems, extreme tiredness, coughing, weight loss, fever, night sweats, and headache.

What Are Some Specific Fungal Infections?

Tinea (TIH-nee-uh) is a general term given to a group of superficial fungal infections that affect the nails, feet (athlete's foot), groin area (jock itch), scalp, or skin (ringworm). *Trichophyton* and *Microsporum* fungi cause these related infections. Ringworm is identified by a red, scaly patch on the skin that looks like an expanding ring around a clearing center. Symptoms of athlete's foot include redness and cracking of the skin between the toes, and infected nails on the hands or feet usually look white and appear to be crumbling.

Candidiasis (kan-dih-DYE-uh-sis) is a superficial fungal infection caused by various strains of *Candida* (CAN-dih-duh) fungi. *Candida* is a yeastlike fungus often found in the mouth and the lining of the intestinal tract of healthy people. In people with weak immune systems, however, it can grow out of control, leading to an infection. A *Candida* infection of the mouth and throat is known as oropharyngeal (or-oh-fair-in-JEE-ul) candidiasis (OPC) or thrush, and infection of the vagina is known as vulvovaginal (vul-vo-VAH-jih-nul) candidiasis (VVC) or vaginal yeast infection. OPC can affect newborns, people with AIDS or diabetes*, and other people with weak immune systems. Its symptoms include white, thick patches on the tongue, mouth, and throat.

KEYWORDS
for searching the Internet and other reference sources

Aspergillosis

Blastomycosis

Candidiasis

Coccidioidomycosis

Cryptococcosis

Fungi

Histoplasmosis

Molds

Mycoses

Mycology

Sporotrichosis

Tinea

Yeasts

* **AIDS**, or acquired immunodeficiency (ih-myoo-no-dih-FIH-shen-see) syndrome, is an infection that severely weakens the immune system; it is caused by the human immunodeficiency virus (HIV).

* **chronic** (KRAH-nik) means continuing for a long period of time.

* **diabetes** (dye-uh-BEE-teez) is a condition in which the body's pancreas does not produce enough insulin or the body cannot use the insulin it makes effectively, resulting in increased levels of sugar in the blood. This can lead to increased urination, dehydration, weight loss, weakness, and a number of other symptoms and complications related to chemical imbalances within the body.

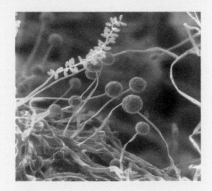

A yeast colony, as seen with an electron microscope, looks like growing vegetation. *Custom Medical Stock Photo, Inc.*

* **sinuses** (SY-nuh-ses) are hollow, air-filled cavities in the facial bones.

* **sputum** (SPYOO-tum) is a substance that contains mucus and other matter coughed out from the lungs, bronchi, and trachea.

* **pulmonary** means referring to or pertaining to the lungs.

* **spores** are a temporarily inactive form of a germ enclosed in a protective shell.

* **feces** (FEE-seez) is the excreted waste from the gastrointestinal tract.

* **liver** is a large organ located beneath the ribs on the right side of the body. The liver performs numerous digestive and chemical functions essential for health.

* **spleen** is an organ in the upper left part of the abdomen that stores and filters blood. As part of the immune system, the spleen also plays a role in fighting infection.

Candida infection commonly occurs in newborns in the form of thrush or diaper rash. VVC is associated with vaginal burning or itching and a thick, cheeselike discharge. In certain situations, *Candida* can enter the bloodstream and spread to internal organs. This is seen most frequently in hospitalized patients who have weak immune systems and have received antibiotics.

Aspergillosis (as-per-jih-LO-sis) is the name for a variety of systemic infections caused by *Aspergillus* (as-per-JIH-lus) fungi. If it is inhaled through the mouth or nose, the fungus can cause a mild allergic reaction or a more serious infection of the sinuses* and lungs. Symptoms of aspergillosis vary and may include fever, cough, chest pain, and wheezing. In severe cases, typically seen in people with weak immune systems, the infection can spread to other organs, including the brain, skin, and bones.

Blastomycosis (blas-toh-my-KO-sis) is a systemic infection caused by the *Blastomyces dermatitidis* fungus commonly found in soil in the southeastern, midwestern, and south-central United States. The disease's symptoms resemble those of the flu: joint and muscle pain, a cough that brings up sputum*, fever, chills, and chest pain. If it progresses, it can lead to chronic pulmonary* infection, causing permanent lung damage, or widespread disease that affects the bones, skin, and genital and urinary tracts. Blastomycosis leads to death in about 5 percent of patients.

Cryptococcosis (krip-toh-kah-KO-sis) is a systemic infection caused by the fungus *Cryptococcus neoformans*, usually found in soil or bird droppings. Typically, the fungus enters the body through the mouth or nostrils when someone inhales fungi spores*, and symptoms of a lung infection, such as cough and chest pain, may develop. Although infection with *Cryptococcus* usually produces no symptoms or only mild symptoms in healthy people, the infection may spread in people who have weak immune systems. If it spreads to the central nervous system, it can cause inflammation of the membranes covering the brain and spinal cord. This is especially common among people with AIDS.

Histoplasmosis (his-toh-plaz-MO-sis) is usually a mild systemic infection caused by *Histoplasma capsulatum*. This fungus is found in the eastern and central United States in soil that contains bird and bat feces*. When the soil is disturbed, the fungal spores may be inhaled. Histoplasmosis can cause flulike symptoms, including body aches, fever, and cough. Most people who become infected do not experience symptoms, but as with other fungal infections, people with weak immune systems are at risk for severe disease. In those cases, the infection affects the lungs and may spread to the liver*, spleen*, bones, and brain.

Sporotrichosis (spo-ro-trih-KO-sis) is a skin infection caused by the *Sporothrix schenckii* fungus, which is found in soil, thorny plants, hay, sphagnum (SFAG-num) moss, and other plant materials. It enters the skin through a small cut or puncture, such as a thorn might make. Soon, small reddish bumps resembling boils* form around the cut and often ulcerate*. In some cases, infection can spread to other parts of the body, such as the lungs or joints.

Coccidioidomycosis (kok-sih-dee-oyd-o-my-KO-sis) is a systemic infection caused by *Coccidioides immitis*, a fungus found in soil in the southwestern United States, Mexico, and South America. Most people with coccidioidomycosis have no symptoms, but 40 percent of patients experience a flulike illness, with fever, rash, muscle aches, and cough. Also know as valley fever, the infection can cause pneumonia* or widespread disease affecting the skin, bones, and membranes covering the brain and spinal cord.

How Common Are Fungal Infections?

Superficial fungal infections, such as athlete's foot and candidiasis, are fairly common. Systemic infections, on the other hand, are rare, appearing in less than one to two people of every 100,000 in the United States, according to the U.S. Centers for Disease Control and Prevention. They are more common in certain populations, such as people with AIDS or those who have had organ transplants.

With the so-called endemic* mycoses, rates of disease are higher in specific geographic areas. For example, coccidioidomycosis occurs in about 15 of every 100,000 people in parts of the southwestern United States (with 10 to 50 percent of the population testing positive for exposure to the fungus). In areas where histoplasmosis is found, up to 80 percent of the population test positive for exposure to *Histoplasma capsulatum*, but the disease develops only in people with weak immune systems.

Are They Contagious?

Some fungal infections, such as candidiasis and ringworm, can spread from person to person through contact with the infected area. Most infections, however, develop from fungi found naturally on the human body or in the environment. Many fungi that cause systemic respiratory disease are found in soil or in the droppings of animals or birds. Usually they are inhaled after the soil or droppings are disturbed, sending dust and fungal spores into the air.

How Do Doctors Make the Diagnosis?

Most superficial fungal infections are diagnosed based on their appearance and location. A doctor also may take a skin scraping to examine under the microscope or to culture* in a laboratory. Some fungi glow with a particular color under ultraviolet light, so a doctor may make the diagnosis by shining such a light on the affected area. Systemic infections can be diagnosed by collecting a sample of blood, urine, cerebrospinal fluid*, or sputum to culture.

Friendly Bacteria

Naturally occurring "friendly" bacteria and fungi live side by side on the human body. Some bacteria help keep fungi in check by preventing them from reproducing uncontrollably and causing disease. From time to time, however, doctors need to prescribe antibiotics to combat not-so-friendly bacteria that cause illness. Most antibiotics kill many types of bacteria, both good and bad, and using them for long periods of time can destroy too many friendly bacteria, allowing fungi to grow unchecked and eventually cause infection. To preserve the bacteria we need, it is important to use antibiotics only when necessary and prescribed by a doctor.

* **boils** are skin abscesses, or collections of pus in the skin.
* **ulcerate** means to become eroded by infection, inflammation, or irritation.
* **pneumonia** (nu-MO-nyah) is inflammation of the lung.
* **endemic** (en-DEH-mik) describes a disease or condition that is present in a population or geographic area at all times.
* **culture** (KUL-chur) is a test in which a sample of fluid or tissue from the body is placed in a dish containing material that supports the growth of certain organisms. Over time, ranging from hours to weeks, the organisms will grow and can be identified.
* **cerebrospinal** (seh-ree-bro-SPY-nuhl) **fluid** is the fluid that surrounds the brain and spinal cord.

*intravenous (in-tra-VEE-nus) means within or through a vein. For example, medications, fluid, or other substances can be given through a needle or soft tube inserted through the skin's surface directly into a vein.

Can Fungal Infections Be Treated?

Most superficial fungal infections are treated at home with antifungal creams or shampoos for 1 to 2 weeks. Oral (taken by mouth) antifungal medication also may be prescribed, if necessary. Some cases of fungal infection last for a while and may need to be treated with medicine for 2 to 4 weeks or even longer. Systemic illnesses often require hospitalization so that the patient can receive intravenous* antifungal drugs and supportive care.

Can Fungal Infections Be Prevented?

Preventing fungal infections can be difficult, because fungi are everywhere. In general, people who are otherwise healthy rarely contract systemic fungal infections. Practicing good hygiene, keeping the skin dry, and changing socks and underwear every day can help prevent superficial skin infections.

Resources

Organization

U.S. Centers for Disease Control and Prevention (CDC), 1600 Clifton Road, Atlanta, GA 30333. The CDC provides fact sheets and other information on fungal infections through its website. Telephone 800-311-3435
http://www.cdc.gov

Website

KidsHealth.org. KidsHealth is a website created by the medical experts of the Nemours Foundation and is devoted to issues of children's health. It contains articles on a variety of health topics, including fungal infections.
http://www.KidsHealth.org

▶ *See also*

Coccidioidomycosis (Valley Fever)

Skin and Soft Tissue Infections

G

Gangrene

Gangrene (GANG-green) is the decay or death of living tissue caused by a lack of oxygen supply to the tissue and/or bacterial infection of the tissue.

KEYWORDS
for searching the Internet
and other reference sources

Clostridium perfringens

Debridement

Frostbite

Hyperbaric chamber

What Is Gangrene?

Gangrene is not a contagious disease. It is a condition in which living tissue (e.g., skin, muscle, or bone) begins to decay and die because blood flow (and oxygen) to an area is blocked or because harmful bacteria invade the body's tissues after entering through a wound or sore. Gangrene most commonly affects the feet, toes, hands, and fingers. Gangrene can also occur inside the body in abdominal organs such as the intestines.

Doctors recognize three major forms of gangrene: dry, wet, and gas gangrene.

Dry gangrene Dry gangrene is the most common form of gangrene, and it occurs most frequently in the feet of people with diabetes*. Dry gangrene results from the gradual loss of blood supply to a part of the body. The tissue slowly dies because it receives little or no oxygen and nutrients from the blood, but it does not become infected. The first symptoms of dry gangrene are often numbness and tingling in the affected area. This is usually followed by severe pain as the condition progresses and the tissue begins to die; the skin temperature drops, and the color of the tissue changes, eventually turning black.

Dry gangrene is most often a complication of diabetes, arteriosclerosis*, or frostbite*. Because this condition usually develops gradually, it may go unnoticed for weeks or months, especially in elderly people. Dry gangrene usually is not life threatening, but it needs to be treated promptly.

Wet gangrene Wet gangrene is caused by a bacterial infection from severe wounds or burns or by a crushing injury that causes blood to stop flowing to a certain part of the body. When blood flow stops, bacteria begin to invade the damaged tissue. In wet gangrene, there is pain, swelling, and blistering of the skin, and the wound gives off a foul smell. Organisms that are commonly involved in wet gangrene include *Streptococcus* (strep-tuh-KAH-kus) and *Staphylococcus* (stah-fih-lo-KAH-kus) bacteria. Without treatment, wet gangrene can be fatal.

* **diabetes** (dye-uh-BEE-teez) is a condition in which the body's pancreas does not produce enough insulin or the body cannot use the insulin it makes effectively, resulting in increased levels of sugar in the blood. This can lead to increased urination, dehydration, weight loss, weakness, and a number of other symptoms and complications related to chemical imbalances within the body.

* **arteriosclerosis** (ar-teer-e-o-sklah-RO-sis) is a condition in which arteries of the body have become narrowed and hardened from the buildup of calcium, cholesterol, and other substances, causing decreased blood flow through these vessels.

* **frostbite** is damage to tissues resulting from exposure to low environmental temperatures. It is also called congelation (kon-jeh-LAY-shun).

People with poor circulation may experience dry gangrene from loss of oxygen and nutrients carried by blood to the extremities. If the tissue turns black and dies, it must be removed surgically. *Photo Researchers, Inc.* ▶

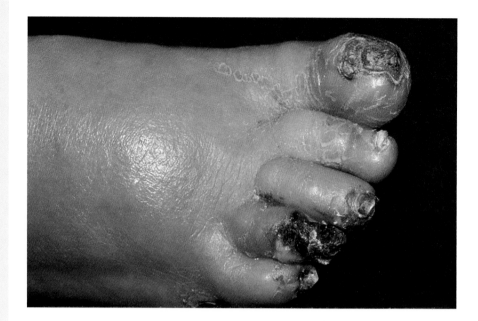

*toxins are poisons that harm the body.

*pus is a thick, creamy fluid, usually yellow or greenish in color, that forms at the site of an infection. Pus contains infection-fighting white cells and other substances.

*amputation (am-pyoo-TAY-shun) is the removal of a limb or other appendage or outgrowth of the body.

Gas gangrene Gas gangrene, which is a form of wet gangrene, involves infection of body tissue by certain types of bacteria (such as *Clostridium perfringens,* klah-STRIH-de-um per-FRING-enz) that are capable of thriving in anaerobic (ah-nuh-RO-bik) conditions (in which there is little or no oxygen). Once present in the tissue, these bacteria release toxins* and gas. Gas gangrene is marked by a high fever, brownish pus*, gas bubbles under the skin, skin discoloration, and a foul odor. It is the rarest form of gangrene, and only 1,000 to 3,000 cases occur in the United States each year. Like wet gangrene, gas gangrene can be fatal if not treated immediately.

How Do Doctors Diagnose and Treat Gangrene?

A doctor will make the diagnosis of gangrene based on a physical examination, the patient's medical history, and the results of blood and other laboratory tests. Cultures from the gangrenous area may be taken and laboratory tests performed to identify the type of bacterial infection and determine the extent to which an infection has spread.

Dead gangrenous tissue must be removed surgically by a procedure called debridement (deh-BREED-ment) so that the wound can heal and healthy new tissue can grow. People with gangrene caused by bacterial infections are treated with antibiotics. In more severe cases, amputation* of a finger, toe, or part of a limb may be necessary. Sometimes patients with gangrene are treated in a hyperbaric chamber, where they are exposed to oxygen at a high pressure to help the affected tissue heal.

The outcome for gangrene is usually favorable if the condition is recognized and treated early. Full recovery and new tissue growth can take several weeks to months. Sepsis, a potentially serious spread of infection through the bloodstream and body, can result from wet and gas gangrene. If left untreated, sepsis can result in shock* or death.

Can Gangrene Be Prevented?

Carefully cleaning and watching wounds for signs of infection can help prevent gangrene. It is wise to seek medical attention for any wounds that are not healing well or look infected. People who are susceptible to dry gangrene, such as those with decreased circulation in their legs and feet from diabetes or arteriosclerosis, are advised to pay attention to any skin infection in those areas (because such infections could lead to the development of wet gangrene) and to avoid smoking (because smoking constricts the blood vessels, further decreasing circulation). Daily foot care and hygiene is very important in people with advanced diabetes. Treatment with antibiotics before and after abdominal surgery has been shown to reduce the rate of infection and the possibility of developing wet or gas gangrene.

Resource

Organization

U.S. National Library of Medicine, 8600 Rockville Pike, Bethesda, MD 20894. The National Library of Medicine has a website packed with information on diseases (including gangrene) and drugs, consumer resources, dictionaries and encyclopedias of medical terms, and directories of doctors and helpful organizations.
Telephone 888-346-3656
http://www.nlm.nih.gov

Gastroenteritis *See* Intestinal Infections

German Measles *See* Rubella (German Measles)

Gonorrhea

Gonorrhea (gah-nuh-REE-uh) is a sexually transmitted disease (STD) spread through all forms of sexual intercourse. It also can be passed from an infected mother to her baby during childbirth. Gonorrhea can affect the genitals, urethra*, rectum*, eyes, throat, joints, and other organs and tissues of the body.

* **shock** is a serious condition in which blood pressure is very low and not enough blood flows to the body's organs and tissues. Untreated, shock may result in death.

▶ *See also*
Sepsis
Staphylococcal Infections
Streptococcal Infections

* **urethra** (yoo-REE-thra) is the tube through which urine passes from the bladder to the outside of the body.

* **rectum** is the final portion of the large intestine, connecting the colon to the anus.

153

* **cervix** (SIR-viks) is the lower, narrow end of the uterus that opens into the vagina.

* **uterus** (YOO-teh-rus) is the muscular, pear-shaped internal organ in a woman where a baby develops until birth.

* **fallopian** (fah-LO-pee-uhn) **tubes** are the two slender tubes that connect the ovaries and the uterus in females. They carry the ova, or eggs, from the ovaries to the uterus.

* **ovaries** (O-vuh-reez) are the sexual glands from which ova, or eggs, are released in women.

* **chlamydial** (kla-MIH-dee-ul) **infection** can occur in various forms in which the bacteria can invade the urinary and genital systems of the body, as well as the eyes and lungs. One of its most common forms is a sexually transmitted disease (STD), usually passed from one person to another through unprotected sexual intercourse.

* **semen** (SEE-men) is the sperm-containing whitish fluid produced by the male reproductive tract.

What Is Gonorrhea?

Gonorrhea is an infection caused by the bacterium *Neisseria gonorrhoeae* (nye-SEER-e-uh gah-no-REE-eye), which can grow in moist areas of the body including the vagina, penis, rectum, eyes, and throat. Gonorrhea may cause a discharge from the penis or vagina and pain while urinating. In women, the infection usually starts within the vagina at the cervix*; if untreated, infection can spread to the uterus* and fallopian tubes* and result in pelvic inflammatory disease (PID); PID refers to an infection of a woman's reproductive organs, including the fallopian tubes, uterus, cervix, and ovaries*, sometimes with spread of infection to other body tissues near these organs. Babies born to mothers who have gonorrhea can develop eye infection which, if untreated, can lead to blindness and other complications.

How Common Is Gonorrhea?

Gonorrhea is the second most commonly reported STD in the United States, according to the U.S. Centers for Disease Control and Prevention (CDC); chlamydial infection* is number one. The CDC reports that the number of cases has been decreasing since the mid-1980s. However, up to 400,000 new cases are reported every year in the United States, and many more go unreported. Some experts estimate that as many as 2 million cases occur per year.

Gonorrhea is most common in highly populated urban areas and in people who have more than one sexual partner, but anyone who has sexual relations with an infected person can contract gonorrhea. Most men who contract the disease are ages 20 to 24; most women are under 21.

Is Gonorrhea Contagious?

Gonorrhea is contagious. When people do not use condoms or other protective measures when having sex or have multiple sexual partners, their risk of contracting the disease increases. From the time someone is infected with the gonorrhea bacterium, that person can spread the disease until properly treated.

The bacteria that cause gonorrhea are spread through body fluids, such as fluid from the vagina or semen*, that are passed from one person to another during vaginal, anal, or oral intercourse. Infected women can pass the infection to their babies during childbirth.

People can infect themselves if they touch an affected area and then rub or scratch their eyes. Gonorrhea can also be spread through kissing if one partner has a cut on the lip, but this way of becoming infected is rare. Sharing towels and sitting on toilet seats that have come in contact with the bacteria do not spread the disease.

How Do People Know They Have Gonorrhea?

Many people who contract gonorrhea do not have any symptoms. For those who do, the symptoms often are mild. Males are much more likely to know they have gonorrhea than females, but up to 20 percent of males do not experience any symptoms at all. Within 2 weeks after being infected, males often feel burning when urinating and have pain or a greenish discharge from the penis. The lymph nodes* in the groin may swell, and the head of the penis may become irritated and red.

Although many women with gonorrhea have mild or no symptoms, those who do develop symptoms usually begin to experience them within 2 to 3 weeks after contact with the bacteria. These include bloody or greenish-yellow discharge from the vagina, pain during urination and/or sexual intercourse, and itching, soreness, or redness in the genital area. Other symptoms, including abdominal* pain, bleeding during or after intercourse, and bleeding between periods may mean a woman has PID.

How Do Doctors Diagnose and Treat Gonorrhea?

Because the symptoms of gonorrhea are similar to those of chlamydial infection, doctors usually test a person experiencing symptoms for both of these STDs.

Diagnosis A sample of genital fluid or discharge from the tip of the penis, vagina, cervix, or rectum can be tested for *Neisseria gonorrhoeae* bacteria by doing a culture. Results are usually known within 48 hours. Another test, polymerase (pah-LIM-er-ace) chain reaction (PCR), can be used to look for DNA* from the bacteria in urine, fluid from the cervix, or from swabs taken from the urethra. This test gives faster, accurate results.

Pharyngeal (fair-un-JEE-ul), or throat, gonorrhea can be detected by doing a throat culture. In newborns at risk for the disease, doctors swab the baby's eye discharge and do a culture to confirm the diagnosis. Gonorrheal eye infection is uncommon in U.S. infants because newborns routinely receive antibiotic eye drops or ointment at birth to prevent infection.

Treatment Gonorrhea is curable when treated with antibiotics, although some strains* of the bacteria are becoming resistant to medication. It is important to stop having sexual relations while infected, and all sexual partners should be told and tested, even if they do not have symptoms. If they have the disease they should also be treated with antibiotics. People who have both gonorrhea and chlamydial infection are treated with a combination of antibiotics. Infected newborns are given antibiotics intravenously (directly into a vein).

With antibiotic treatment, gonorrhea usually clears up within 2 weeks. It is important to take the full course of medication even if the symptoms get better, and to contact the doctor if they do not. When treated early, there are usually no long-term complications.

Complications If a person has had gonorrhea before, it does not reduce the chances of becoming infected again. In fact, it increases the likelihood that complications may occur. In women, untreated gonorrhea can lead to PID, which can cause ectopic pregnancy* and sometimes lead

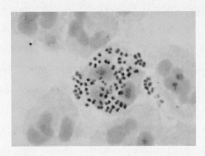

Neisseria gonorrhoeae bacteria can be seen in this microscopic image of discharge from the urethra, the tube through which urine passes from the bladder to the outside of the body. *Visuals Unlimited, Inc.*

* **lymph** (LIMF) **nodes** are small, bean-shaped masses of tissue that contain immune system cells that fight harmful microorganisms. Lymph nodes may swell during infections.

* **abdominal** (ab-DAH-mih-nul) refers to the area of the body below the ribs and above the hips that contains the stomach, intestines, and other organs.

* **DNA**, or deoxyribonucleic acid (dee-OX-see-ry-bo-nyoo-klay-ik AH-sid), is the specialized chemical substance that contains the genetic code necessary to build and maintain the structures and functions of living organisms.

* **strains** are various subtypes of organisms, such as viruses or bacteria.

* **ectopic** (ek-TAH-pik) **pregnancy** is an abnormal pregnancy in which the fertilized egg develops outside the uterus, usually within one of the fallopian tubes.

to infertility (the inability to become pregnant). Ectopic pregnancies require emergency surgery; an ectopic pregnancy that bursts can cause massive bleeding and even death.

Without treatment, gonorrhea can spread throughout the body, through the blood, and to the joints, heart, and brain, although this rarely occurs in young people who are in good health. Newborns who are not treated for gonorrheal eye infection are at risk for blindness. People with untreated gonorrhea are more likely to contract HIV* if they have unprotected sex with someone who is HIV-positive.

Can Gonorrhea Be Prevented?

The best way to avoid contracting or spreading gonorrhea is to abstain from sexual intercourse. For those who do have sex, using a latex condom properly during all forms of intercourse is important. Doctors advise women who are sexually active to have a yearly gynecological exam with STD screening. They also recommend that people with any symptoms of gonorrhea or who are at risk for STDs see a doctor. If a person is found to have gonorrhea, all sexual partners also need to be tested and treated.

Resources

Organizations

U.S. National Institute of Allergy and Infectious Diseases (NIAID), Building 31, Room 7A-50, 31 Center Drive MSC 2520, Bethesda, MD 20892-2520. The NIAID posts fact sheets about many STDs, including gonorrhea, at its website.
Telephone 301-496-5717
http://www.niaid.nih.gov

Planned Parenthood Federation of America, 810 Seventh Avenue, New York, NY 10019. Planned Parenthood posts information about sexually transmitted infections at its website.
Telephone 212-541-7800
http://www.plannedparenthood.org

Website

KidsHealth.org. KidsHealth is a website created by the medical experts of the Nemours Foundation and is devoted to issues of children's health. It contains articles on a variety of health topics, including gonorrhea and other STDs.
http://www.KidsHealth.org

*HIV, or the human immunodeficiency (HYOO-mun ih-myoo-no-dih-FIH-shen-see) virus, is the virus that causes AIDS (acquired immunodeficiency syndrome).

▶ See also
AIDS and HIV Infection
Chlamydial Infections
Sexually Transmitted Diseases
Syphilis

H

Hantavirus Pulmonary Syndrome

Hantavirus pulmonary syndrome (HAN-tuh-vy-rus PUL-mo-nar-ee SIN-drome) is a lung disease that causes respiratory distress (breathing difficulty) and, in some cases, death. Hantavirus, the virus that causes the disease, is carried by rodents.

KEYWORDS
for searching the Internet
and other reference sources

Hantavirus

Pulmonary system

Sin Nombre virus

Viral zoonoses

What is Hantavirus Pulmonary Syndrome?

Hantavirus pulmonary syndrome, or HPS, is a potentially deadly disease that attacks the lungs. A family of viruses called hantavirus causes HPS. These viruses live in rodents but do not make them sick. The Sin Nombre virus (SNV) hantavirus causes most HPS in the United States, but some cases have come from the Bayou, the New York, and the Black Creek Canal viruses.

Rodents, usually mice and rats, shed hantavirus in their saliva, urine, and droppings. Humans catch the virus when they disturb dried droppings (by sweeping, for example) and inhale the particles that are sent into the air. People can also contract hantavirus by touching an infected animal or its droppings and then touching their nose or mouth. Eating food or drinking water contaminated by rodent droppings is another source of infection. Rodent bites, although rare, can also spread the disease.

The most common carriers of hantavirus are deer mice (found almost everywhere in North America), cotton rats and rice rats (found in the southeastern United States and Central and South America), and white-footed mice (found in most parts of the United States and Mexico). Cats and dogs do not carry hantavirus and they cannot catch it from rodents. However, cats and dogs can spread hantavirus to humans if they bring an infected rodent into a home or other buildings where people live or work.

Is HPS Common?

HPS is rare. Health authorities first recognized the disease in the United States in 1993, and the U.S. Centers for Disease Control and Prevention (CDC) recorded only 333 reported cases through early 2003. Although HPS occurs in people throughout North and South America, most cases in the United States appear in the Southwest and in places that are infested with rodents.

Camp with Care

The great outdoors is home for most rodents, and many of them carry hantavirus. Campers can help keep camping and hiking trips safe by following a few simple precautions:

- using a tent with a built-in floor and pitching it away from woodpiles or any rodent nests or burrows

- sleeping on a raised surface, at least 12 inches off the floor

- airing out cabins that have not been used for a half hour or more, then checking for rodent droppings

- using water and disinfectant to wipe out the area (no sweeping!)

- keeping all food in rodent-proof containers

- burying or burning trash

- using bottled water for drinking, cooking, and all washing

- staying away from mice, rats, chipmunks, and all other rodents.

157

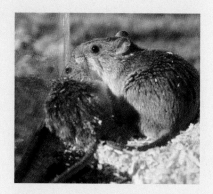

▲

Mice and rats shed hantavirus in their saliva, urine, and droppings. The rice rat (seen here) primarily inhabits the southeastern United States and carries the Bayou virus, a form of the disease that has been found in Louisiana.

* **abdominal** (ab-DAH-mih-nul) refers to the area of the body below the ribs and above the hips that contains the stomach, intestines, and other organs.

* **shock** is a serious condition in which blood pressure is very low and not enough blood flows to the body's organs and tissues. Untreated, shock may result in death.

* **antibodies** (AN-tih-bah-deez) are protein molecules produced by the body's immune system to help fight specific infections caused by microorganisms, such as bacteria and viruses.

* **strains** are various subtypes of organisms, such as viruses or bacteria.

* **ultrasound**, also called a sonogram, is a diagnostic test in which sound waves passing through the body create images on a computer screen.

People of every age, sex, and race can contract HPS, but it is not contagious and cannot be spread by sneezing, coughing, kissing, or having other bodily contact.

What Are the Symptoms of HPS?

The first symptoms of HPS usually appear 1 to 5 weeks after a person has been exposed to the virus. HPS can be difficult to diagnose because the early signs, such as fever, tiredness, and body aches, are similar to those of the flu. About half of the people who catch HPS also may experience dizziness, chills, nausea, vomiting, abdominal* pain, or headaches.

From 2 to 5 days after the first symptoms, a person infected with hantavirus starts coughing and experiences shortness of breath. The disease quickly becomes more severe, and people who do not receive immediate treatment may become extremely ill and go into shock*, needing intensive care in a hospital.

How Do Doctors Diagnose HPS?

A doctor may suspect HPS if a person with flulike symptoms complains about difficulty breathing, especially if the person has been exposed to rodents or rodent droppings. To confirm the diagnosis, the doctor uses blood tests to see if the person has developed antibodies* to a strain* of hantavirus. Chest X rays or ultrasound* images can help the doctor check the condition of a person's heart and lungs.

How Is HPS Treated?

HPS is a serious disease, and someone who has it needs treatment in a hospital's intensive care unit. There he might be given fluids, have his blood pressure monitored, and have a tube inserted in his throat to help him breathe. Because a virus causes HPS, antibiotics do not work against it, although an antiviral drug may help some patients. According to the CDC, 38 percent of reported cases of HPS have been fatal.

Doctors today know more about the disease and are quicker to get patients into treatment. The earlier people with HPS receive help, the better their chances of survival. Recovery from HPS is fairly fast, although patients may feel worn out for several months.

Can HPS Be Prevented?

There is no vaccination available for HPS. The best way to avoid contracting the virus is to get rid of possible sources of infection, which means avoiding woodpiles and other places where rodents live outdoors and keeping homes and workplaces free of mice and rats. Experts also recommend sealing holes where rodents can enter (they can squeeze through spaces as small as .25 inch in diameter) and wearing a mask and gloves when cleaning out areas with rodent droppings.

Resources

Organization

National Center for Infectious Diseases, U.S. Centers for Disease Control and Prevention, Mailstop C-14, 1600 Clifton Road, Atlanta, GA 30333. The website for this government agency provides an extensive look at HPS, including advice on preventing the disease.
Telephone 800-311-3435
http://www.cdc.gov/ncidod

Website

Discovery Online. *Death in the Desert.* This article, which can be found through the site's Plague Patrol page, describes how researchers found hantavirus in the American Southwest in 1993, solving several mysterious deaths.
http://www.discovery.com/stories/science/infectious/infectious.html

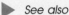 See also
Public Health

Zoonoses

Helicobacter Pylori Infection (Peptic Ulcer Disease)

Helicobacter pylori (HEEL-ih-ko-bak-ter pie-LOR-eye) infection, the major cause of peptic ulcer disease, is a bacterial infection that can lead to inflammation and ulcers* in the lining of the stomach and the upper part of the small intestine*.

KEYWORDS
for searching the Internet and other reference sources

Digestive system

Duodenum

Gastroenterology

Peptic ulcer

Small intestine

Stomach

What Is *H. pylori* Infection?

For years scientists and doctors thought that stomach and intestinal ulcers were caused by stress, eating spicy foods, or drinking too much alcohol. But in 1982 two Australian doctors, Barry Marshall and Robin Warren, discovered that *H. pylori,* a bacterium that lives in the lining of the stomach, can cause what is known as peptic ulcer disease. *H. pylori* infection is found in about 90 percent of people with ulcers in the duodenum (do-uh-DEE-num), the upper part of the small intestine. *H. pylori* infection is also responsible for most gastric (GAS-trik), or stomach, ulcers. Although *H. pylori* bacteria are responsible for most peptic ulcers, ulcers also can be caused by regularly taking certain medications, such as aspirin or ibuprofen; long-term smoking or alcohol use; infection with certain viruses; and, rarely, tumors in the pancreas or small intestine that lead to overproduction of stomach acid.

 H. pylori infection also can cause gastritis (gah-STRY-tis), or inflammation of the lining of the stomach, in adults and children. Even

* **ulcers** are open sores on the skin or the lining of a hollow body organ, such as the stomach or intestine. They may or may not be painful.

* **small intestine** is the part of the intestines—the system of muscular tubes that food passes through during digestion—that directly receives the food when it passes through the stomach.

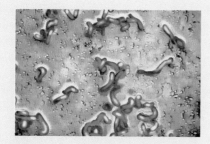

▲

As early as the nineteenth century, people had seen particular bacteria among the cells of the mucous lining of the stomach, particularly around ulcers. No one had ever been able to isolate the organisms until Barry Marshall and Robin Warren accidentally left cultures in an incubator over the Easter weekend, thus extending the usual incubation period. It turned out that the *Helicobacter* bacteria grow much more slowly than other types of bacteria. *Custom Medical Stock Photo, Inc.*

* **esophagus** (eh-SAH-fuh-gus) is the soft tube that, with swallowing, carries food from the throat to the stomach.

though infection with *H. pylori* can cause disease, most people who have the bacteria in their stomach or intestines never experience any symptoms. In fact, the presence of *H. pylori* bacteria appears to lessen the risk that a person will get another serious disease, cancer of the esophagus*.

How Common Is *H. pylori* Infection?

According to the U.S. Centers for Disease Control and Prevention (CDC), about two-thirds of the world's population is infected with *H. pylori*, but most people will never experience any symptoms. In the United States, *H. pylori* infection is more common among older adults, people from lower socioeconomic groups, and Hispanics and African Americans. Each year between 500,000 and 850,000 new cases of ulcer disease are diagnosed in the United States.

Is the Infection Contagious?

H. pylori infection may be contagious, but it is not known how it spreads. Some doctors suspect that the infection can be spread when an infected person passes the bacterium in feces (FEE-seez), or bowel movements. When another person comes into contact with the infected feces, whether by changing a diaper, cleaning a bathroom, or doing someone's laundry, he or she could become infected with the bacterium. Mouth-to-mouth contact also may contribute to the spread of *H. pylori* infection. Some research has found *H. pylori* bacteria in saliva, leading researchers to suggest that kissing is one way that the bacteria spread. In addition, coming into contact with food, water, or vomited material that contains *H. pylori* bacteria also may put a person at risk of infection.

What Are the Signs and Symptoms of *H. pylori* Infection?

H. pylori infection can cause a variety of symptoms, but the most common one is abdominal pain. A person with peptic ulcer disease may feel a gnawing or burning pain below the ribs and above the navel. Abdominal pain from an ulcer usually occurs when the stomach is empty, typically several hours after eating or in the morning or evening hours. Eating food, drinking milk, or taking antacids may make the pain subside for a short while.

Other symptoms of peptic ulcer disease may include:

- frequently feeling sick to the stomach (nausea, NAW-zee-uh)
- loss of appetite
- frequent burping
- sudden, sharp abdominal pain
- weight loss
- vomiting
- bloody or black stools

How Do Doctors Make the Diagnosis?

If a person has lasting abdominal pain or other symptoms of peptic ulcer disease, there are several methods a doctor can use to make a diagnosis. One of the most common ways to check for ulcers is with endoscopy (en-DOS-ko-pee). For this procedure, a person is given medication to relax and numb the throat. Then a doctor gently inserts an endoscope, a thin, flexible tube with a camera and light on the end, down the throat, through the esophagus, and into the stomach and intestines. The camera on the end of the endoscope allows the doctor to view the digestive system and take pictures of it. In addition, the doctor can perform a biopsy, removing a small amount of tissue for study. The biopsy tissue can be sent to a laboratory for further testing and to check for evidence of *H. pylori* infection.

A person suspected of having *H. pylori* infection also might undergo a breath test. During a breath test, a person drinks a liquid containing a carbon marker known as carbon-13 (^{13}C). The person then provides a breath sample by blowing up a balloon or blowing bubbles. The sample is checked for the presence of the ^{13}C marker. If the person has *H. pylori* infection, there will be traces of ^{13}C present in the carbon dioxide gas molecules of the person's breath. Although it is less helpful than endoscopy, another test that may be used to check for ulcers is an upper gastrointestinal* series, a set of X rays of the gastrointestinal system. A person taking the test first drinks a white, chalky liquid called barium, which helps highlight the ulcer and makes it visible on the X ray. A person's blood also can be checked for the presence of antibodies* to *H. pylori*, indicating infection.

How Is *H. pylori* Infection Treated?

Years ago people who had ulcers were given medication to lessen the production of stomach acid. This treatment minimized pain by allowing the ulcer to heal, but it did not treat the infection causing the inflammation. It was not uncommon for ulcers to return after this treatment was stopped.

Today, peptic ulcer disease usually is treated for 2 weeks with a combination of two or three antibiotic medicines that kill *H. pylori* bacteria, in addition to about a month of other prescribed medications that limit acid production as the ulcer heals. Treatment with antibiotics greatly lessens the chance that peptic ulcers will recur. After treatment is completed, tests sometimes are done to check that *H. pylori* infection has been eliminated from the body. Together with medication, eating regular small meals to prevent having an empty stomach for long periods of time may help decrease the pain associated with ulcers. A doctor also may advise avoiding ibuprofen or other medications that can cause stomach irritation.

With the recommended treatment, ulcers can take a few weeks to heal. Without antibiotic treatment to get rid of the bacteria, the infection can return, and the painful ulcers may not go away. Sometimes

How Ulcers Form

How exactly does *H. pylori* cause ulcers? Doctors think that *H. pylori* bacteria first weaken the protective coating of the stomach and duodenum. Then the acid in the stomach that assists in digestion can irritate the sensitive tissues of the digestive system. Finally, acid and bacteria from the stomach come in direct contact with the digestive system lining, resulting in the sores called ulcers.

* **gastrointestinal** (gas-tro-in-TES-tih-nuhl) means having to do with the organs of the digestive system, the system that processes food. It includes the mouth, esophagus, stomach, intestines, colon, and rectum and other organs involved in digestion, including the liver and pancreas.

* **antibodies** (AN-tih-bah-deez) are protein molecules produced by the body's immune system to help fight specific infections caused by microorganisms, such as bacteria and viruses.

*anemia (uh-NEE-me-uh) is a blood condition in which there is a decreased amount of oxygen-carrying hemoglobin in the blood and, usually, fewer than normal numbers of red blood cells.

antibiotic treatment needs to be repeated over the course of a few months to eliminate the infection.

Are There Complications of *H. pylori* Infection?

A person who has untreated *H. pylori* infection has an increased risk of developing stomach cancer later in life. Long-term loss of blood from the gastrointestinal tract due to ulcers can cause anemia*. Severe untreated ulcers can lead to a perforation, or a hole, when the sore erodes all the way through the lining of the stomach or intestine. Perforations can cause sudden severe bleeding that, in some cases, can be fatal.

Can *H. pylori* Infection Be Prevented?

Although doctors are not sure how *H. pylori* is spread, they believe that washing the hands often with warm, soapy water, especially after using the bathroom and before eating, may help prevent the spread of the infection.

Because water and food can be contaminated with *H. pylori,* it is important to ensure that any water used for drinking or preparation of food comes from a safe source. It also is advisable to heat foods to proper temperatures and to wash utensils and dishes in hot, soapy water.

Because smoking and heavy drinking of alcoholic beverages have been associated with the development of peptic ulcers, avoiding these habits may help prevent the disease.

At present, there is no vaccine against *H. pylori* infection.

Resources

Organizations

The Helicobacter Foundation was founded by Dr. Barry Marshall in 1994 and provides information about the diagnosis and treatment of *H. pylori* infection at its website.
http://www.helico.com

U.S. Centers for Disease Control and Prevention (CDC), 1600 Clifton Road, Atlanta, GA 30333. The CDC posts English and Spanish fact sheets about *H. pylori* and peptic ulcers at its website.
Telephone 800-311-3435
http://www.cdc.gov

U.S. National Digestive Diseases Information Clearinghouse, National Institute of Diabetes and Digestive and Kidney Diseases (NIDDK), National Institutes of Health, 2 Information Way, Bethesda, MD 20892. The NIDDK publishes brochures and posts fact sheets about *H. pylori* and peptic ulcers at its website.
http://www.niddk.nih.gov

► *See also*
Intestinal Infections

Hepatitis, Infectious

Hepatitis (heh-puh-TIE-tis) is an inflammation of the liver*. It can have several different causes, most commonly viral infection.

What Is Infectious Hepatitis?

The liver plays many important roles in the body. It filters out toxins* and other harmful substances from the blood, stores vitamins and nutrients, regulates cholesterol* production, and helps in the production of many other substances the body needs to function normally. Long-term drug or alcohol abuse, exposure to harmful chemicals or other toxins, various infections, trauma*, and certain medications all can damage the liver and lead to hepatitis. Viruses usually cause infectious hepatitis, although other organisms, such as bacteria or parasites, sometimes can be the culprit as well.

Several different viruses can bring about acute* hepatitis, including at least five known hepatitis viruses (A through E). Among these viruses, hepatitis B (HBV) and C (HCV) cause the most serious disease. Most of the time, people recover fully from viral hepatitis. But in some people HBV and HCV cause chronic* hepatitis, in which the infection remains in the body and the liver does not recover completely from the inflammation. Chronic hepatitis eventually can lead to severe liver damage, liver cancer, and sometimes cirrhosis* of the liver. Other viral infections, such as infectious mononucleosis* or "mono," which usually is caused by the Epstein-Barr (EP-steen BAR) virus, can produce short-lived, mild hepatitis.

Types of Viral Hepatitis

Hepatitis A   Among the five major types, hepatitis A virus (HAV) causes the most common and least serious form of hepatitis. It typically spreads through eating food or drinking water contaminated with feces* from someone who is infected. Parts of the world with poor sanitation are at greatest risk for outbreaks of the disease. In the United States, cases of HAV infection sometimes arise when food handlers fail to practice good hygiene, such as regularly washing their hands. HAV also can be transmitted during unprotected sexual intercourse.

Hepatitis B   HBV infection can lead to chronic hepatitis in up to 10 percent of infected adults and older children, in up to 30 percent of infected children younger than 6 years old, and in up to 90 percent of infants who contract the virus from their infected mothers at birth. It is a more serious form of hepatitis because it can cause long-term or permanent liver inflammation and scarring, liver cancer, and liver failure.

KEYWORDS
for searching the Internet and other reference sources

Alpha-interferon

Cirrhosis

Liver disease

Sexually transmitted diseases

* **liver** is a large organ located beneath the ribs on the right side of the body. The liver performs numerous digestive and chemical functions essential for health.

* **toxins** are poisons that harm the body.

* **cholesterol** (ko-LES-ter-ol) is a fatlike substance found in the blood and body tissues.

* **trauma** is severe injury to the body.

* **acute** describes an infection or other illness that comes on suddenly and usually does not last very long.

* **chronic** (KRAH-nik) means continuing for a long period of time.

* **cirrhosis** (sir-O-sis) is a condition that affects the liver, involving long-term inflammation and scarring, which can lead to problems with liver function.

* **mononucleosis** (mah-no-nu-klee-O-sis) is an infectious illness caused by a virus that often leads to fever, sore throat, swollen glands, and tiredness.

* **feces** (FEE-seez) is the excreted waste from the gastrointestinal tract.

* **semen** (SEE-men) is the sperm-containing whitish fluid produced by the male reproductive tract.

* **vaginal** (VAH-jih-nul) refers to the vagina, the canal in a woman that leads from the uterus to the outside of the body.

* **transfusions** (trans-FYOO-zhunz) are procedures in which blood or certain parts of blood, such as specific cells, are given to a person who needs them because of illness or blood loss.

* **kidney** is one of the pair of organs that filter blood and remove waste products and excess water from the body in the form of urine.

* **dialysis** (dye-AL-uh-sis) is a process that removes waste, toxins (poisons), and extra fluid from the blood. Usually dialysis is done when a person's kidneys are unable to perform these functions normally.

* **circumcision** is a surgical procedure in which the fold of skin covering the end of the penis is removed.

HBV can pass easily from person to person through direct contact with infected blood and other body fluids, including semen*, vaginal* fluids, and sometimes saliva. It most often is spread through unprotected sexual intercourse, injection of drugs with contaminated needles, blood transfusions*, kidney* dialysis*, organ transplants, or from a mother to her child during birth. HBV also can be transmitted if improperly sterilized equipment is used during body piercing, tattooing, or circumcision*. Health care workers are advised to take precautions to avoid accidental sticks from needles used in the care of patients, because patients might be infected with the virus.

Hepatitis C Like HBV, HCV can spread through direct contact with infected body fluids, especially blood. HCV most often is transmitted through the sharing of needles by injection drug users. In the United States, up to 90 percent of cases occur this way. Patients receiving long-term dialysis for kidney failure are also at relatively higher risk of HCV infection. The infection can result in long-lasting complications. About 80 percent of those who contract HCV may develop chronic hepatitis, which can put them at risk for other forms of serious liver disease. HCV infection is the most common reason for liver transplants in the United States.

Hepatitis D Hepatitis D virus (HDV) infection is found only in those who also have been infected with HBV. HDV is passed from person to person in the same way as HBV. Co-infection can transform a mild HBV infection or an infection that has no symptoms at all into a more serious, rapidly progressing disease. HDV usually spreads through contact with infected blood, most often from injection drug use with contaminated needles.

Hepatitis E Like HAV, hepatitis E virus (HEV) is transmitted through drinking water contaminated with infected feces. HEV infection occurs most often in underdeveloped countries with poor sanitation.

How Common Is Viral Hepatitis?

Infectious hepatitis is common all over the world. Each year HAV infects up to 1.4 million people worldwide, including about 250,000 Americans. Most cases in the United States are seen in children less than 10 years of age. According to the U.S. Centers for Disease Control and Prevention (CDC), at least 80,000 people in the United States are infected with HBV each year, and about 5,000 die from the disease annually. Africa and parts of South America and Asia, especially the Middle East, all have high rates of HAV and HBV infection. The World Health Organization (WHO) estimates that there are 170 million people infected with HCV around the globe, with 3 million to 4 million new cases appearing annually. About 4 million people in the United States have HCV, with about 25,000 new cases diagnosed each year.

What Are the Signs and Symptoms of Hepatitis?

Common symptoms of all forms of acute infectious hepatitis include extreme tiredness, loss of appetite, fever, headache, muscle and joint aches, nausea, vomiting, diarrhea, jaundice*, and stomach pain. Bowel movements may look pale in color, and urine may become dark, so that it looks like tea. Children infected with HAV frequently have few or no signs of illness, and people with HCV infection often show no symptoms or have only mild symptoms like those of the flu until the disease has caused serious liver damage.

How Do Doctors Make the Diagnosis?

Hepatitis is diagnosed by blood tests, which can show that the liver is inflamed and indicate how well it is working. Blood tests can also reveal which type of hepatitis virus is causing the disease. When a person is very ill from hepatitis or remains sick for a long time, a biopsy* of the liver may be done to determine whether the liver is becoming damaged or scarred.

What Is the Treatment for Hepatitis?

Treatment for viral hepatitis depends on its cause and how sick the patient is.

Hepatitis A and E   People with HAV and HEV infection usually recover completely without needing hospitalization. They can take care of themselves at home by making sure they get enough rest and drink plenty of fluids. Doctors advise avoiding alcohol and drugs, because these substances can stress an already inflamed liver.

Hepatitis B and C   Most of the time, HBV and HCV infection can be monitored with blood tests that look for liver inflammation and measure liver function. In severe cases of viral hepatitis, hospitalization may be necessary, especially when the liver is damaged and stops working well. Medications, including alpha-interferon (AL-fa in-ter-FEER-on) injections, may be given to help the body's immune system fight chronic hepatitis B, C, and D. It is recommended that people who have chronic infectious hepatitis live a healthy lifestyle by avoiding alcohol, getting enough sleep, exercising regularly, and eating a nutritious diet. These measures reduce stress on the liver and can prevent or slow the progression of long-term liver disease.

What to Expect

People typically recover completely from HAV or HEV infection within about 2 months, but sometimes it takes longer. Those infected with HBV or HCV usually recover within 6 months. Cases of chronic viral hepatitis can last for decades or even a lifetime. HBV and HCV can lead to scarring of the liver, liver cancer, liver failure, and sometimes death. A liver transplant may be required in cases that progress to liver failure.

* **jaundice** (JON-dis) is a yellowing of the skin, and sometimes the whites of the eyes, caused by a buildup in the body of bilirubin, a chemical produced in and released by the liver. An increase in bilirubin may indicate disease of the liver or certain blood disorders.

* **biopsy** (BI-op-see) is a test in which a small sample of body tissue is removed and examined for signs of disease.

*vaccine (vak-SEEN) is a preparation of killed or weakened germs, or a part of a germ or product it produces, given to prevent or lessen the severity of the disease that can result if a person is exposed to the germ itself. Use of vaccines for this purpose is called immunization.

*immune globulin (ih-MYOON GLAH-byoo-lin), also called gamma globulin, is the protein material that contains antibodies.

How Can Hepatitis Be Prevented?

A vaccine* exists for HAV, but it is not used routinely in the United States, except in areas where the number of cases is consistently high, as seen in several western states. The vaccine is recommended for certain laboratory workers, anyone who has more than one sexual partner or who engages in other high-risk types of behavior, or people traveling to underdeveloped areas of the world with poor sanitation. People who come into contact with HAV can be treated with immune globulin*, which is more than 85 percent effective in preventing HAV infection if treatment begins within 2 weeks after exposure to the virus. The best way to prevent HAV and HEV is to practice good hygiene, such as frequent hand washing. Avoiding areas of poor sanitation and unwashed or uncooked food, particularly while traveling, can limit the risk of infection as well.

Today, infants in the United States typically are vaccinated against HBV by age 2 years. Infants born to mothers with HBV infection generally are given immediate injections of HBV immune globulin and receive their first dose of the HBV vaccine within 12 hours of birth. It is recommended that all teens and adults who are at high risk of exposure to infected body fluids, such as health care workers, receive the HBV vaccine. Since HDV infects only those who already have HBV, vaccination against HBV can prevent HDV as well. Using latex condoms for all forms of sexual intercourse also can help protect against HBV. Avoiding intravenous drug use and sharing of razors, toothbrushes, or needles, even for tattoos or body piercing, can help prevent both HBV and HCV. Since 1992 blood banks in the United States have screened donated blood for HBV and HCV. Currently, there is no vaccine for HCV.

Resources

Organizations

American Liver Foundation, 75 Maiden Lane, Suite 603, New York, NY 10038. The American Liver Foundation is a national nonprofit organization dedicated to the prevention, treatment, and cure of hepatitis and other liver diseases. It posts articles on liver health at its website.
Telephone 800-465-4837
http://www.liverfoundation.org

Hepatitis Foundation International, 504 Blick Drive, Silver Spring, MD 20904. The Hepatitis Foundation International offers information on hepatitis at its website, as well as counseling via its toll-free hotline.
Telephone 800-891-0707
http://www.hepfi.org

KidsHealth.org. KidsHealth is a website created by the medical experts of the Nemours Foundation and is devoted to issues of children's health. It contains articles on a variety of health topics, including hepatitis.
http://www.KidsHealth.org

Herpes Simplex Virus Infections

Herpes simplex (HER-peez SIM-plex) virus is a virus that can cause several types of infections, including sores on the skin, usually around the mouth or in the genital* area.

What Is Herpes Simplex Virus?

There are two types of the herpes simplex virus (HSV): HSV-1 and HSV-2. Both are part of the herpesvirus (her-peez-VY-rus) family, a group of viruses with similar traits that also includes the varicella zoster (var-uh-SEH-luh ZOS-ter) virus, which causes chicken pox, and the Epstein-Barr (EP-steen BAR) virus, which causes infectious mononucleosis.

HSV-1 causes small, clear blisters (also known as cold sores, fever blisters, or oral herpes) on the skin. Cold sores usually occur on the face, particularly around the mouth and nose, but they can pop up anywhere on the skin or mucous membranes*. They may show up one at a time or in groups. The painful blisters can break, bleed, and crust over, leaving red spots of healing skin. When the sores appear, this is known as a herpes outbreak.

High-school and college wrestlers sometimes develop herpes blisters on their shoulders and back from close contact with one another and from virus-contaminated mats, a condition called herpes gladiatorum. Rugby players also commonly pass along HSV-1 through close physical contact during matches, with the blisters nicknamed "scrum pox." Small HSV-1 sores known as herpetic whitlow can appear on the fingers, especially in children who bite their nails or suck their fingers, which spreads the virus from the mouth to the hands. HSV-1 infection can occur in other situations as well when the virus comes in contact with broken skin.

Although the HSV-1 virus occasionally causes blisters in the genital area, it is usually HSV-2, also known as genital herpes, that causes sores on the penis in sexually active males and on the vulva*, vagina, and cervix* in sexually active females. Both sexes can develop herpes blisters around the anus and on the buttocks. HSV-2 occasionally produces sores on other parts of the body, such as the mouth or throat. Having genital herpes also increases a person's risk of getting HIV (the virus that

▶ *See also*
Mononucleosis, Infectious
Sexually Transmitted Diseases

KEYWORDS
for searching the Internet and other reference sources
Cold sores
Fever blisters
Genital herpes
Herpes gladiatorum
Herpes keratitis
Herpes labialis
Herpes simplex
Herpesvirus family
Herpetic whitlow
HSV-1
HSV-2
Oral herpes

* **genital** (JEH-nih-tul) refers to the external sexual organs.

* **mucous membranes** are the moist linings of the mouth, nose, eyes, and throat.

* **vulva** (VUL-vuh) refers to the organs of the female genitals that are located on the outside of the body.

* **cervix** (SIR-viks) is the lower, narrow end of the uterus that opens into the vagina.

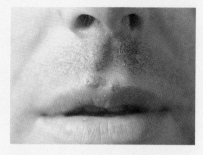

▲

Herpes simplex virus type 1 causes small, clear blisters to appear around the mouth and nose. Also called cold sores, fever blisters, or sun blisters, they typically unite to form a larger sore. *Custom Medical Stock Photo, Inc.*

** **AIDS,** or acquired immunodeficiency (ih-myoo-no-dih-FIH-shensee) syndrome, is an infection that severely weakens the immune system; it is caused by the human immunodeficiency virus (HIV).*

causes AIDS*) if he or she has unprotected sex with a person who is HIV-positive.

When the herpes simplex virus enters the body for the first time, this is called a primary infection. Once primary infection occurs, HSV-1 and HSV-2 remain in the body for life. The virus travels to the body's nerve cells and lies dormant (inactive) until it reactivates, as during a herpes outbreak. Emotional or physical stresses (like exhaustion or an illness), sun exposure, menstruation, or fever can all trigger such an outbreak, but sometimes active herpes infection returns for no apparent reason. These outbreaks are known as recurrent infections. Recurrent infections often appear close to or at the area where the primary infection occurred. For example, repeated outbreaks of HSV-1 may cause cold sores in the same spot along the outer border of the lips, but they also can occur anywhere around the mouth.

How Common Is Herpes Simplex Virus?

Both HSV-1 and HSV-2 are common. Between 50 and 80 percent of adults in the United States are infected with oral herpes by age 30. It is estimated that every year up to 1 million people in the United States become infected with genital herpes, and the disease is on the rise among sexually active adults. According to the U.S. Centers for Disease Control and Prevention, at least 45 million people, or about one in five adolescents and adults, in the United States now have genital herpes.

How Is Herpes Simplex Virus Spread?

Both types of herpes simplex virus are contagious, which means they can be passed from person to person. Both types can spread when someone comes into direct contact with an infected person's skin or saliva. Many people with oral herpes first became infected when they were children, perhaps from contact with a family member. Kissing or sharing dishes or eating utensils with someone who has oral herpes can lead to HSV-1 infection.

If a person has unprotected vaginal, oral, or anal sex with someone infected with HSV-2 (whether or not sores are present on the skin at the time of sexual contact), that person is at risk for contracting genital herpes. HSV-2 does not spread from toilet seats or hot tubs.

People with either HSV-1 or HSV-2 can pass the virus to others even when they do not have an active herpes outbreak. Research suggests that at least 60 percent of new cases of herpes simplex are acquired when the person transmitting the infection has no noticeable blisters or sores.

What Happens When Someone Has Herpes Simplex Virus?

Signs and symptoms Symptoms of an active HSV-1, or oral herpes, infection may include:

- tenderness, tingling, or itching in the spot where the blister eventually appears
- blisters or sores (which are often painful) on the lips, face, neck, and shoulders
- fever or symptoms like those of the flu

Symptoms of an active HSV-2, or genital herpes, infection may include:
- fever or symptoms like those of the flu
- reddish rash
- itching or tingling of the genitals
- swollen glands (lymph nodes)
- burning feeling during urination
- muscle aches
- discharge from the vagina or penis
- blisters or sores (which are often painful)

Diagnosis Doctors can often diagnose outbreaks of HSV-1 or HSV-2 based upon the appearance and location of the sores. Sometimes, however, sores in the genital region may be difficult to recognize, as they can resemble those of other sexually transmitted infections.

Tests to positively diagnose herpes simplex infection involve scraping the blister and culturing* the sample to see if the herpes virus grows. Sometimes, doctors use a Tzanck preparation, a scraping of a blister examined under a microscope to look for signs of the virus, to help quickly confirm a diagnosis. A doctor may also take a sample of a person's blood to look for antibodies* to the herpes virus or to test for evidence of herpes DNA* in the blood.

Treatment There is no cure for either type of the herpes simplex virus. Currently, antiviral medications can help control outbreaks of herpes virus and are used to treat genital herpes or sometimes recurrent cold sores from HSV-1. Some over-the-counter ointments or creams may help reduce the pain of cold sores, but they do not necessarily speed healing or prevent the sores from returning. For painful herpes simplex outbreaks, applying ice to the area, drinking cold drinks, or taking over-the-counter pain medication such as acetaminophen (uh-see-teh-MIH-noh-fen) can ease discomfort. People with active cold sores may also want to avoid acidic foods such as tomatoes, lemons, and oranges because these can irritate open sores on the lips or in the mouth.

Both HSV-1 and HSV-2 remain in the body for life and can cause future outbreaks, the severity of which varies greatly from person to person. When someone develops a primary infection, the symptoms may last from 2 to 4 weeks. The course of recurrent herpes infections is usually shorter than the primary one.

Don't Confuse Canker Sores and Cold Sores

What is the difference between cold sores and canker sores? Canker sores are small, red sores inside the mouth that turn white. Unlike cold sores, canker sores are not caused by the herpes simplex virus. Doctors and scientists think that stress may cause canker sores, but they are not sure. Both canker sores and cold sores are painful, but canker sores only appear inside the mouth, not on the face, lips, or neck, where cold sores occur.

* **culturing** (KUL-chur-ing) means subjecting to a test in which a sample of fluid or tissue from the body is placed in a dish containing material that supports the growth of certain organisms. Typically, within days the organisms will grow and can be identified.

* **antibodies** (AN-tih-bah-deez) are protein molecules produced by the body's immune system to help fight specific infections caused by microorganisms, such as bacteria and viruses.

* **DNA**, or deoxyribonucleic acid (dee-OX-see-ry-bo-nyoo-klay-ik AH-sid), is the specialized chemical substance that contains the genetic code necessary to build and maintain the structures and functions of living organisms.

On average, people with genital herpes experience 4 to 5 outbreaks of herpes each year. Although the virus will always be in the body, over time the number of outbreaks usually decreases.

Complications   People with either type of herpes simplex infection may experience pain, embarrassment, or emotional stress when they have an outbreak, although the infections usually are not dangerous.

In rare cases, however, (usually in people with weakened immune systems) herpes can infect the skin surrounding the eye. The virus then can enter the eye's cornea*, causing a condition called herpes keratitis. This may lead to scarring of the eye and blindness if left untreated.

Infants born to women with genital herpes are at risk for serious complications from HSV-2 infection as they pass through the birth canal during delivery, particularly if the woman has an outbreak of sores. People who have immune systems weakened by disease, such as people with cancer or AIDS, or those with an organ transplant can also become very ill and may die from herpes simplex infection. The virus can spread throughout the body, causing life-threatening infections in the lungs, liver*, and other organs. In some cases, herpes simplex may also infect the brain, causing a dangerous inflammation known as viral encephalitis (en-seh-fuh-LYE-tis).

Can Infection with Herpes Simplex Virus Be Prevented?

There is no vaccine* against either HSV-1 or HSV-2, but researchers are working to develop one. Because so many people have oral herpes and because HSV-1 can be spread even when people do not have visible blisters, it is difficult to prevent. To reduce the risk of getting oral herpes, experts recommend not kissing someone with active cold sores and not sharing lipstick, towels, razors, silverware, food, glasses, or utensils with anyone, especially someone who has had cold sores or currently has them.

Using sunscreen when outside, especially on areas prone to blisters, may reduce the likelihood of an outbreak of cold sores in anyone infected with HSV-1. Experts advise that people with active cold sores around the mouth always wash their hands before touching the genitals or buttocks.

Ways of reducing the risk of getting genital herpes include practicing abstinence (not having sex) or by always using a latex condom, because someone with genital herpes is contagious even if no blisters are visible. A condom does not protect all of the skin in the genital region, so anyone with known genital herpes should not have sex during outbreaks of blisters.

* **cornea** (KOR-nee-uh) is the transparent circular layer of cells over the central colored part of the eyeball (the iris) through which light enters the eye.

* **liver** is a large organ located beneath the ribs on the right side of the body. The liver performs numerous digestive and chemical functions essential for health.

* **vaccine** (vak-SEEN) is a preparation of killed or weakened germs, or a part of a germ or product it produces, given to prevent or lessen the severity of the disease that can result if a person is exposed to the germ itself. Use of vaccines for this purpose is called immunization.

Resources

Organizations

American Social Health Association (ASHA), P.O. Box 13827, Research Triangle Park, NC 27709. The ASHA provides information about herpes symptoms and prevention methods in its National Herpes Resource Center. The ASHA also operates the National Herpes Hotline, to provide referrals and information to anyone with questions about herpes.
Telephone 919-361-8488
http://www.ashastd.org

U.S. Centers for Disease Control and Prevention (CDC), 1600 Clifton Road, Atlanta, GA 30333. The CDC is the U.S. government authority for information about infectious and other diseases. The CDC's division of STD prevention offers information about genital herpes and how to prevent it and other sexually transmitted diseases, as well as a hotline to call for questions about herpes and other STDs.
Telephone 800-227-8922
http://www.cdc.gov/std

Website

KidsHealth.org. KidsHealth is a website created by the medical experts of the Nemours Foundation and is devoted to issues of children's health. It contains articles on a variety of health topics, including herpes.
http://www.KidsHealth.org

▶ *See also*

AIDS and HIV Infection

Encephalitis

Mononucleosis, Infectious

Sexually Transmitted Diseases

Varicella (Chicken Pox) and Herpes Zoster (Shingles)

HPV (Human papillomavirus) *See* Warts

I

Immune Deficiencies

Immune deficiencies (ih-MYOON dih-FIH-shen-seez) are conditions that impair the body's immune system so that it is less capable of fighting infection.

What Are Immune Deficiencies?

Immune deficiencies arise when one or more of the parts of the immune system are missing or not working correctly, leaving the body less able to fight disease-causing agents. There are two types of these deficiencies: primary, or inherited, immune deficiencies and secondary, or acquired, immune deficiencies.

The immune system has many parts that work together to protect the body from foreign invaders, such as microorganisms* and toxins*. When any segment of the immune system is absent or breaks down, it can lead to an immune deficiency. With so many elements of the immune system, there are more than 80 different types of primary immune deficiencies. They range from those that have severe and sometimes fatal effects to mild diseases that cause people few, if any, problems. About half a million people in the United States have some type of primary immune deficiency, with more boys than girls affected by these conditions.

Secondary immune deficiencies are much more common than inherited deficiencies. Unlike patients with primary immune deficiencies, people with secondary immune deficiencies are born with a healthy immune system, but sometime later in life the system becomes weakened or damaged. Both primary and secondary deficiencies typically lead to frequent infections and sometimes to additional medical problems, including certain cancers. These people often experience a variety of skin, respiratory, and bone problems as well, and they are more likely to have autoimmune diseases*.

Overview of the Immune System

The immune system consists of a group of organs, cells, and a specialized system called the lymphatic (lim-FAH-tik) system that helps clear infectious agents from the body. Together, they guard the body against infectious diseases. The lymphatic system is a key part of the immune system: it consists of lymphatic vessels, lymph nodes*, and the thymus (THY-mus) and spleen. Lymph nodes and lymphatic vessels transport

KEYWORDS
for searching the Internet
and other reference sources

Acquired immunodeficiency syndrome (AIDS)

Human immunodeficiency virus (HIV)

Hypogammaglobulinemia

Immune response

Immune system

Primary immune deficiencies

Secondary immune deficiencies

Selective IgA deficiency

Severe combined immunodeficiency disease (SCID)

X-linked agammaglobulinemia

* **microorganisms** are tiny organisms that can be seen only using a microscope. Types of microorganisms include fungi, bacteria, and viruses.

* **toxins** are poisons that harm the body.

* **autoimmune** (aw-toh-ih-MYOON) **diseases** are diseases in which the body's immune system attacks some of the body's own normal tissues and cells.

* **lymph** (LIMF) **nodes** are small, bean-shaped masses of tissue that contain immune system cells that fight harmful microorganisms. Lymph nodes may swell during infections.

lymph, a clear fluid that contains white blood cells called lymphocytes (LIM-fo-sites), throughout the body. The lymphocytes mature in the thymus, a gland located behind the breastbone. The spleen, an organ that is the center of certain immune system activities, is found in the upper-left side of the abdomen. Lymphatic tissue also is found in other locations throughout the body, including the tonsils* and the appendix*.

When a foreign substance or microorganism enters the body, phagocytes (FAH-go-sites) often are the first cells on the scene. These large scavenger white blood cells patrol the bloodstream, looking for possible invaders. When they find one, they engulf, digest, and destroy the intruder.

Other components of the immune response react when presented with specific antigens*. The most important players in this fight are two types of lymphocytes that learn to "recognize" and destroy the foreign invaders.

B cells, the first type, are white blood cells that produce antibodies*, which circulate in the blood and lymph streams. The first time B cells encounter a new foreign substance, they make antibodies in response to the intruder's antigens. When the antibodies come across that specific antigen again, they attach themselves to it, marking it (and with it, the entire foreign substance or microorganism) for destruction by other cells. Antibodies also summon phagocytes and body chemicals, such as complement proteins*, to the site of an infection and move them into action against the antigens.

T cells, the second type, are specialized white blood cells that have several roles. They monitor and coordinate the entire immune response, which includes recruiting many different cells to take part in that response. Some T cells, the T helper cells, signal the B cells to start making antibodies. Other T cells, the T killer cells, attack and destroy substances that they recognize as foreign. Once the foreign antigens have been defeated, cleanup crews of scavenger phagocytes called neutrophils (NU-tro-fils), a type of white blood cell that can surround and destroy invading organisms, and macrophages (MAH-kro-fay-jez), another form of engulf-and-destroy cell, arrive to clear up remains of the infection.

Primary Immune Deficiencies

A genetic* abnormality in any type of cell of the immune system can lead to a primary immune deficiency. Some of these deficiencies produce no symptoms, whereas others cause severe symptoms and may even be fatal. Although primary immune deficiencies are present at birth, some patients do not begin to show signs of the condition until later in childhood or even beyond childhood.

There are several well-known primary immune deficiencies. About 1 person in 600 is born with selective IgA deficiency, a mild disease that most often affects those of European ancestry. People with this condition lack immunoglobulin (ih-myoo-no-GLAH-byoo-lin) A (IgA), a

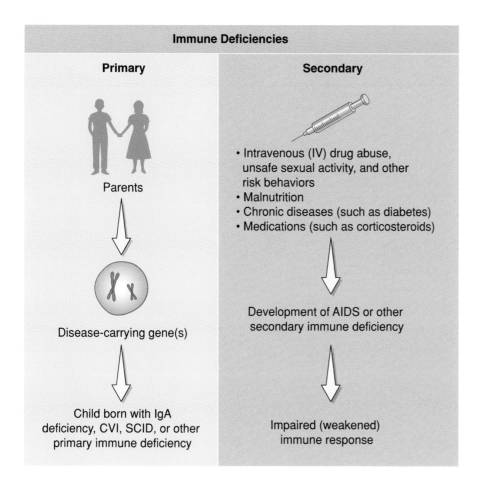

Immune Deficiencies

Primary

Parents

Disease-carrying gene(s)

Child born with IgA
deficiency, CVI, SCID, or other
primary immune deficiency

Secondary

• Intravenous (IV) drug abuse,
unsafe sexual activity, and other
risk behaviors
• Malnutrition
• Chronic diseases (such as diabetes)
• Medications (such as corticosteroids)

Development of AIDS or other
secondary immune deficiency

Impaired (weakened)
immune response

The SCID Mouse

To gain a better understanding of the human immune system, scientists developed a laboratory mouse that lacks an enzyme* necessary for its immune system to function properly. Like people with severe combined immunodeficiency disease, these "SCID" mice cannot fight infections.

Another very useful mouse model was developed in the 1980s, when scientists transplanted parts of the human immune system into the mouse. This gave an opportunity to researchers to study the workings of the human immune response more easily, as well as the impact of drugs and viruses on the immune system. This mouse has been described as a "living test tube."

* **enzyme** (EN-zime) is a protein that helps speed up a chemical reaction in the body.

---

class of antibodies that fight organisms that can infect the mucous membranes that line the mouth, airways, and digestive system*. Many patients with this disorder experience few symptoms, but some may have frequent infections.

The effects of common variable immunodeficiency, also known as hypogammaglobulinemia (hi-po-gah-muh-gloh-byoo-lih-NEE-me-uh), can range from mild to severe. Its symptoms occasionally affect infants but often do not appear until early adulthood. Those symptoms include frequent bacterial infections of the ears, sinuses*, bronchi*, or lungs brought on by low levels of various immunoglobulins, including IgA and IgG.

Caused by defective genes on the X chromosome*, X-linked agammaglobulinemia (a-gah-muh-gloh-byoo-lih-NEE-me-uh) is uncommon and affects only males. Patients have very low levels of mature B cells as well as low levels of immunoglobulins, which can result in pus* collections in the lungs, sinuses, and ears in addition to other infections.

Severe combined immunodeficiency (ih-myoo-no-dih-FIH-shen-see), also known as SCID or the "bubble boy" disease, strikes about 1 in a

* **sinuses** (SY-nuh-ses) are hollow, air-filled cavities in the facial bones.

* **bronchi** (BRONG-kye) are the larger tube-like airways that carry air in and out of the lungs.

* **chromosome** is a unit or strand of DNA, the chemical substance that contains the genetic code to build and maintain a living being. Humans have 23 pairs of chromosomes, for a total of 46.

* **pus** is a thick, creamy fluid, usually yellow or greenish in color, that forms at the site of an infection. Pus contains infection-fighting white cells and other substances.

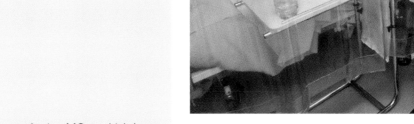

Organisms that typically do not cause problems in a person with a healthy immune system may produce an "opportunistic infection" in a person with an immune deficiency. A person particularly at risk for such infections might be placed in isolation in a sterile environment. *Custom Medical Stock Photo, Inc.* ▶

* **pneumonia** (nu-MO-nyah) is inflammation of the lung.

* **sepsis** is a potentially serious spreading of infection, usually bacterial, through the bloodstream and body.

* **meningitis** (meh-nin-JY-tis) is an inflammation of the meninges, the membranes that surround the brain and the spinal cord. Meningitis is most often caused by infection with a virus or a bacterium.

* **chronic** (KRAH-nik) means continuing for a long period of time.

* **diabetes** (dye-uh-BEE-teez) is a condition in which the body's pancreas does not produce enough insulin or the body cannot use the insulin it makes effectively, resulting in increased levels of sugar in the blood. This can lead to increased urination, dehydration, weight loss, weakness, and a number of other symptoms and complications related to chemical imbalances within the body.

* **cirrhosis** (sir-O-sis) is a condition that affects the liver, involving long-term inflammation and scarring, which can lead to problems with liver function.

million people. This group of immune disorders is marked by major deficiencies in B cells and T cells, low levels of white blood cells, and decreased levels of IgA, IgG, and IgM antibodies. Such massive defects in the immune system can leave patients open to many serious infections, including pneumonia*, sepsis*, and meningitis*, which can lead to death.

Other primary immune deficiency diseases may involve other components of the immune system, including neutrophils and phagocytes. There may be fewer of these cells produced, as occurs in a condition known as neutropenia (nu-tro-PEE-nee-uh) that is marked by low levels of neutrophils in the blood. Chronic* granulomatous (gran-yoo-LO-muh-tus) disease is an immune disorder in which bacteria-fighting phagocytes are present but do not work properly. Genetic defects also can impair the complement system, a series of 20 or more proteins that come together during the body's immune response to "complement," or support, the work of antibodies. These conditions and defects in other parts of the complex immune system cause problems with the body's immune response, often making a person more susceptible to a variety of infections.

Secondary Immune Deficiencies

Secondary immune deficiencies are acquired, rather than inherited, disorders. Many chronic conditions, such as diabetes*, cancer, and cirrhosis* of the liver, make a person more likely to have infections. Patients who have had their spleens removed or whose spleens do not work properly, as occurs in sickle-cell disease*, for example, are especially vulnerable to infection by certain bacteria that the spleen normally fights. In addition, some medications, particularly corticosteroids* and drugs used to treat cancer, may limit the immune system. Malnutrition, especially when there is a lack of protein in the diet, also may weaken a person's immune response.

The human immunodeficiency virus (HIV), a virus that attacks the immune system and is the cause of acquired immunodeficiency syndrome (AIDS), is responsible for a sharp increase in the number of people with secondary immune deficiencies. HIV destroys T cells, which are crucial to the normal functioning of the human immune system. This can lead to overwhelming infections. People can contract the virus through contact with blood, semen*, vaginal* secretions, and breast milk.

What Are the Signs and Symptoms of Immune Deficiencies?

Immune deficiencies may be characterized by frequent, recurrent, or prolonged infections. In some cases, there may be an overwhelming or unusual infection. In others, organisms that typically do not cause problems in a person with a healthy immune system may produce an opportunistic infection* in a person with an immune deficiency. These infections are seen in people infected with HIV and often mark the onset of AIDS.

Other immune deficiencies are characterized by chronic opportunistic infections. Depending on the condition, patients may experience recurrent lung and sinus infections, weakness, tiredness, a lingering cough, diarrhea (dye-uh-REE-uh), skin rashes, and hair loss. Many patients simply look sick. Signs of immune deficiencies also include poor response to treatments, incomplete or slow recovery from illness, fungal or yeast infections that keep coming back, and certain specific infections, such as pneumonia caused by *Pneumocystis carinii* (nu-mo-SIS-tis kah-RIH-nee-eye).

How Do Doctors Make the Diagnosis?

Although symptoms of opportunistic infections may suggest an immune deficiency, laboratory tests are needed to diagnose the specific deficiency. These include blood tests to measure levels of white blood cells, red blood cells, and platelets* and to measure the presence of specific types of cells, such as B cells and T cells. Other blood tests can measure the levels or function of antibodies (such as IgA, IgG, and IgM) and complement proteins. Skin tests may be done to check the responses of T cells. Other, more specific tests of the immune system's competency depend on the type of deficiency suspected.

How Are Immune Deficiencies Treated?

The primary goal of treating immune deficiencies is to prevent infections. Although it is a good idea for some people who have immune deficiencies to avoid contact with people who have infections, this is not always practical. Many patients take daily medication to prevent certain infections, and patients with antibody deficiencies may receive regular

** **sickle-cell disease** is a hereditary condition in which the red blood cells, which are usually round, take on an abnormal crescent shape and have a decreased ability to carry oxygen throughout the body.

* **corticosteroids** (kor-tih-ko-STIR-oyds) are chemical substances made by the adrenal glands that have several functions in the body, including maintaining blood pressure during stress and controlling inflammation. They can also be given to people as medication to treat certain illnesses.

* **semen** (SEE-men) is the sperm-containing whitish fluid produced by the male reproductive tract.

* **vaginal** (VAH-jih-nul) refers to the vagina, the canal in a woman that leads from the uterus to the outside of the body.

* **opportunistic infections** are infections caused by infectious agents that usually do not produce disease in people with healthy immune systems but can cause widespread and severe illness in patients with weak or faulty immune systems.

* **platelets** (PLATE-lets) are tiny disk-shaped particles within the blood that play an important role in clotting.*

* **bone marrow** is the soft tissue inside bones where blood cells are made.

doses of the immunoglobulins they lack. People who have HIV or AIDS take combinations of drugs to keep the virus from making more copies of itself and destroying more T cells. Bone marrow* transplantation, to replace the absent or poorly functioning immune system cells of the affected person, is necessary for some patients with severe immune deficiencies, such as SCID. Prompt recognition and treatment of infections, including opportunistic infections, is essential.

Resources

Organizations

Immune Deficiency Foundation, 40 W. Chesapeake Avenue, Suite 308, Towson, MD 21204. The Immune Deficiency Foundation offers information on primary immune deficiencies and an overview of the immune system just for kids at its website.
Telephone 800-296-4433
http://www.primaryimmune.org

Jeffrey Modell Foundation, 747 Third Avenue, New York, NY 10017. The Jeffrey Modell Foundation is a nonprofit research foundation devoted to primary immune deficiencies.
Telephone 212-819-0200
http://www.jmfworld.org

▶ *See also*
AIDS and HIV Infection
Body Defenses
Meningitis
Pneumonia
Sepsis

KEYWORDS
for searching the Internet and other reference sources

Pandemic

Respiratory infection

Spanish flu

Vaccination

Viral infection

Influenza

Influenza (in-floo-EN-zuh), also known as the flu, is a contagious viral infection that attacks the respiratory tract, including the nose, throat, and lungs.

What Is Influenza?

The respiratory infection influenza, commonly known as the flu, causes symptoms that include fever, muscle aches, sore throat, and a cough. Once inhaled, flu germs quickly multiply and take over healthy cells. In its early stages, influenza sometimes is confused with the common cold because both affect similar body parts, but the flu is more severe, lasts longer, and can cause dangerous complications.

Flu viruses come in three varieties: types A, B, and C. Types A and B cause large flu outbreaks or epidemics* each year, whereas the less common Type C flu virus causes only mild symptoms. Usually, if people have been infected by a virus or are vaccinated against the virus, their bodies build up immunity* that defends them from being infected by that particular virus again. Flu viruses, however, can cause epidemics be-

* **epidemics** (eh-pih-DEH-miks) are outbreaks of diseases, especially infectious diseases, in which the number of cases suddenly becomes far greater than usual. Usually, epidemics that involve worldwide outbreaks are called pandemics.

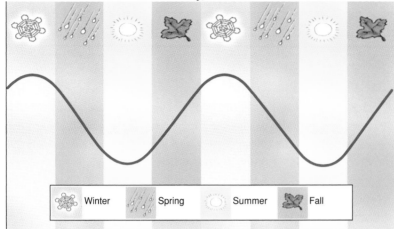

Pneumonia and Influenza Mortality, Winter Peaks and Summer Lows

Pneumonia- and Influenza-related Deaths

| Winter | Spring | Summer | Fall |

Seasons

Source: Centers for Disease Control and Prevention (CDC)

Cases of influenza virus infection typically peak in the fall and winter and decrease in the warmer months. During the 1918 pandemic, the virus killed more than 33,000 people in New York City alone, just over 1% of the city's population.

cause they have the ability to mutate (change) so that new strains of viruses appear regularly. This is why people who are at risk for complications of flu need to get a flu vaccination every year.

How Common Is Influenza?

Millions of Americans of all ages contract the flu each year, but the people most at risk of severe illness are people over 65 years of age, children under age 5, and anyone with a serious medical condition. Flu season is November through April in the United States.

Influenza is extremely contagious, mostly because people (especially school children) often spread it before they even know that they are sick. Also, those with the infection usually remain contagious for about a week after first showing symptoms.

When an infected person sneezes, coughs, or talks too closely to others, the flu virus is passed through tiny drops of fluid that are launched into the air and can be breathed in by someone else. The virus can also be left on surfaces that a person with the flu has touched, such as doorknobs, desks, and keyboards, so people who forget to wash their hands after touching these things can easily become infected by rubbing their eyes or touching their mouth.

How Do People Know They Have the Flu?

Flu symptoms are usually worse than those seen with a cold. Symptoms include:

- sneezing, runny nose, and congestion (stuffed-up nose)
- high fever

* **immunity** (ih-MYOON-uh-tee) is the condition of being protected against an infectious disease. Immunity often develops after a germ is introduced to the body. One type of immunity occurs when the body makes special protein molecules called antibodies to fight the disease-causing germ. The next time that germ enters the body, the antibodies quickly attack it, usually preventing the germ from causing disease.

What Is the Stomach Flu?

When people complain about the stomach flu, what they actually are describing is gastroenteritis (gas-tro-en-ter-EYE-tis). The stomach cramps, nausea, and vomiting that accompany a bout of gastroenteritis usually only last a day or two and are different from the group of symptoms seen with influenza virus infection.

* abdominal (ab-DAH-mih-nul) refers to the area of the body below the ribs and above the hips that contains the stomach, intestines, and other organs.

* bronchitis (brong-KYE-tis) is a disease that involves inflammation of the larger airways in the respiratory tract, which can result from infection or other causes.

* pneumonia (nu-MO-nyah) is inflammation of the lung.

* chronic (KRAH-nik) means continuing for a long period of time.

* asthma (AZ-mah) is a condition in which the airways of the lungs repeatedly become narrowed and inflamed, causing breathing difficulty.

- headache
- chills
- dry-sounding cough
- muscle aches
- abdominal* pain and poor appetite
- tiredness

Most people have symptoms of the flu for 7 to 14 days. The high fever and body aches usually disappear within a few days, but those symptoms may be quickly replaced by a sore throat, runny nose, and lingering cough. In some cases, fever may even return for a brief period. Feelings of tiredness and exhaustion can last several days or weeks in some people with the flu. Trying to return to a normal routine too quickly can cause symptoms, especially exhaustion, to reoccur.

Sometimes people with the flu develop bronchitis* or pneumonia*. Pneumonia can be a serious complication of the flu. It usually occurs when bacteria infect lung tissue that is already inflamed by the flu virus. This complication can be life threatening in young infants and in elderly people. Influenza can also worsen the symptoms of other common heart and lung diseases, such as congestive heart failure, chronic* bronchitis, and asthma*.

The flu can knock even the healthiest people off their feet for a couple of weeks. Most people recover with time and rest, but for some people with chronic medical conditions, the flu can pose a severe health risk and can even be deadly. Hundreds of thousands of Americans are hospitalized every year due to the virus, and about 20,000 die from the flu or its complications.

Because the flu can go from bad to worse very quickly, doctors recommend that people with the flu seek medical care immediately if they experience any of the following:

FLU ON THE FRONT LINES

In 1918, the world was blindsided by the most catastrophic flu outbreak of all time. In the midst of World War I, the flu virus spread to nations around the globe through soldiers traveling by boat or gathering in trenches. In less than 2 years, the flu killed over 20 million people worldwide. This pandemic (a worldwide outbreak of disease) came to be known as the Spanish Flu because Spain lost the most people to the deadly infection, nearly 8 million.

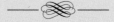

- a fever that lasts longer than 5 days
- any breathing difficulty, including wheezing (WEE-zing), a whistling sound that occurs while breathing or coughing
- a continuous cough that makes it difficult to breathe
- a cough that brings up blood or thick green or dark yellow mucus

How Is Influenza Diagnosed and Treated?

To diagnose the flu, a doctor performs a physical examination and asks the patient questions about symptoms to find out if influenza is the culprit or if a cold or another kind of respiratory problem is to blame. A small cotton swab may be used to collect some of the fluid from the back of the nose. This fluid sample can then be tested to see if the flu virus is present. The doctor also will make sure that the person is not experiencing any complications of the flu, such as bronchitis or pneumonia.

Like all viral infections, the flu will not respond to antibiotics, although in some cases they may be helpful for treating bacterial infections, such as pneumonia, that can occur as complications of the flu. The best medicine for the flu is lots of rest. Taking an over-the-counter, non-aspirin medication such as acetaminophen (uh-see-teh-MIH-noh-fen) to ease fever and muscle aches, drinking plenty of liquids, and using a humidifier to keep the air cool, moist, and easier to breathe can help people with the flu feel better as they recover.

Occasionally, doctors will prescribe antiviral flu medications, such as amantadine (uh-MAN-ta-deen) or rimantadine (rih-MAN-tuh-deen). These medications do not offer a cure but can reduce the length and severity of the illness. They must be taken within 48 hours of the start of flu symptoms in order to work.

Can the Flu Be Prevented?

Getting a flu shot can help prevent a person from contracting some strains of the flu. The vaccine contains particles from killed influenza viruses of the types expected to cause flu outbreaks during the upcoming season. After the shot, the body builds up a defense against these particular influenza virus strains. Although the flu shot does not guarantee that a person will not contract the flu, it does reduce the chance of becoming sick by 80 to 90 percent. Despite popular belief, the flu shot cannot give a person the flu. The elderly, people with certain heart and lung diseases, and workers in places such as hospitals, schools, and daycare centers should get a flu shot every year before the flu season begins in November. More recently, flu vaccination has been recommended for infants and children from age 6 months to 2 years because children in this age group are at high risk for respiratory complications of the flu.

Because the highly contagious flu virus is easily passed from person to person through the air, the virus can be lurking almost anywhere.

Soup's on!

It turns out that Mom's chicken soup does more than just warm you up. The steamy soup naturally clears congestion and relieves stuffy noses and dry coughs. Researchers also have discovered that compounds found in chicken soup slow down the activity of the white blood cells that cause inflammation (and discomfort) in the respiratory tract during an infection.

Experts recommend that hands be washed thoroughly with warm, soapy water for at least 15 to 30 seconds after using a public restroom and before eating or touching the face.

Avoiding contact with people who have the flu can also lower the risk of catching it. By avoiding close contact in large crowds, especially at schools or in malls, and by not touching used tissues or sharing drinks, a person can reduce the chance of becoming sick.

Resources

Organization

American Lung Association, 61 Broadway, 6th floor, New York, NY 10006. The American Lung Association offers guidelines on its website for the treatment and prevention of influenza.
Telephone 212-315-8700
http://www.lungusa.org

Website

KidsHealth.org. KidsHealth is a website created by the medical experts of the Nemours Foundation and is devoted to issues of children's health. It contains articles on a variety of health topics, including influenza.
http://www.KidsHealth.org

Intestinal Infections

As the name indicates, intestinal infections affect the gastrointestinal* tract, often causing diarrhea (dye-uh-REE-uh). Gastroenteritis (gas-tro-en-ter-EYE-tis), an inflammation of the stomach and intestines*, frequently accompanies such infections.

What Are Intestinal Infections and Gastroenteritis?

Viruses, bacteria, parasites, or other pathogens (PAH-tho-jens, microscopic organisms that cause disease) can cause infections in the stomach and small and large intestines, which often lead to gastroenteritis.

When people get sick because they eat food or drink water that has been contaminated with disease-causing organisms or toxins (poisons that harm the body), it is called food poisoning or foodborne illness. Food poisoning usually affects the stomach and/or the intestines. Occasionally, however, the organism or toxin behind the illness can travel through the bloodstream and cause various symptoms in other parts of the body,

▶ *See also*
Bronchitis, Infectious
Common Cold
Laryngitis
Pneumonia
Vaccination (Immunization)

KEYWORDS
for searching the Internet and other reference sources

Campylobacter

Campylobacteriosis

Clostridium

E. coli

Enteroviruses

Foodborne illnesses

Food poisoning

Hepatitis A

Listeria

Listeriosis

Rotaviruses

Salmonella

Salmonellosis

Shigella

Shigellosis

Staphylococcus aureus

Typhoid fever

182

such as the liver*. Some types of food poisoning can harm the fetus* carried by a pregnant woman.

Intestinal infections can be spread in many ways. Some people become infected by eating contaminated shellfish, raw or undercooked meat, or unpasteurized* dairy products, or from drinking or swimming in contaminated water. Others get sick after touching a surface (such as a kitchen counter) or bowel movement (when changing a diaper or doing laundry, for example) contaminated with an infectious organism. If they forget to wash their hands, they can carry the organism to their mouths on their hands or on food that they eat. Outbreaks of intestinal infections occur when many people eat or drink the same contaminated food or water.

Intestinal infections are very common, particularly in developing parts of the world. The World Health Organization (WHO) estimates that about 2 million children worldwide die each year from diseases that cause diarrhea. Children, the elderly, and people who have weak immune systems are most likely to contract intestinal infections.

What Bacteria Cause Intestinal Infections or Food Poisoning?

Not all bacteria that grow in the intestines are bad. In fact, some are necessary, and many aid the body with digestion and actually help fight infection. However, other types are less welcome.

Salmonella   Several different strains of *Salmonella* (sal-muh-NEH-luh) bacteria can cause illness. The *Salmonella typhi* (sal-muh-NEH-luh TIE-fee) bacterium causes the most serious illness, typhoid (TIE-foyd) fever, which is common in developing countries. The National Center for Infectious Diseases reports an estimated 12.5 million cases of typhoid fever worldwide each year. In the United States, about 400 cases occur each year, most in people who have traveled to undeveloped countries. Typhoid fever spreads when people eat or drink food or water contaminated with the bacteria. People who are infected may have a high fever, headache, extreme tiredness or weakness, stomach pain, loss of appetite, and sometimes a flat, red rash. A vaccination* for travelers can help prevent typhoid fever, and antibiotics can help patients who become sick.

Salmonellosis (sal-muh-neh-LO-sis) is a more common but less serious illness caused by *Salmonella* bacteria. The U.S. Centers for Disease Control and Prevention (CDC) reports 40,000 cases in the United States each year and estimates that 20 times that number may go undiagnosed. As many as 1,000 people in the United States die from the disease each year. Eating food from contaminated animals, such as eggs, poultry, and meat, can cause salmonellosis. Symptoms start 12 to 72 hours after infection and include nausea (NAW-zee-uh), vomiting, diarrhea, fever, and stomach cramps. The disease usually runs its course in 4 to 7 days. Only infants, young children, the elderly, and people with weakened immune

* **gastrointestinal** (gas-tro-in-TES-tih-nuhl) means having to do with the organs of the digestive system, the system that processes food. It includes the mouth, esophagus, stomach, intestines, colon, and rectum and other organs involved in digestion, including the liver and pancreas.

* **intestines** are the muscular tubes that food passes through during digestion after it exits the stomach.

* **liver** is a large organ located beneath the ribs on the right side of the body. The liver performs numerous digestive and chemical functions essential for health.

* **fetus** (FEE-tus) is the term for an unborn human after it is an embryo, from 9 weeks after fertilization until childbirth.

* **unpasteurized** (pas-CHUR-ized) refers to foods that have not undergone the process of pasteurization (pas-chu-rih-ZAY-shun), in which food is heated to a certain temperature over a period of time to kill organisms and help make the food safer to consume.

* **vaccination** (vak-sih-NAY-shun), also called immunization, is giving, usually by an injection, a preparation of killed or weakened germs, or a part of a germ or product it produces, to prevent or lessen the severity of a disease.

systems typically require treatment. (Antibiotic treatment can actually prolong the time that it takes for *Salmonella* bacteria to leave the body.)

Shigella   Shigellosis (shih-geh-LO-sis), caused by *Shigella* (shih-GEH-luh) bacteria, inflames the lining of the small intestine. In the United States, about 18,000 cases are reported to the CDC each year, although the actual number may be 20 times higher. Young children are especially at risk for contracting the infection because shigellosis is transmitted through feces (FEE-seez, or bowel movements). The disease can produce complications in this age group, including seizures*.

Symptoms of shigellosis include diarrhea (sometimes with blood or mucus*), fever, vomiting, nausea, and abdominal* cramping. Most people recover without treatment, usually within a week, although doctors may prescribe antibiotics to patients to keep the disease from spreading.

Escherichia coli   Although there are hundreds of types of *Escherichia coli* (commonly referred to as *E. coli*) bacteria, only five are known to cause illness in people. In the United States, the CDC estimates that there are 73,000 cases of *E. coli* infection, leading to about 60 deaths, each year.

The most dangerous strain* of *E. coli*, 0157:H7, is found in the intestines of cattle. People usually become infected with the bacteria from eating undercooked ground beef, although contaminated water, unpas-

* **seizures** (SEE-zhurs) are sudden bursts of disorganized electrical activity that interrupt the normal functioning of the brain, often leading to uncontrolled movements of the body and sometimes a temporary change in consciousness.

* **mucus** (MYOO-kus) is a thick, slippery substance that lines the insides of many body parts.

* **abdominal** (ab-DAH-mih-nul) refers to the area of the body below the ribs and above the hips that contains the stomach, intestines, and other organs.

* **strain** is a subtype of an organism, such as a virus or bacterium.

TYPHOID MARY

An Irish immigrant cook, Mary Mallon, infected as many as 22 people in New York City with typhoid fever between 1900 and 1907. Mallon, who became known later as "Typhoid Mary," was a carrier of the disease. This means that she had no symptoms and was otherwise healthy but could spread the infection to others. (This was before antibiotics were available, which may have been able to kill the bacteria in her body.)

Although she committed no crime, city authorities held Mallon in an isolation cottage on an island in New York's East River from 1907 to 1910, and then again from 1915 (after it was discovered that she was responsible for another outbreak of typhoid fever that infected 25 people) until her death in 1938. She was confined as a threat to public health.

Many decades later, this case still raises an important and difficult question: how far should health authorities go in restricting individual rights to protect the general welfare of the public?

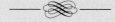

teurized dairy products and juices, and even fruits and vegetables can be sources of infection.

E. coli infection can cause abdominal cramps and bloody diarrhea, which last about 5 days. Most people do not need treatment, although those with weak immune systems, children, and the elderly will need to be hospitalized if they develop a serious infection.

Campylobacter   Campylobacteriosis (kam-pee-lo-bak-teer-e-O-sis), caused by *Campylobacter* (kam-pee-lo-BAK-ter) bacteria, is the most common type of bacterial diarrhea in the United States. *Campylobacter jejuni* (je-JOO-nee) causes about 99 percent of these cases. The CDC estimates that more than 2 million people, or almost 1 percent of the U.S. population, contract the infection each year.

Campylobacter lives in animals, especially birds. Humans become infected after eating poultry that has not been thoroughly cooked. Outbreaks also have occurred after people drank contaminated water or unpasteurized milk.

Symptoms of illness begin 2 to 5 days after infection and include diarrhea (often bloody), abdominal cramping and pain, and fever. Most people recover on their own within 2 to 5 days.

Clostridium difficile *infection* and Clostridium perfringens *food poisoning*   *Clostridium difficile* (klos-TRIH-dee-um DIH-fih-seel) bacteria often live in the intestinal tracts of infants and young children without causing disease. In adults, however, especially the elderly, *C. difficile* can produce fever, watery diarrhea, abdominal pain, and loss of appetite. Risk factors for infection include taking antibiotics, a hospital stay, gastrointestinal surgery, and having another serious illness. Health care workers often spread the bacteria when they touch infected feces or contaminated surfaces, then touch patients or give them medicine without first washing their hands. *C. difficile* infection that causes symptoms most often occurs in people receiving long courses of antibiotics that limit the growth of the harmless bacteria that are usually present in the intestine.

Perfringens poisoning is caused by the *Clostridium perfringens* bacterium and is one of the most common types of food poisoning in the United States. Some *C. perfringens* bacteria may remain in food even after it has been cooked, then multiply when the food is cooled slowly and left at room temperature. People who eat contaminated food may develop intense abdominal cramps, diarrhea, and flatulence (excessive gas), usually within 8 to 22 hours. Most people recover from perfringens poisoning within a day or two, although symptoms can last longer in older people. Quickly refrigerating uneaten cooked food and reheating leftovers to 165 degrees or higher can help prevent perfringens poisoning.

Listeria   Listeriosis (lis-teer-e-O-sis) is caused by the *Listeria monocytogenes* bacterium, which is found in the soil and in the intestinal tracts of animals and humans. People contract listeriosis from eating vegetables grown in contaminated soil or raw or undercooked meat, or from drinking water or unpasteurized milk and milk products.

Symptoms of illness include fever, headache, nausea, and diarrhea. The bacteria also can spread into the bloodstream or nervous system, leading to meningitis*. Pregnant women are at the greatest risk for listeriosis, and the disease can cause miscarriage*, stillbirth*, or serious illness in the newborn. Infants, older people, and people with weak immune systems are also at risk.

Staphylococcus   Toxins produced by certain strains of *Staphylococcus aureus* (stah-fih-lo-KAH-kus ARE-ree-us) bacteria can cause food poisoning. When people who are infected with the bacteria handle food such as meat, poultry, egg products, or dishes containing mayonnaise or cream, they may spread the bacteria to the food. The toxins build up when the food sits for long periods of time at room temperature. When a person becomes infected, symptoms come on quickly, within 2 to 8 hours, and last less than 12 hours. They include severe nausea and vomiting and sometimes abdominal cramping, diarrhea, and headache.

What Are the Major Types of Viral Intestinal Infections?

Rotaviruses   Rotaviruses (RO-tuh-vy-ruh-sez) can infect people of all ages, but infants and young children are infected most often. Outbreaks occur most frequently from November to April in the United States, with about 1 million children affected each year. Of those, between 55,000 and 70,000 require hospitalization. Deaths from the illness are rare in the United States, but worldwide there are more than 600,000 deaths among children each year from rotavirus infection, according to WHO.

Rotaviruses spread when people come into contact with infected human feces. The disease is most common in daycare centers, hospital pediatric wards, and homes with young children. Symptoms appear about 2 days after infection. They include fever, vomiting, and abdominal pain, which last for 2 to 3 days, and diarrhea, which can linger for up to 8 days. Most people do not require treatment.

Enteroviruses   Enteroviruses (en-tuh-ro-VY-ruh-sez) are a group of viruses that attack the intestinal tract and cause a wide range of illnesses, including intestinal infections. People who are infected may experience mild diarrhea, vomiting, fever, and abdominal pain. Most get better on their own without treatment from a doctor.

Hepatitis A   The hepatitis (heh-puh-TIE-tis) A virus is found in water contaminated by sewage, in shellfish from contaminated water, and in fruits and vegetables grown in contaminated soil. The virus can spread

*meningitis (meh-nin-JY-tis) is an inflammation of the meninges, the membranes that surround the brain and the spinal cord. Meningitis is most often caused by infection with a virus or a bacterium.

*miscarriage is the ending of a pregnancy through the death of the embryo or fetus before birth.

*stillbirth is the birth of a dead fetus.

when people eat or drink contaminated food or water or from person to person during sexual intercourse. Infected people who handle or prepare food can transmit the virus if they touch food after going to the bathroom and not washing their hands thoroughly.

Some people with hepatitis A infection show no signs of illness, but those who do may experience fever, extreme tiredness, loss of appetite, nausea, and vomiting. The patient's liver enlarges and the skin may appear yellowish, a condition known as jaundice*. The disease can lead to permanent liver damage, although this is rare. Symptoms appear 2 to 4 weeks after infection and may last several weeks to months. A vaccine is available to protect people at high risk from hepatitis A infection.

Other Causes of Intestinal Infection

Parasites are the culprits behind many intestinal infections. Amebiasis (ah-mih-BYE-uh-sis), caused by *Entamoeba histolytica* (en-tuh-ME-ba his-toh-LIH-tih-kuh); giardiasis (jee-ar-DYE-uh-sis), the work of the *Giardia intestinalis* protozoa*; and infection with *Cyclospora cayetanensis* (sy-klo-SPORE-uh kye-uh-tuh-NIN-sis) are all common parasitic infections that lead to intestinal symptoms such as cramping and diarrhea.

How Do Doctors Diagnose Intestinal Infections and Food Poisoning?

Many cases of intestinal infection are so mild that they go unnoticed. Others get better without the patient ever seeing a doctor. The symptoms of gastroenteritis, namely nausea, vomiting, abdominal pain, diarrhea, and loss of appetite, are common to many intestinal infections and some other diseases as well. When patients go to a doctor, they may be diagnosed with an intestinal infection or food poisoning based on a physical exam and their history of symptoms and food intake.

Mild cases likely will not require any laboratory tests, and the actual cause of the infection may never be known. In more severe cases of illness, however, doctors may collect samples of a bowel movement to examine under the microscope and send to be cultured* in order to identify the organism involved.

How Are Intestinal Infections Treated?

Most intestinal infections do not require treatment, and patients get better on their own. People with diarrhea and other signs of intestinal infections should talk to their doctors if the symptoms do not clear up in a few days.

In most cases, patients can remain at home and maintain a relatively normal schedule. Children sometimes need to stay out of daycare until the illness resolves. While they recover, patients must be sure to drink plenty of fluids to avoid dehydration*. Doctors also advise that they avoid anti-diarrhea medicine because it may keep the infectious agent in the body longer. More severe cases of intestinal infections sometimes require

jaundice (JON-dis) is a yellowing of the skin, and sometimes the whites of the eyes, caused by a buildup in the body of bilirubin, a chemical produced in and released by the liver. An increase in bilirubin may indicate disease of the liver or certain blood disorders.

protozoa (pro-tuh-ZOH-uh) are single-celled microorganisms (tiny organisms), some of which are capable of causing disease in humans.

cultured (KUL-churd) means subjected to a test in which a sample of fluid or tissue from the body is placed in a dish containing material that supports the growth of certain organisms. Typically, within days the organisms will grow and can be identified.

dehydration (dee-hi-DRAY-shun) is a condition in which the body is depleted of water, usually caused by excessive and unreplaced loss of body fluids, such as through sweating, vomiting, or diarrhea.

*intravenous (in-tra-VEE-nus) fluids are fluids injected directly into a vein.

*AIDS, or acquired immunodeficiency (ih-myoo-no-dih-FIH-shen-see) syndrome, is an infection that severely weakens the immune system; it is caused by the human immunodeficiency virus (HIV).

*paralysis (pah-RAH-luh-sis) is the loss or impairment of the ability to move some part of the body.

*arthritis (ar-THRY-tis) refers to any of several disorders characterized by inflammation of the joints.

*abscesses (AB-seh-sez) are localized or walled off accumulations of pus caused by infection that can occur anywhere within the body.

*kidney is one of the pair of organs that filter blood and remove waste products and excess water from the body in the form of urine.

*anemia (uh-NEE-me-uh) is a blood condition in which there is a decreased amount of oxygen-carrying hemoglobin in the blood and, usually, fewer than normal numbers of red blood cells.

hospitalization so patients can receive intravenous fluids*, antibiotics, or other treatment. In most cases, people should feel better within days to a week, although it may be several more weeks before their gastrointestinal tracts recover completely.

Can Intestinal Infections Cause Other Medical Complications?

In otherwise healthy people, intestinal infections rarely cause complications. Mild dehydration is the most common consequence. Infants and the elderly are most at risk for severe dehydration. For people with weak immune systems (such as patients undergoing chemotherapy or people with HIV or AIDS*), the infectious agent may spread throughout the body, causing widespread disease and even death. In infants and young children, cases of long-lasting illness occasionally lead to malnutrition or a failure to grow properly because the infections interfere with their nourishment.

More specific complications from intestinal infections vary. Salmonellosis and shigellosis can lead to Reiter (RYE-ter) syndrome, which is characterized by joint pain, eye inflammation, and difficulty and pain with urination. Campylobacter infection may trigger Guillain-Barre (GEE-yan bah-RAY) syndrome, a nerve inflammation that causes muscle weakness or paralysis*. Salmonella infection can result in arthritis*, meningitis, brain abscesses*, and bone infections. *Escherichia coli* can cause hemolytic uremic syndrome, a disease that can progress to kidney* failure and severe anemia*.

How Can People Prevent Intestinal Infections?

Practicing good hygiene is the best way to prevent intestinal infection. That includes frequently and thoroughly washing hands, especially after changing diapers, after going to the bathroom, and before handling food or eating.

Travelers who plan to visit developing countries need to make sure they have any recommended vaccinations (such as the one for typhoid fever) before they leave. Once there, experts advise that they drink only bottled water and avoid eating raw fruits and vegetables, food from street vendors, and unpasteurized dairy products. To be safe, all food should be eaten steaming hot.

In the United States, a rotavirus vaccine used in the late 1990s caused bowel problems in some infants and is no longer recommended. Work continues on the development of a new vaccine.

Resources

Organizations

U.S. Centers for Disease Control and Prevention (CDC), 1600 Clifton Road, Atlanta, GA 30333. The CDC is the U.S. government

authority for information about infectious and other diseases. It has fact sheets on many types of intestinal infections on its website.
Telephone 800-311-3435
http://www.cdc.gov

U.S. Food and Drug Administration, Center for Food Safety and Applied Nutrition (CFSAN), 5100 Paint Branch Parkway, College Park, MD 20740. CFSAN has an online "Bad Bug Book" that gives facts and figures on various foodborne illnesses.
Telephone 888-723-3366
http://www.cfsan.fda.gov

Intestinal Parasites

Intestinal parasites* are organisms that live in the gastrointestinal* tract of animals, including humans. They can cause diarrhea (dye-uh-REE-uh) and other symptoms.

What Are Intestinal Parasites?

In humans, three types of intestinal parasites may live in the small and large intestines: tapeworms, roundworms (or nematodes, NEE-muh-todes), and protozoa (pro-tuh-ZOH-uh). Certain types remain in the intestines; others travel outside the intestines to invade other organs. Some are so small they can only be seen under a microscope; others can be many feet long. Most tapeworms and roundworms develop in the human body and lay their eggs there. The eggs then pass out of the body through feces (FEE-seez, or bowel movements) and can infest others.

Intestinal parasites exist throughout the world. The World Health Organization (WHO) estimates that 3.5 billion people worldwide are infested with some type of intestinal parasite, and as many as 450 million of them are sick as a result. Children are most frequently infected with these parasites.

Intestinal parasites spread in areas with poor sanitation and are most common in tropical developing countries on the African, Asian, and South American continents. They are not a large problem in the United States, and Americans are most likely to get intestinal parasites when they travel to remote areas.

How Are Intestinal Parasites Spread?

Intestinal parasites can be acquired in many ways. Some parasites can live in the soil for extended periods. They may penetrate the body through the skin or if contaminated soil is ingested accidentally. Other parasites live in animals, such as pigs and cows. People can become infested with

▶ *See also*
Hepatitis, Infectious
Intestinal Parasites
Staphylococcal Infections
Travel-related Infections
Vaccination (Immunization)

KEYWORDS
for searching the Internet and other reference sources

Amebas

Amebic dysentery

Hookworms

Nematodes

Pinworms

Protozoa

Roundworms

Tapeworms

* **parasites** (PAIR-uh-sites) are organisms such as protozoa (one-celled animals), worms, or insects that must live on or inside a human or other organism to survive. An animal or plant harboring a parasite is called its host. Parasites live at the expense of the host and may cause illness.

* **gastrointestinal** (gas-tro-in-TES-tih-nuhl) means having to do with the organs of the digestive system, the system that processes food. It includes the mouth, esophagus, stomach, intestines, colon, and rectum and other organs involved in digestion, including the liver and pancreas.

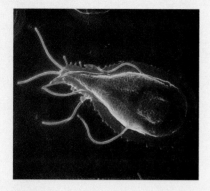

▲

Both public water supplies and natural water sources can become contaminated with human or animal waste (mainly from dogs and beavers) harboring the parasite (shown here) that causes giardiasis. The disease causes stomach upset and diarrhea when the parasite attaches itself to the lining of the digestive system, where it interferes with the body's ability to absorb fats and carbohydrates. *Custom Medical Stock Photo, Inc.*

*infestations** refer to illnesses caused by multi-celled parasitic organisms, such as tapeworms, roundworms, or protozoa.

*small intestine** is the part of the intestine between the stomach and large intestine.

these by eating undercooked meat or drinking unpasteurized milk (milk that has not been processed with heat to kill parasites and bacteria).

The eggs of some intestinal parasites pass through an infested person's gastrointestinal tract and into feces. The parasite then can spread to other people through unintentional contact with the feces. Depending on the type of parasite, a person may become infested by touching his or her mouth after contact with feces that contain the organism (when changing a diaper or doing laundry, for example) or a contaminated area. Parasites can spread when a person eats contaminated food (such as unwashed raw fruits or vegetables, which can carry parasites from the soil or from people who have handled them) or drinks water contaminated by feces. Swimming in contaminated water also may result in infestation by certain parasites.

Parasitic intestinal infestations* often occur in outbreaks, when several people have symptoms at the same time. This is especially likely if many people come into contact with the same supply of contaminated food or water.

What Are Some Common Intestinal Parasites?

Ascariasis   Ascariasis (as-kuh-RYE-uh-sis) is caused by *Ascaris lumbricoides*, an intestinal roundworm. It is one of the most common intestinal parasites, affecting people in all parts of the world, especially in areas with poor sanitation. In the United States, ascariasis is rare, but it occurs most frequently in the rural parts of the Southeast. The worm also can infest pigs.

The life cycle of *Ascaris lumbricoides* begins when an adult worm lays its eggs in the intestines of an infected person. The eggs leave the body through the feces and can live in soil for up to 2 years. When people eat raw food containing this contaminated soil, they may swallow the worm's eggs, which hatch in the stomach as larvae (LAR-vee, or immature worms). The larvae migrate through the blood to the lungs and then to the throat, where they are swallowed. Eventually, they pass into the intestines, where they begin the cycle again. The adult worms, which can grow to be more than 12 inches long, can live 1 to 2 years in the small intestine*. Ascariasis is not contagious, and a person can become infested only by ingesting the worm's eggs.

Ascariasis usually causes no symptoms or only mild stomachaches or bloating. If a person is heavily infested, he or she may experience more severe pain. Some people also may have a cough or breathing problems when the larvae move through their lungs.

People often discover they have ascariasis when a worm passes in their bowel movements, or when they cough up a worm or it crawls out through the nose. This can be frightening, but the ascaris worm usually does not cause permanent damage to the body. Because of the relatively large size of adult ascaris worms, they can partially block the intestinal tract as well as the ducts leading from the biliary tract* and pancreas*. In rare cases, surgery may be needed to remove them.

Strongyloidiasis   Strongyloidiasis (stron-juh-loy-DYE-uh-sis) is caused by another roundworm, *Strongyloides stercoralis*. This common infestation can be especially dangerous in people with weakened immune systems. If a person comes into contact with contaminated soil, the larva of the parasite can burrow through the skin. It travels to the lungs and then, in a manner similar to ascaris, is swallowed and ends up in the intestines, where the worm grows to adulthood and begins laying eggs. What is special about this parasite is that the eggs can hatch inside the intestines and the worms can continue to cycle through many generations (called the auto-infective cycle), causing an infestation that can last for decades.

In people with weakened immune systems, particularly those taking drugs such as corticosteroids*, strongyloidiasis can become overwhelming, and huge numbers of larvae can invade the lungs and other organs. This problem is called the hyperinfection syndrome and, although rare, it can be fatal.

Giardiasis   Giardiasis (jee-ar-DYE-uh-sis) is the most common waterborne parasitic infection in the United States. Caused by *Giardia intestinalis*, a single-cell protozoan (also known as *Giardia lamblia*), this infection can lead to diarrhea, cramping, and an upset stomach.

Giardia intestinalis lives in humans and animals. People become infected by drinking or swimming in contaminated water or by touching the feces of an infected person, or a contaminated surface, and then their mouths. People can spread the parasite if they do not wash their hands properly. Giardiasis occurs most frequently in settings where contaminated feces can be spread easily, such as in children in diapers, especially those in daycare centers, and in people who live in institutional settings such as nursing homes. Some people who are infected do not become sick but still can pass the infection on to others.

In people who do develop symptoms, stomach pain and watery diarrhea usually start 1 to 2 weeks after infection. About half the people who are infected also lose weight. The illness lasts 2 to 6 weeks, or longer in people who are sick with another disease.

Hookworm   Hookworms (a type of roundworm) are another common intestinal parasite. The U.S. Centers for Disease Control and Prevention (CDC) estimates that 1 billion people worldwide have hookworm infestations, although improved sanitation has reduced the number of cases in the United States.

Two species, *Ancylostoma duodenale* and *Necator americanus*, infest humans. The worms' eggs hatch into larvae in warm, moist soil. Hookworms can penetrate human skin, so many people become infested when they walk barefoot in or touch contaminated soil. They also can become infested when they eat such soil (on unwashed raw fruit or vegetables,

* **biliary** (BIH-lee-ah-ree) **tract** refers to the organs and ducts, including the liver and gallbladder, that produce, store, and transport bile, a substance which aids in digestion.

* **pancreas** (PAN-kree-us) is a gland located behind the stomach that produces enzymes and hormones necessary for digestion and metabolism.

* **corticosteroids** (kor-tih-ko-STIR-oyds) are chemical substances made by the adrenal glands that have several functions in the body, including maintaining blood pressure during stress and controlling inflammation. They can also be given to people as medication to treat certain illnesses. People being treated with corticosteroid medication, particularly with high doses, may have a reduced ability to fight certain infections.

for example). The hookworm larvae travel to the lungs via the bloodstream; the larvae then travel to the throat and are swallowed, in a similar fashion to the ascaris worm. When they reach the small intestine, the larvae latch onto the intestinal walls and suck blood. There they mature and eventually lay eggs, which pass out of the body in feces. Hookworms can live for 1 to 2 years in the body.

A rash or itching at the site where the larvae entered the skin may signal hookworm infestation, followed by mild cramping and diarrhea. Heavily infested people may lose their appetite, lose weight, and have abdominal* pain. Hookworms can cause serious problems, including malnutrition and anemia* from intestinal bleeding. Newborns, young children, pregnant women, and malnourished people are most susceptible to these complications.

Dogs and cats sometimes carry their own types of hookworms (*Ancylostoma ceylanicum* and *Ancylostoma braziliense*), and these occasionally infest humans who come into contact with soil contaminated with cat or dog feces. In this type of infestation, called cutaneous larva migrans (kyoo-TAY-nee-us LAR-vuh MY-granz) or creeping eruption, the worm larvae burrow into the skin and cause severe itching but do not invade deeper into the body. The condition resolves without treatment after several weeks or months.

Amebiasis   Amebiasis (ah-mih-BYE-uh-sis) is caused by a single-cell parasite called *Entamoeba histolytica*. It occurs mainly in areas with poor sanitary conditions. Cases in the United States usually are seen in people who have recently arrived from or traveled in remote areas.

Amebiasis spreads when people touch infected feces or contaminated surfaces and then touch their mouths, or when they eat or drink contaminated food or water. It also can spread through certain types of sexual contact. Symptoms such as mild diarrhea and stomach pain may occur 1 to 4 weeks after infection, but only 1 infected person in 10 becomes sick and develops symptoms.

Amebic dysentery (uh-ME-bik DIH-sen-ter-e), a more severe form of the illness, causes bloody diarrhea, extreme stomach pain, and fever. Rarely, the infection spreads to other body organs, particularly the liver*, where the parasite can form large abscesses*. Because of the risk of amebic dysentery, *Entamoeba histolytica* is one of the most dangerous intestinal parasites, and infection with it can be fatal.

Other forms of amebas, including *Entamoeba coli*, *Entamoeba dispar*, and *Entamoeba hartmanni*, infect humans but cause no illness. These amebas can live in the human body for months or years without causing problems.

Cyclosporiasis and Cryptosporidiosis   Scientists identified cyclosporiasis (sy-klo-spoh-RYE-uh-sis), caused by the protozoan *Cyclospora cayetanensis*, in 1979. The infection is found worldwide, most

* **abdominal** (ab-DAH-mih-nul) refers to the area of the body below the ribs and above the hips that contains the stomach, intestines, and other organs.

* **anemia** (uh-NEE-me-uh) is a blood condition in which there is a decreased amount of oxygen-carrying hemoglobin in the blood and, usually, fewer than normal numbers of red blood cells.

* **liver** is a large organ located beneath the ribs on the right side of the body. The liver performs numerous digestive and chemical functions essential for health.

* **abscesses** (AB-seh-sez) are localized or walled off accumulations of pus caused by infection that can occur anywhere within the body.

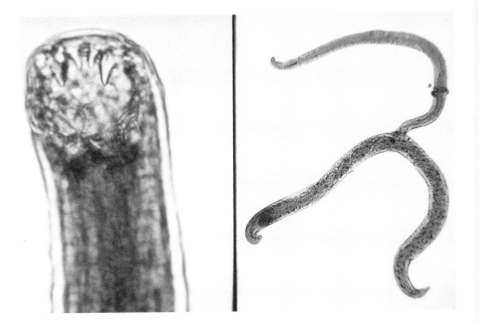

Two species of hookworm, *Ancylostoma duodenale* (left) and *Necator americanus* (right), can infect humans. *Custom Medical Stock Photo, Inc.*

frequently in developing countries, although there have been outbreaks in the United States and Canada.

Because *Cyclospora cayetanensis* must spend some time outside the human body to become infectious, it is not contagious from person to person. Infection usually results from ingesting contaminated water or soil or fresh produce grown in them.

Symptoms, which appear 1 week after infection and last from 1 to several weeks, may include diarrhea with frequent, watery, and sometimes explosive bowel movements; loss of appetite; stomach cramps; bloating; nausea (NAW-zee-uh); fever; vomiting; and weight loss. The diagnosis can be made by examining a sample of the patient's bowel movements under a microscope to view the organism. If the illness is not treated, its symptoms may return.

Cryptosporidiosis (krip-toh-spor-id-e-O-sis) is an intestinal infection with symptoms similar to cyclosporiasis caused by the protozoan *Cryptosporidium parvum* that can live in people and animals. People can pick up the parasite through person-to-person contact or through water contaminated by the feces of infected animals.

Initially, it was thought that only people with weak immune systems, such as those with AIDS, contracted the infection. It is now known that the organism can infect people with normal immune systems and that cryptosporidiosis is one of the most common causes of protozoal diarrhea in the world. The infection goes away on its own in most people, but antibiotics and other treatments may be necessary for people with weak immune systems who contract cryptosporidiosis.

Enterobiasis   Enterobiasis (en-tuh-roh-BY-uh-sis), also known as pinworm infestation, is caused by a staple-size worm known as *Enterobius* *vermicularis.* It is the most common worm infestation in the United States and is found primarily in children. Outbreaks of pinworm often occur in schools and daycare centers. From there, infested children may spread the worms to their family members.

Enterobius vermicularis lives in the rectum, the last part of the large intestine*, and comes out at night to lay eggs on the perineum (per-ih-NEE-um), the area around the anus and genitals. These eggs become contagious in a few hours and can spread to sheets and clothing, where they can remain contagious for about 2 weeks. Infestation occurs when people touch a contaminated area and then their mouths.

Itching of the perineum is the most common symptom of pinworm. This can lead to sleeplessness and irritability. Frequently, however, people show no signs of infestation.

Human tapeworm Human tapeworm infestations usually are caused by eating meat or fish contaminated with worm larvae. Like other intestinal parasites, these worms frequently cause infestations in areas with poor sanitation, where livestock animals are exposed to contaminated soil or fish to contaminated water.

There are three common species of tapeworms: *Taenia solium* (pork tapeworm), *Taenia saginata* (beef tapeworm), and *Diphyllobothrium latum* (fish tapeworm). After someone eats contaminated meat or fish, tapeworm larvae travel to the intestines, where they latch onto the lining of the intestines and gradually grow into adults. The largest tapeworms can reach amazing sizes, measuring more than 20 feet long in some cases. The worms shed their eggs into the feces, from which they find their way into soil and water and are ingested by animals or fish. Humans ingest the larvae when they eat the contaminated meat or fish. Symptoms of a tapeworm infestation are often mild or nonexistent but can include abdominal pain, diarrhea, and malnutrition.

Two other diseases in humans can be traced to tapeworms that usually infest animals. In echinococcosis (ih-kye-nih-kah-KO-sis), large cysts* can develop in the liver, lungs, and other organs; in cysticercosis (sis-tuh-sir-KO-sis), the parasites can invade the muscles, brain, and eyes. Both echinococcosis and cysticercosis can occur when people eat food contaminated with the eggs of tapeworms that are found in the droppings of certain animals.

Trichinosis Trichinosis (trih-kih-NO-sis) arises from several varieties of *Trichinella* roundworms. Although once very common, it is now relatively rare in the United States, with the CDC reporting an average of just 38 cases per year. Trichinosis is more common in developing countries, however.

Trichinella larvae live in cysts in pigs and wild animals. When people eat their meat raw or undercooked, the cysts travel to the stomach, where acid dissolves the walls of the cysts and releases the immature

* **large intestine** is the part of the intestine that contains the colon and rectum.

* **cysts** (SISTS) are shell-like enclosures that contain small organisms in a resting stage.

worms. They move to the small intestine, mature, and lay eggs. Once the eggs hatch, the worms travel through the bloodstream to muscles, where they burrow in, forming cysts. This ends the cycle in humans.

The first symptoms of trichinosis, which include stomach pain, extreme tiredness, nausea, diarrhea, vomiting, and fever, appear 1 or 2 days after people eat infested meat. Headaches, chills, swelling of the eyes, cough, muscle aches and pains, and constipation (infrequent bowel movements) may follow. People with severe infestations also may have heart problems or trouble breathing.

How Are Intestinal Parasitic Diseases Diagnosed?

Doctors use samples of feces, sometimes taken a day or two apart, to diagnose intestinal parasitic diseases. The feces are examined for evidence of parasites, such as eggs, larvae, or adults. Blood samples can be taken to check for antibodies* to specific parasites, and doctors may use a medical instrument called an endoscope* to examine the intestines for infection.

To detect pinworms, doctors often request that patients take a "tape test." For this test, patients briefly apply a piece of transparent tape to the skin around the anus in the early morning, after the worm has laid its eggs. The tape is removed and examined at the doctor's office for any eggs that might be sticking to it.

How Are Intestinal Parasitic Diseases Treated?

Some cases require little or no treatment, and the parasites eventually disappear on their own. People with diarrhea and other signs of intestinal parasitic disease should talk to a doctor if their symptoms last more than a few days.

Medication used to treat the illnesses varies with the type of infection. Doctors may use antibiotics or antiparasitic medicines. In most cases, patients can remain at home and maintain a normal schedule. Children must stay out of daycare until they have been treated adequately and can no longer spread the infection. While they recover, patients are advised to drink plenty of fluids to avoid dehydration*. Antidiarrhea medicine is not recommended because it may keep the parasites in the body longer. More severe cases may require treatment in the hospital.

In most cases, patients who have symptoms should feel better within 1 to 2 weeks, although it may be several more weeks before their bowel movements are completely back to normal.

Can Intestinal Parasitic Diseases Cause Medical Complications?

Dehydration is the most common general complication of intestinal parasite infections. Infants and young children are particularly vulnerable to dehydration and nutrition problems when they become infected. In

* **antibodies** (AN-tih-bah-deez) are protein molecules produced by the body's immune system to help fight specific infections caused by microorganisms, such as bacteria and viruses.

* **endoscope** (EN-doh-skope) is a tool for looking inside parts of the body. It consists of a lighted tube and optical fibers and/or lenses.

* **dehydration** (dee-hi-DRAY-shun) is a condition in which the body is depleted of water, usually caused by excessive and unreplaced loss of body fluids, such as through sweating, vomiting, or diarrhea.

Microorganisms	Usual Sources	Preventive Measures
Bacteria		
Salmonella bacteria	• Eggs, poultry, and meat	
Staphylococcus aureus bacteria	• Contaminated meat, poultry, and egg products left at room temperature	
Shigella bacteria	• Food contaminated with contaminated feces	
Campylobacter jejuni bacteria	• Undercooked poultry, contaminated water, and unpasteurized milk	Wash hands frequently, especially before cooking, after changing diapers, and after using the bathroom.
E. coli bacteria	• Undercooked ground beef and vegetables, contaminated water, unpasteurized dairy products, and juices	
Clostridium difficile bacteria	• Contaminated feces and surfaces	
Listeria monocytogenes bacteria	• Vegetables grown in contaminated soil, raw or undercooked meat, contaminated water, unpasteurized milk, and milk products	Promptly refrigerate cooked foods.
Clostridium perfringens bacteria	• Contaminated food stored without sufficient refrigeration	
Viruses		
Rotavirus	• Contaminated feces	
Hepatitis A virus	• Water contaminated by sewage, shellfish from contaminated water, and fruits and vegetables grown in contaminated soil	Cook foods to recommended temperatures and reheat leftovers to at least 165 degrees Fahrenheit.
Parasites/Protozoa		
Entamoeba histolytica parasite	• Contaminated food, water, and feces	
Giardia intestinalis protozoa	• Contaminated water and feces	When traveling in developing countries, drink only bottled water. Avoid eating raw fruits and vegetables, food from street vendors, and unpasteurized dairy products. Before traveling, check with a doctor about recommended vaccines.
Cyclospora cayetanensis parasite	• Foods grown in contaminated soil or water	

people with weak immune systems (such as people undergoing chemo-therapy), infants, and the elderly, these infections can be fatal.

Some infections cause specific complications: amebiasis can affect the liver, lungs, and brain; parasites migrating through the lungs may cause difficulty breathing; and hookworm infestation can cause anemia and malnutrition, which can affect growth and development in children.

How Can Infection with Intestinal Parasites Be Prevented?

Good hygiene is the best defense against intestinal parasites. This in-cludes frequent and thorough hand washing, especially after changing diapers, after going to the bathroom, and before handling food.

Doctors advise that travelers to undeveloped countries drink and brush their teeth with bottled water and avoid eating raw fruits and veg-etables, food from street vendors, and unpasteurized dairy products. In addition, cooking all food until it is steaming hot kills parasites. Always wearing shoes and avoiding swimming in bodies of fresh water such as ponds, rivers, and lakes can minimize the risk of contact with contami-nated soil and water.

Resources

Organizations

U.S. Centers for Disease Control and Prevention (CDC), 1600 Clifton Road, Atlanta, GA 30333. The CDC is the U.S. government authority for information about infectious and other diseases. It has fact sheets for the most common types of intestinal parasite infesta-tions at its website.
Telephone 800-311-3435
http://www.cdc.gov

U.S. Food and Drug Administration, Center for Food Safety and Ap-plied Nutrition (CFSAN), 5100 Paint Branch Parkway, College Park, MD 20740. CFSAN has an online "Bad Bug Book" that gives facts and figures on many foodborne parasites and illnesses.
Telephone 888-723-3366
http://www.cfsan.fda.gov

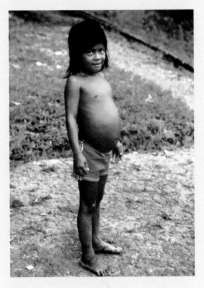

▲

Symptoms of late-stage hookworm infestation are an enlarged abdomen and diarrhea. Worms can live up to 15 years in the human body, and females can lay 10,000 to 25,000 eggs every day. In severe cases the number of parasites may grow so large that the intestines become blocked. *Photo Researchers, Inc.*

 See also
Intestinal Infections
Pinworm Infestation
Trichinosis

197

K

Kawasaki Disease

Kawasaki disease is an inflammatory illness in children that involves the body's blood vessels. The hallmarks of the disease are high fever, swollen glands, and a rash, and it may lead to complications affecting the heart.

What Is Kawasaki Disease?

For children in the United States, Kawasaki disease is the leading cause of acquired heart disease, that is, heart disease that is not present at birth but develops later in life. In 1967, the Japanese pediatrician Tomisaku Kawasaki first described the illness. He called it mucocutaneous (myoo-ko-kyoo-TAY-nee-us) lymph node syndrome, but today, it is better known as Kawasaki disease. Even after many years of research, the cause of this disease remains unknown, but doctors suspect that an infectious microorganism* may trigger the onset of inflammation in the body. Kawasaki disease sometimes occurs in outbreaks, often in late winter or spring, and can resemble diseases like measles or scarlet fever*, which suggests a possible link to an infectious organism.

Kawasaki disease can cause inflammation of blood vessels, mucous membranes (moist linings of the mouth, nose, eyes, and throat), lymph nodes*, and the heart. Although it eventually clears up on its own, if left untreated it can damage the blood vessels that supply the heart muscle. Kawasaki disease is associated with a 1 in 5 risk of coronary aneurysms*. This blood vessel damage can lead to a heart attack, especially in very young children.

How Common Is It?

As many as 3,500 children are hospitalized with Kawasaki disease each year in the United States. Four out of five children who get the disease are less than 5 years old, and it is extremely rare in children older than 15. Kawasaki disease develops in boys about twice as often as in girls. It is more common in children of Asian descent, though it occurs in all races.

Is It Contagious?

The disease itself has not been proved to be contagious. Doctors suspect, however, that an infectious microorganism may trigger it and that the organism might be contagious. Nonetheless, it is rare for more than one child in a family to have Kawasaki disease.

KEYWORDS
for searching the Internet and other reference sources

Coronary aneurysm

Coronary artery

Gamma globulin

Heart attack

Heart disease

Myocardial infarction

Myocarditis

* **microorganism** is a tiny organism that can be seen only using a microscope. Types of microorganisms include fungi, bacteria, and viruses.

* **scarlet fever** is an infection that causes a sore throat and a rash.

* **lymph** (LIMF) **nodes** are small, bean-shaped masses of tissue that contain immune system cells that fight harmful microorganisms. Lymph nodes may swell during infections.

* **coronary aneurysm** (KOR-uh-nair-e AN-yuh-rih-zum) is an abnormal stretching and weakening of a blood vessel that supplies blood to the heart. If it breaks open, it may cause serious damage to the heart, sometimes leading to death.

* **platelets** (PLATE-lets) are tiny disk-shaped particles within the blood that play an important role in clotting (the body's way of thickening blood to stop bleeding).

* **echocardiogram** (eh-ko-KAR-dee-uh-gram) is a diagnostic test that uses sound waves to produce images of the heart's chambers and valves and blood flow through the heart.

* **coronary arteries** (KOR-uh-nair-e AR-tuh-reez) are the blood vessels that directly supply blood to the heart.

* **blood clots** are thickenings of the blood into a jelly-like substance that helps stop bleeding. Clotting of the blood within a blood vessel can lead to blockage of blood flow.

* **gamma globulin** (GAH-muh GLAH-byoo-lin) is a type of protein in the blood that contains the antibodies produced by the cells of the body's immune system that help defend the body against infection-causing germs, such as bacteria and viruses.

* **Reye syndrome** (RYE SIN-drome) is a rare condition that involves inflammation of the liver and brain, and sometimes appears after illnesses such as chicken pox or influenza. It has also been associated with taking aspirin during certain viral infections.

* **angiogram** (AN-jee-o-gram) is a test in which X rays are taken as dye is injected into the body, showing the flow of blood through the heart and blood vessels.

* **stress test** measures the health of a person's heart while the heart is intentionally stressed by exercise or medication.

What Are the Signs and Symptoms of the Disease?

Kawasaki disease has distinctive features. A high fever, often more than 104 degrees Fahrenheit, usually appears first and lasts for at least 5 days. Afterward, signs of Kawasaki disease show up in stages and may include a red rash over the entire body, cracked lips, inflamed lining of the mouth, and a red, swollen tongue. Infected children also may have reddened and swollen hands, feet, fingers, and toes, with peeling skin; conjunctivitis in both eyes; sore, stiff joints; and swollen lymph nodes in the neck. Some children experience abdominal pain and diarrhea as well. The earliest phase of the disease, including fever and rash, usually lasts 10 to 14 days. The later phase, with peeling skin and slowly easing joint pain, can persist up to 2 months. Heart problems, if they occur, are more likely to show up during this time.

Making the Diagnosis

No single laboratory test can identify Kawasaki disease, so doctors make the diagnosis based on the child's symptoms and a physical examination: 5 days of high fever, accompanied by most of the associated telltale signs mentioned earlier. Blood tests help support the diagnosis and include tests to determine the numbers of white blood cells (cells that respond to infection) and platelets* and tests that detect inflammation in the body. Echocardiograms* and chest X rays are done to look for evidence of damage to the heart and coronary arteries*.

How Do Doctors Treat Kawasaki Disease?

Kawasaki disease is treated in the hospital. Children typically are given high doses of aspirin to decrease inflammation, prevent blood clots* in the heart's blood vessels, and lessen fever and joint pain. A one-time dose of intravenous gamma globulin* also is given to lower the risk of heart problems, particularly coronary aneurysms. (Even though aspirin is an important part of the treatment for Kawasaki disease, children normally are not given aspirin for minor fever or pain, because Reye syndrome*, a dangerous condition, has been linked to aspirin use in children.)

Much of the treatment for Kawasaki disease focuses on keeping the patient comfortable while the illness runs its course. After the disease clears up, children still need follow-up testing to make sure it has not caused heart disease. They may have additional echocardiograms or angiograms* to examine the heart for damage and sometimes a stress test* to check the heart's function.

What Are the Possible Complications of Kawasaki Disease?

Up to 25 percent of children with untreated Kawasaki disease may experience complications that involve the heart and coronary arteries. With treatment, that risk goes down to less than 5 percent. Babies younger than 1 year and children older than 9 years have the greatest risk of heart problems. By far the most serious complication of Kawasaki disease is coronary aneurysm. If an aneurysm clots or, more rarely, bursts in a blood vessel supplying the heart muscle, it can cause a heart attack or even death. Kawasaki disease can affect the heart in other ways as well, leading to myocarditis* or an irregular heartbeat.

Can Kawasaki Disease Be Prevented?

Because little is known about its cause, there are no proven ways to prevent Kawasaki disease.

Resources

Organizations

American Heart Association, National Center, 7272 Greenville Avenue, Dallas, TX 75231. The American Heart Association provides information about Kawasaki disease and related heart problems at its website.
Telephone 800-242-8721
http://www.americanheart.org

U.S. National Library of Medicine, 8600 Rockville Pike, Bethesda, MD 20894. The National Library of Medicine's website provides general information for the public on a variety of health topics, including Kawasaki disease.
Telephone 888-346-3656
http://www.nlm.nih.gov

* **myocarditis** (my-oh-kar-DYE-tis) is an inflammation of the muscular walls of the heart.

 See also
Conjunctivitis
Myocarditis/Pericarditis

L

Laryngitis

Laryngitis (lair-in-JY-tis) is an inflammation of the vocal cords that causes hoarseness or a temporary loss of voice.

The vocal cords are the two bands of muscle found inside the larynx (LAIR-inks), or voice box, located between the base of the tongue and the top of the trachea*. As they let air into and out of the lungs, the vocal cords are relaxed. When a person talks, however, the vocal cords tighten as air passes through them, causing the cords to vibrate and thereby produce sound.

People who lose their voice after cheering too much at a hockey game or who begin to sound hoarse or raspy when they have a bad cold probably have laryngitis. Laryngitis refers to inflammation or irritation of the vocal cords. Inflammation causes swelling, which prevents the vocal cords from working properly, and the sounds they produce can seem strange or be hard to hear. Although laryngitis can make it difficult to communicate, it is rarely serious.

Why Do People Get Laryngitis?

Almost everyone gets laryngitis at some point, whether it is a low raspy whisper or a complete loss of voice. Overusing the voice, such as yelling, speaking too loudly or for too long, and even singing, can lead to laryngitis. People who use their voice constantly, such as radio announcers, politicians, and singers, get laryngitis more often than other people do. The larynx is located along the respiratory tract*, which is why respiratory infections such as the flu (influenza) and the common cold can easily spread to the voice box and cause laryngitis. People who have allergies or who develop polyps* on the vocal cords may also experience laryngitis. Smoking, heavy drinking, inhaling harmful fumes, and acid reflux* all irritate and inflame the vocal cords and can result in long-term or chronic laryngitis.

What Are the Signs and Symptoms of Laryngitis?

The most obvious symptoms of laryngitis are a hoarse or low voice, the inability to speak above a whisper, a raw feeling or sensation of having a lump in the throat, difficulty swallowing, and the need to clear the throat often. When laryngitis is caused by an infection such as the flu,

KEYWORDS
for searching the Internet and other reference sources

Hoarseness

Larynx

Loss of voice

Respiratory infections

Vocal cords

Voice disorders

* **trachea** (TRAY-kee-uh) is the windpipe, the firm, tubular structure that carries air from the throat to the lungs.

* **respiratory tract** includes the nose, mouth, throat, and lungs. It is the pathway through which air and gases are transported down into the lungs and back out of the body.

* **polyps** (PAH-lips) are bumps or growths, usually on the lining or surface of a body part (such as the nose or intestine). Their size can range from tiny to large enough to cause pain or obstruction. They may be harmless, but they also may be cancerous.

* **acid reflux** is a condition in which stomach acid flows upward into the esophagus, often causing a burning sensation (so-called "heartburn") in the upper abdomen or chest.

Hand Washing 101

Hand washing is one of the best ways to prevent the respiratory infections that lead to laryngitis. What is the best way to wash hands? Rubbing the hands together, front and back, with warm, soapy water for at least 15 to 30 seconds is much better at preventing the spread of germs than just a quick rinse.

a person may also experience sneezing, coughing, runny nose, headache, and fever.

Severe laryngitis can sometimes lead to breathing problems, especially in young children. Anyone with laryngitis who develops difficulty breathing or high fever or who is not getting better after a few days needs medical care.

How Is Laryngitis Diagnosed and Treated?

A doctor will ask about a person's symptoms and voice use to help determine whether laryngitis is the result of a respiratory infection or some other cause. In some cases, a doctor might take a close look at the vocal cords by holding a small mirror at the back of the throat. To get an even better view, a doctor might use a tiny camera on a long, thin tube that goes through the mouth or nose. This method allows the doctor to watch the vocal cords in action.

How a doctor treats laryngitis depends on what is causing it. If the cause is a viral infection, antibiotics will not help and the laryngitis will go away on its own. The doctor may recommend certain medicines to help relieve symptoms. Other tips that can help a person to feel better sooner are:

- resting the voice for several days (this means barely even a whisper) to help the vocal cords heal
- using a humidifier at home or sitting in the bathroom while a steamy shower is running; both put moisture into the air that can help to soothe an inflamed larynx
- drinking plenty of liquids
- getting lots of rest
- avoiding smoking or drinking alcohol

Laryngitis usually disappears after a few days, but it can last much longer and happen more often in people who are smokers or heavy drinkers or who use their voices for hours at a time in their jobs. It may take weeks of voice rest before their voices return to normal. Such long-term hoarseness might cause complications that require speech therapy to help prevent further damage. If growths have formed on the vocal cords over time, surgery may be needed.

Preventing Laryngitis

Laryngitis is not contagious, but colds, flu, and other infections that cause it are. Doing what is possible to avoid these infections (such as frequent hand washing) decreases a person's chances of getting laryngitis.

Following these prevention basics can help maintain a healthy voice for life:

- not shouting or talking too loudly for too long

- staying away from cigarette smoke, which irritates the entire respiratory system
- keeping vocal cords from getting dry by drinking enough water every day

Resources

Websites

KidsHealth.org. KidsHealth is a website created by the medical experts of the Nemours Foundation and is devoted to issues of children's health. It contains articles on a variety of health topics, including laryngitis.
http://www.KidsHealth.org

The National Center for Voice and Speech website offers self-help for better vocal health.
http://www.ncvs.org/lifelong/strategies.html

▶ *See also*
Bronchitis, Infectious
Influenza

Legionnaire's Disease

Legionnaire's (lee-juh-NAIRS) disease, also known as legionellosis (lee-juh-nel-O-sis), is a bacterial infection that can lead to a serious form of pneumonia (nu-MO-nyah), or inflammation of the lungs.

What Is Legionnaire's Disease?

In 1976 more than 200 people attending an American Legion convention at the Bellevue-Stratford Hotel in Philadelphia, Pennsylvania, suddenly came down with a mysterious illness that caused high fever, chills, and a cough. Thirty-four people died from severe pneumonia. The illness, later named Legionnaire's disease in memory of the convention attendees, was caused by a previously undiscovered bacterium that scientists called *Legionella pneumophila,* (lee-juh-NEL-uh new-MOH-fee-luh). The bacteria were found to be living in the hotel's air-conditioning system. Since the initial outbreak, several other species of *Legionella* bacteria have been discovered, some of which can cause a very similar but less serious disease. Although we often hear about outbreaks of Legionnaire's disease in public places that affect many people at once, such outbreaks actually occur more frequently on a much smaller scale. The disease can even break out in homes.

How Common Is It?

Between 8,000 and 18,000 cases of Legionnaire's disease occur in the United States every year. It is believed that many more may go undiagnosed because the symptoms are so mild that people do not seek

KEYWORDS
for searching the Internet and other reference sources
Legionella pneumophila

Legionellosis

Pneumonia

Pontiac fever

Respiratory infections

* **chronic** (KRAH-nik) means continuing for a long period of time.

* **emphysema** (em-fuh-ZEE-mah) is a lung disease in which the tiny air sacs in the lungs become permanently damaged and are unable to maintain the normal exchange of oxygen and other respiratory gases with the blood, often causing breathing difficulty.

* **AIDS**, or acquired immunodeficiency (ih-myoo-no-dih-FIH-shen-see) syndrome, is an infection that severely weakens the immune system; it is caused by the human immunodeficiency virus (HIV).

treatment. An outbreak is most likely to occur in summer or early fall, but it can happen at any time. The disease can affect people of all ages, but people who are middle age or older, who smoke cigarettes, or who have chronic* lung conditions, such as emphysema*, may be at especially high risk. People with weakened immune systems, such as those who have AIDS* or cancer, or those who have undergone organ transplantation, also are at greater risk of contracting the disease.

How Does Legionnaire's Disease Spread?

Legionnaire's disease is not spread from person to person. *Legionella* bacteria live and grow in warm, stagnant (still) water, such as that found in air-conditioning systems, hot-water tanks, or whirlpool spas. People might become infected by breathing in the mist from contaminated water sources (for example, the vents of air conditioners at a hotel or the showers at a gym).

Signs and Symptoms

Symptoms of *Legionella* infection can range from mild to severe. In fact, some people infected with the bacteria may show no symptoms at all. Those who do might experience high fever, chills, and a cough that usually produces sputum (SPYOO-tum), a mixture of thick, slippery mucus (MYOO-kus) and other material coughed up from the inflamed lungs and windpipe. Some people also have extreme tiredness, muscle aches, headache, shortness of breath, stomach pain, diarrhea, and loss of appetite. Symptoms typically begin within 2 to 10 days of exposure to the bacterium. Kidney problems also may occur. *Legionella* bacteria also have been found to cause a less serious disease called Pontiac fever, which is characterized by mild flulike symptoms, without signs of pneumonia.

How Do Doctors Diagnose and Treat the Disease?

Legionnaire's disease can be difficult to distinguish from other types of pneumonia. There are very specific tests for it, but before ordering these tests, doctors need to learn as much as possible about a patient. First, doctors will ask patients about their general health and recent activities. This history will help determine whether the patient might have been exposed to *Legionella* bacteria. Doctors then will perform a physical examination of the patient and take chest X rays to look for signs of pneumonia in the lungs. If a doctor suspects Legionnaire's disease at this time, more specific laboratory tests might be ordered, including blood tests, to determine whether the patient's body is producing antibodies* to *Legionella* bacteria. Cultures of fluids from the patient's lungs may be done. To perform a culture, a person's sputum is placed on special material called a culture medium. If *Legionella* bacteria are present in the sputum,

* **antibodies** (AN-tih-bah-deez) are protein molecules produced by the body's immune system to help fight specific infections caused by microorganisms, such as bacteria and viruses.

the medium will help them grow so that the bacterium can be identified. A urine test also can help confirm the presence of infection. The disease is treated with antibiotics and usually requires a stay in the hospital. In the hospital, patients receive supportive care, such as oxygen if they are having trouble breathing and extra fluids to replace what has been lost during periods of high fever.

What Are the Complications of Legionnaire's Disease?

Some people with *Legionella* infection experience only mild symptoms of illness, whereas others may be hospitalized for several weeks. Afterward, they may continue to be very tired for several more months. Most people who become ill with Legionnaire's disease recover, but in people with chronic lung problems, *Legionella* can make the condition worse, leading to severe illness. Up to 15 percent of cases of Legionnaire's disease are fatal.

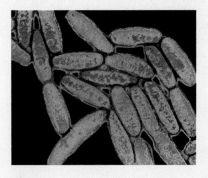

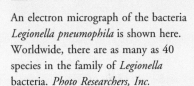

An electron micrograph of the bacteria *Legionella pneumophila* is shown here. Worldwide, there are as many as 40 species in the family of *Legionella* bacteria. *Photo Researchers, Inc.*

THE CDC IN ACTION

When Legionnaire's disease broke out at the American Legion convention in Philadelphia in the summer of 1976, theories about its cause ranged from swine flu to chemical poisoning to communist conspiracies against American veterans. As fears mounted, the U.S. Centers for Disease Control and Prevention (CDC) in Atlanta, Georgia, in cooperation with other federal, state, and local authorities, launched one of the largest joint disease investigations in history. Investigators looked at the possible sources of the outbreak and the ways the infection could have spread. Survivors were examined, bodies were autopsied, and specimens of air, water, soil, and various hotel materials were tested. Comparing tissue samples from people who had become infected with samples held in storage at the CDC, investigators were even able to link the Philadelphia cases to unidentified cases of illness dating back as far as the 1940s. Finally, in 1977, doctors isolated the culprit bacterium from the hotel's cooling tower, and federal authorities put in place new hygiene safeguards to limit future problems. The CDC continues to work today in disease prevention and control, addressing such wide-ranging topics as air pollution, water contamination, and unsafe working conditions and implementing educational programs and various other strategies to protect the health of Americans.

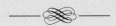

Can the Disease Be Prevented?

There is little that people can do to avoid becoming infected with *Legionella*. In public places, better maintenance of plumbing and air-conditioning systems, including regular inspection and cleaning, can help limit the growth of the bacteria. If there is an outbreak, government health teams step in to decontaminate the suspected source of the bacteria.

Resource

Organization

National Center for Infectious Diseases, U.S. Centers for Disease Control and Prevention, Office of Health Communication, Mailstop C-14, 1600 Clifton Road, Atlanta, GA 30333. The website for the National Center for Infectious Diseases offers information on various infectious illnesses, including Legionnaire's disease.
Telephone 800-311-3435
http://www.cdc.gov/ncidod

▶ *See also*
Pneumonia

Leishmaniasis

Leishmaniasis (leesh-muh-NYE-uh-sis) is a parasitic infection spread by sand flies. It causes symptoms ranging from sores on the skin to damage to internal organs.

What Is Leishmaniasis?

The disease occurs when a person becomes infected with any of several types of *Leishmania* parasites*. They spread to people through the bite of female sand flies and can cause different forms of illness, all of which are called leishmaniasis. Cutaneous (kyoo-TAY-nee-us) leishmaniasis affects the skin; mucocutaneous (myoo-ko-kyoo-TAY-nee-us) leishmaniasis attacks the mucous membranes* in the mouth, nose, and throat; and visceral (VIH-suh-rul) leishmaniasis (also known as systemic leishmaniasis or kala azar) damages internal organs, such as the liver* and spleen*.

Cutaneous and mucocutaneous infections can lead to severe scarring and permanent disfigurement. In patients with a mucocutaneous infection, the disease can destroy soft tissue in the mouth and nose, drastically deforming the face. The visceral form of the disease is considered the most dangerous. It can grow worse over time and is usually fatal if not treated. Leishmaniasis damages the immune system so that it cannot fight off infections; these infections are generally the cause of death, not leishmaniasis itself. In some countries, visceral disease has been found

KEYWORDS
for searching the Internet and other reference sources

Kala azar

Parasitic infections

Sand fly

Travel-related illnesses

*** parasites** (PAIR-uh-sites) are organisms such as protozoa (one-celled animals), worms, or insects that must live on or inside a human or other organism to survive. An animal or plant harboring a parasite is called its host. Parasites live at the expense of the host and may cause illness.

*** mucous membranes** are the moist linings of the mouth, nose, eyes, and throat.

*** liver** is a large organ located beneath the ribs on the right side of the body. The liver performs numerous digestive and chemical functions essential for health.

208

with increasing frequency in people who also have human immunodeficiency virus* infection.

How Common Is the Disease?

The infection is most common in tropical and subtropical regions, such as countries in South America, Africa, and Asia, and the number of areas where it occurs continues to grow. The U.S. Centers for Disease Control and Prevention (CDC) estimates that one and a half million people around the world contract cutaneous leishmaniasis each year and half a million people experience the more serious visceral form of the disease. Ninety percent of the visceral cases are found in just five countries: India, Nepal, Bangladesh, Sudan, and Brazil. Leishmaniasis is exceptionally rare in the United States, although a few cutaneous cases have been diagnosed in rural southern Texas.

Is It Contagious?

People cannot get leishmaniasis directly from other people. Instead, the disease spreads through the bite of blood-sucking sand flies. A fly bites an infected animal or person and takes in the parasite with its meal of blood. The *Leishmania* parasites reproduce in the fly, which can spread them when it bites another person. Sand flies are quite small—about a third of the size of a mosquito—and fly silently, so people often do not even know the flies are nearby. Less often, the disease can be transmitted through contaminated blood in a transfusion*, by sharing or reusing needles for injecting drugs, or from a mother to her baby during pregnancy or birth.

What Are the Signs and Symptoms of Leishmaniasis?

Cutaneous leishmaniasis is marked by sores that often look like volcanoes: they have a central pit and a raised rim. They can be painful or painless and may be covered by scabs. The sores tend to appear on the face, arms, and legs, and some people have as many as 200 of them. Patients with cutaneous leishmaniasis also may have swollen lymph nodes* near the sores. In mucocutaneous cases, the lesions appear in the mouth, nose, and throat and gradually destroy the soft tissues in those areas.

The visceral form of the disease can cause lack of appetite, serious weight loss, fever (which can last from 2 weeks to 2 months), and increasing weakness. It also can lead to an enlarged spleen and liver and sometimes swollen lymph nodes. Blood tests may show that the patient has low levels of white blood cells, red blood cells, or platelets*. As the disease progresses, the skin can become dark and dry—a symptom that gave the disease the name kala azar (meaning "black fever"). In children, visceral leishmaniasis often begins suddenly, with fever, diarrhea, and cough.

*__spleen__ is an organ in the upper left part of the abdomen that stores and filters blood. As part of the immune system, the spleen also plays a role in fighting infection.

*__human immunodeficiency__ (HYOO-mun ih-myoo-no-dih-FIH-shen-see) __virus__, or HIV, is the virus that causes AIDS (acquired immunodeficiency syndrome).

*__transfusion__ (trans-FYOO-zhun) is a procedure in which blood or certain parts of blood, such as specific cells, are given to a person who needs them because of illness or blood loss.

*__lymph__ (LIMF) __nodes__ are small, bean-shaped masses of tissue that contain immune system cells that fight harmful microorganisms. Lymph nodes may swell during infections.

*__platelets__ (PLATE-lets) are tiny, disk-shaped particles within the blood that play an important role in clotting.

Cutaneous leishmaniasis affects the skin, causing sores that may look like volcanoes: they have a central pit and a raised rim. The disease can destroy tissue and lead to permanent scarring. *AP/Wide World Photos* ▶

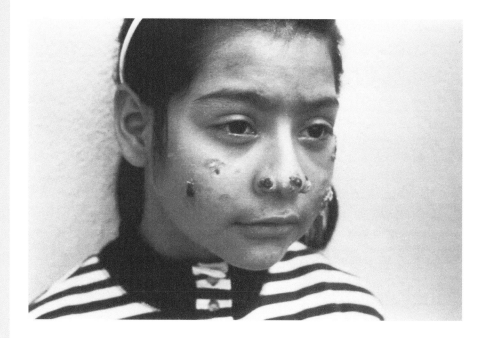

* **cultured** (KUL-churd) means subjected to a test in which a sample of fluid or tissue from the body is placed in a dish containing material that supports the growth of certain organisms. Over time, ranging from hours to weeks, the organisms will grow and can be identified.

* **antibodies** (AN-tih-bah-deez) are protein molecules produced by the body's immune system to help fight specific infections caused by microorganisms, such as bacteria and viruses.

* **biopsies** (BI-op-seez) are tests in which a small sample of skin or other body tissue is removed and examined for signs of disease.

* **antimony** (AN-tih-mo-nee) is an element that has properties of both metals and nonmetals and can kill or inhibit the growth of certain bacteria.

How Do Doctors Make the Diagnosis?

A key to making the diagnosis is learning whether the patient has traveled to a country where leishmaniasis occurs. During the physical examination, the doctor also checks the patient's body for the types of sores seen with the infection. The doctor may take blood samples and tissue samples from any sores that are found. These samples will be cultured*, examined for signs of the parasite, or tested for antibodies* to the parasite. For suspected cases of visceral infection, biopsies* of the abnormal tissue may be done.

What Is the Treatment?

Doctors treat the infection with prescription medications; many of these medicines contain antimony*. Cutaneous cases usually can be treated at home, but visceral disease may require hospitalization and supportive care, such as intravenous* fluids. Patients who have severe disfigurement from cutaneous, and especially mucocutaneous, leishmaniasis often need reconstructive surgery to regain a normal appearance. However, such extensive (and expensive) treatment is not available to vast numbers of people in developing countries who contract this disease.

How Long Does the Disease Last?

Although some cases of cutaneous leishmaniasis clear up on their own, most cases of mucocutaneous and visceral infection will not get better without treatment. Left untreated, visceral disease typically leads to death within 2 years. Cutaneous cases may take several months to heal, even with treatment, and may return after the treatment has been completed.

What Are the Complications of Leishmaniasis?

The cutaneous and mucocutaneous forms of leishmaniasis often cause widespread scarring. In mucocutaneous cases, destruction of tissue in the mouth and nose can lead to facial deformity. Visceral disease can damage the immune system to the point that it is unable to fight off other infections. Some patients may need to have the spleen removed if it is trapping and destroying too many of the person's blood cells, and advanced cases of disease often result in death.

Can the Disease Be Prevented?

Avoiding sand fly bites is the best way to limit the spread of leishmaniasis. In areas where the flies live, people are advised to stay inside from dusk until dawn, when the insects are most active. Wearing long-sleeved shirts, long pants, and socks and tucking pants into socks can reduce the amount of bare skin that is vulnerable to fly bites. Using insect repellent, staying in screened-in or air-conditioned areas, sleeping under mosquito netting, and spraying living areas with an insecticide to kill flies also can help lessen the risk of being bitten.

Resources

Organizations

U.S. Centers for Disease Control and Prevention (CDC), 1600 Clifton Road, Atlanta, GA 30333. The CDC provides a fact sheet and other information on leishmaniasis at its website.
Telephone 800-311-3435
http://www.cdc.gov

World Health Organization (WHO), Avenue Appia 20, 1211 Geneva 27, Switzerland. WHO tracks disease outbreaks around the world and offers information about leishmaniasis at its website.
Telephone 011-41-22-791-2111
http://www.who.int

Leprosy

Leprosy (LEH-pro-see) is a chronic*, infectious disease that damages the skin, peripheral nerves*, and mucous membranes* of the mouth, throat, and eyes. Leprosy also is known as Hansen disease.

What Is Leprosy?

His equipment was inadequate and his colleagues thought his theories were laughable. Still, Gerhard Henrik Armauer Hansen (1841–1912)

* **intravenous** (in-tra-VEE-nus) means within or through a vein. For example, medications, fluid, or other substances can be given through a needle or soft tube inserted through the skin's surface directly into a vein.

▶ *See also*
Travel-related Infections
Trypanosomiasis
West Nile Fever

KEYWORDS
for searching the Internet and other reference sources

Hansen disease

Lepromatous leprosy

Multibacillary Hansen disease

Mycobacterium leprae

Paucibacillary Hansen disease

Tuberculoid leprosy

spent day after day bent over his microscope, determined to prove that leprosy was caused by bacteria. And he did. In 1873 the Norwegian physician identified the rod-shaped bacterium *Mycobacterium leprae* (my-ko-bak-TEER-e-um LEH-pray) as the cause of the illness. Hansen's discovery was immensely valuable in the treatment of leprosy, and it was a scientific milestone—the first proof that bacteria could cause human disease. Today, the use of the word "leper" is considered insulting, because it defines a person by the disease he or she has. Many advocates for people with leprosy prefer to call it Hansen disease.

The name paucibacillary (paw-sih-BAH-sih-lair-e) Hansen disease comes from the Latin word *pauci,* meaning few, and is used to describe a mild form of leprosy. Paucibacillary Hansen disease begins in the peripheral nerves and spreads to the skin, causing patches of skin to become numb and hypopigmented, which means that the skin has lost its coloring and appears white. Multibacillary (mul-tie-BAH-sih-lair-e) Hansen disease is a more severe form of the disease. Multibacillary Hansen disease also causes skin lesions (LEE-zhuns), or patches of damaged tissue; nodules, or lumps; and thickening of the skin. Without treatment, this type of leprosy can worsen over time, resulting in severe skin and tissue damage and disfigurement.

3,000 YEARS OF LEPROSY

Leprosy has left a trail of pain, suffering, and death that dates back thousands of years. Archeologists have uncovered skeletal remains with erosion in the bones of the nose that is characteristic of leprosy. Researchers translating from ancient Indian and Chinese texts have found descriptions of the disease. As men and armies roamed the globe in search of conquest, the germ that causes leprosy traveled with them. Researchers believe that in the first century B.C., Roman soldiers fighting in Egypt carried the disease home to Italy. In the Middle Ages, the disease spread from Italy throughout Europe. During the Crusades, a series of "holy wars" spanning the eleventh to the thirteenth centuries, European soldiers and pilgrims carried the disease as far as Jerusalem in the Middle East. The disease continued to follow the paths of conquering armies. The Spanish conquistadors and the slave trade brought the disease to the American continents, and European colonists probably spread the disease to islands in the Pacific Ocean.

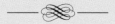

How Common Is Leprosy?

Throughout human history leprosy has caused untold suffering. Even after Hansen's groundbreaking discovery, the disease remained unchecked in many parts of the world. In 1991, the World Health Organization (WHO) began a global campaign to reduce the number of cases of leprosy. A decade later the organization announced that it had reached its goal and estimated that there were at that time 600,000 to 750,000 cases of leprosy worldwide. The disease is most common in tropical and subtropical regions, and in 2001, it remained a particular problem in Brazil, India, Madagascar, Mozambique, Nepal, and Myanmar. Leprosy is most common in densely populated areas with poor sanitation and health care, and children are at greater risk than adults of getting the disease. In the United States about 100 cases are reported each year, many of them in people who have recently immigrated.

Is the Disease Contagious?

Leprosy is contagious but does not spread easily. Researchers believe that *Mycobacterium leprae* is transmitted from person to person via respiratory droplets, bits of moisture that leave the mouth or nose when a person laughs, talks, sneezes, or coughs. Most people seem to have a natural immunity* that enables them to resist the disease. Of those in whom leprosy is diagnosed, most have had prolonged and close contact with someone who has an active infection. Once a person with leprosy has been taking medication for 3 or 4 days, the disease is no longer active or contagious.

What Are the Signs and Symptoms?

Leprosy begins as an infection in the nerve endings and spreads gradually; the skin near the infected nerves may become numb and hypopigmented. In severe cases, these skin lesions become wider and thicker. The muscles in the hands and feet can become weak or paralyzed (unable to move) because of damage to the peripheral nerves. That loss of sensation can lead to accidental injury, because a person loses the withdrawal reflex that helps protect against injury from hot or sharp objects. Left unchecked, the most severe form of the disease can progress, producing large, disfiguring nodules and enlarged facial features that give a person the lionlike appearance associated with severe leprosy.

How Is Leprosy Diagnosed?

Leprosy is not difficult to diagnose once it is suspected. A procedure in which a tiny piece of skin is scraped or cut away and then examined usually reveals the presence of *Mycobacterium leprae* in the multibacillary form of leprosy. (The bacteria may not be found using this method in milder, paucibacillary disease.) The procedure can be done quickly and relatively painlessly in a doctor's office or clinic. It is an important part

*immunity (ih-MYOON-uh-tee) is the condition of being protected against an infectious disease. Immunity often develops after a germ is introduced to the body. One type of immunity occurs when the body makes special protein molecules called antibodies to fight the disease-causing germ. The next time that germ enters the body, the antibodies quickly attack it, usually preventing the germ from causing disease.

As long ago as biblical times, people with the disfiguring signs of leprosy were cast out of their homes and villages and made to live together in isolated colonies. Even in modern times such colonies were established in the Western world, for example, on Penikese Island off Massachusetts and on the Hawaiian island of Molokai. *Corbis Corporation (Bellevue)* ▶

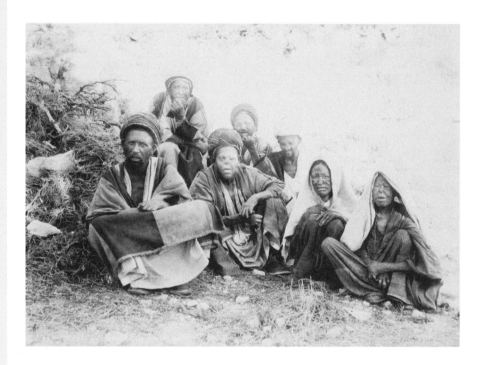

* **neurocutaneous** (nur-o-kyoo-TAY-nee-us) means affecting the skin and nerves.

of the diagnosis, because in the early stages of the disease leprosy lesions look very much like skin damage caused by other neurocutaneous* diseases. The presence of the characteristic lesions, accompanied by a history of living in areas where the disease is common, is what usually causes doctors to suspect the diagnosis.

Can Leprosy Be Treated?

Early diagnosis and treatment are key to stopping the spread of leprosy to other people and preventing long-term damage to the patient. Doctors most often prescribe multidrug therapy (MDT), combining two or three drugs that kill the bacteria: dapsone (DAP-sone), rifampicin (rye-FAM-pih-sin), and clofazimine (klo-FAY-zuh-meen). The MDT approach has been preferred since the early 1980s, when researchers noticed that the bacterium was becoming resistant to some treatments. Patients may take the drugs for as little as 6 months or as long as 2 years. Patients who have become disfigured or who experience disabilities may need surgery to correct these problems.

What Are the Complications and Course of Leprosy?

With MDT, paucibacillary Hansen disease can be cured within 6 to 12 months and multibacillary Hansen disease within 2 years. Untreated, leprosy can cause blindness, permanent nerve damage, and deformity. People may lose the use of their hands or feet, because, over time, the decreased sensation may result in repeated injuries to the limbs.

How Can Leprosy Be Prevented?

Despite centuries in which people with leprosy were vilified, shunned, and even isolated in far-off "leper colonies," there is no need to separate people with leprosy from the rest of society to avoid the spread of infection. MDT treatment is more effective and far more humane, and it has been determined that leprosy is much less contagious than once was believed. Hand washing, disinfection, and monitoring of close contacts are recommended to help prevent the spread of the disease.

Resources

Book

Eynikel, Hilde. *Molokai: The Story of Father Damien.* Translated by Lesley Gilbert. New York: Alba House, 1999. This is the story of the Belgian priest who cared for thousands of people with leprosy who were banished to the remote island of Molokai in the Hawaiian Islands. The book was made into a movie by the same name that is available on DVD.

Organization

World Health Organization (WHO), Avenue Appia 20, 1211 Geneva 27, Switzerland. The WHO tracks efforts to eradicate leprosy and has links to fact sheets and information on the prevention and control of the disease on its website.
Telephone 011-41-22-791-2111
http://www.who.int

▶ *See also*
Public Health

Lockjaw   *See* Tetanus (Lockjaw)

Lyme Disease

Lyme (LIME) disease is a bacterial infection that is spread to humans by the bite of an infected tick. It begins with a distinctive rash and/or flulike symptoms and, in some cases, can progress to a more serious disease with complications affecting other body organs.

Lyme disease was first described in 1977 when a group of children in and around Lyme, Connecticut, became ill with arthritis. In its early stage, Lyme disease produces flulike symptoms; if untreated, the disease

KEYWORDS
*for searching the Internet
and other reference sources*

Arthropod-borne infections

Black-legged tick

Borrelia burgdorferi

Borreliosis

Deer tick

Erythema migrans

Ixodes tick

Tick-borne infections

Zoonoses

The life cycle of a tick takes 2 years to complete. In the spring, eggs hatch into larvae, which feed on mice, birds, and small mammals until the fall, when they become dormant. The following spring they molt into nymphs, which feed through the summer and then become adults in the fall. At any of these stages of growth, ticks may become infected with Lyme disease bacteria by feeding on infected animals; as adults they may feed on humans and transmit the bacteria that cause the disease.

can progress to affect the joints, heart, and nervous system, especially in adults.

Lyme disease is caused by a corkscrew-shaped bacterium called *Borrelia burgdorferi* (buh-REEL-e-uh burg-DOR-fe-ree). It is most commonly carried by very small, immature ticks of the *Ixodes* (iks-O-deez) group called deer ticks or black-legged ticks. Deer ticks spread Lyme disease in the northeast, midwest, and some other parts of the United States; another kind of *Ixodes* tick, the western black-legged tick, is the source of Lyme disease in the western United States. Lyme disease also occurs in other countries such as China, Japan, and some countries in Europe.

Lyme disease is not spread from person to person. It is spread by ticks that become infected with *Borrelia burgdorferi* after feeding on an animal, usually a mouse. Ticks then pass the bacteria to humans while attached to the person's skin and feeding on blood. To infect a human, the tick must be attached for at least 24 hours. Just because people are bitten by a tick does not mean that they will get Lyme disease; most tick bites do not cause disease.

Do Many People Get Lyme Disease?

More than 16,000 cases of Lyme disease occur each year in the United States, according to the U.S. Centers for Disease Control and Prevention (CDC). Although cases of Lyme disease have been reported in nearly every state, most cases are reported from the northeastern states, including New York, Connecticut, Massachusetts, Rhode Island, New Hampshire, Pennsylvania, New Jersey, Delaware, and Maryland, and from Minnesota, Wisconsin, and California. These areas contain natural habitats of *Ixodes* ticks.

People who live, play, or work in tick-infested wooded areas or overgrown brush are most at risk of getting the disease. Lyme disease is most common during the late spring and summer months in the United States (May through September), when ticks are most active and people are frequently outdoors.

What Happens When a Person Has Lyme Disease?

Signs and symptoms Within a few days to weeks after being bitten by an infected tick, about 80 percent of people develop a red circular rash known as erythema migrans (air-uh-THEE-muh MY-granz) at the site of the bite. The center of the rash may clear as it grows, giving the appearance of a bull's-eye pattern. The rash may feel warm, but it is usually not painful or itchy. Other symptoms in the early stage of Lyme disease may include tiredness, fever, chills, joint pain, muscle aches, headache, stiff neck, and swollen lymph nodes* (glands). Some people have no noticeable symptoms or only have the non-specific, flulike symptoms such as fever and headache.

Did You Know?

Immature *Ixodes* ticks (called nymph ticks) are about the size of a poppyseed. Adult ticks are only the size of a sesame seed.

*****lymph** (LIMF) **nodes** are small, bean-shaped masses of tissue that contain immune system cells that fight harmful microorganisms. Lymph nodes may swell during infections.

217

As is evident in this map showing the occurrence of Lyme disease in the United States for the year 2000, most of the cases came from the northeastern, north-central, and mid-Atlantic states. In all, 95 percent were identified in Connecticut, Rhode Island, New Jersey, New York, Massachusetts, Delaware, Pennsylvania, Maryland, Wisconsin, Minnesota, New Hampshire, and Vermont. ▶

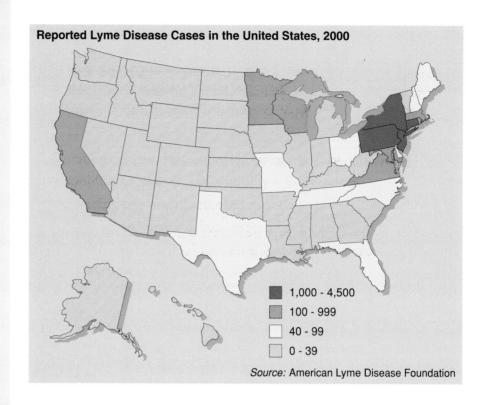

Reported Lyme Disease Cases in the United States, 2000

■ 1,000 - 4,500
■ 100 - 999
□ 40 - 99
□ 0 - 39

Source: American Lyme Disease Foundation

* **paralysis** (pah-RAH-luh-sis) is the loss or impairment of the ability to move some part of the body.

* **Bell's palsy** (PAWL-zee) is a condition in which there is weakness or loss of function of muscles on one side of the face.

* **meningitis** (meh-nin-JY-tis) is an inflammation of the meninges, the membranes that surround the brain and the spinal cord. Meningitis is most often caused by infection with a virus or a bacterium.

* **chronic** (KRAH-nik) means continuing for a long period of time.

* **antibodies** (AN-tih-bah-deez) are protein molecules produced by the body's immune system to help fight specific infections caused by microorganisms, such as bacteria and viruses.

If untreated, Lyme disease can progress to the next stage, called the early disseminated stage, as the infection spreads and starts to affect certain body functions. This more advanced stage appears a few weeks to as long as 3 months after a bite by an infected tick. Symptoms may include two or more areas of rash, severe headache, severe tiredness, stiffness (especially in the joints and neck), one-sided facial paralysis* (Bell's palsy*), tingling or numbness in the legs and arms, irregular heartbeat, fever, and meningitis*.

A late stage of Lyme disease may develop weeks to years later if the disease remains untreated. In this stage, symptoms can include chronic* Lyme arthritis (episodes of pain and swelling in the joints, especially in the arms and legs), memory loss (which is rare in children and teens), and numbness in the hands, arms, legs, and feet.

Diagnosis Diagnosing Lyme disease can be difficult because the symptoms often look like those of other diseases. A known recent tick bite or the erythema migrans rash are often key to the diagnosis of Lyme disease. Following a physical examination and medical history that includes asking about exposure to tick-infested areas, the doctor may order blood tests that look for the presence of antibodies* to *Borrelia burgdorferi.* If any joints are swollen or signs of meningitis are present, joint fluid or spinal fluid is sometimes tested for Lyme disease.

Some blood tests for Lyme disease can give false negative results, particularly if done within the first month after infection. False positive test results can also occur. Because of this, doctors may have difficulty interpreting Lyme disease test results and confirming the diagnosis.

Treatment Lyme disease is usually treated with antibiotics taken for 3 to 4 weeks. Antibiotics are usually taken by mouth, but in severe or advanced cases of Lyme disease they may be given by injection. If treatment begins at the early stage of the disease, a complete cure is likely; it generally takes a few weeks or months for the symptoms to go away. Sometimes symptoms recur, making it necessary for a patient to take another course of antibiotics. If treatment is not started until later in the progression of the disease (at the early disseminated or late stage), antibiotics still work but recovery may take longer; the patient's symptoms may last for months or even years. Children usually recover from Lyme disease faster and with fewer complications than do adults.

Is Lyme Disease Preventable?

The best way to prevent Lyme disease is to prevent tick bites. Experts recommend avoiding areas that are likely to be infested with ticks, particularly in the spring and summer when nymph (immature) ticks feed. For any activity in tick-infested areas, it is wise to:

- Wear light-colored clothing so that ticks can be spotted easily.
- Keep arms and legs covered.
- Wear high rubber boots, because ticks usually are found close to the ground.
- Tuck shirts into pants and pants into socks or boots to help keep ticks from reaching the skin.
- Wear a hat and keep long hair pulled back.
- Shower and wash clothing after being in tick-infested areas.
- Inspect pets for ticks after they have been in the woods.

Applying insect repellents containing 10 percent DEET (n,n-diethyl-m toluamide), which is safe to use on children and adults, on both clothes and exposed skin, and permethrin (per-ME-thrin) (which kills ticks on contact) on clothes, may also help reduce the risk of tick attachment. If ticks are found attached to skin, they should be carefully removed with tweezers or forceps. A vaccine to prevent Lyme disease has been developed but is not currently available for use while it is being evaluated for possible side effects.

Resources

Book

Monroe, Judy. *Lyme Disease*. Mankato, MN: Capstone Press, 2001.

The Safe Way to Remove a Tick

- First, stay calm.
- Second, using tweezers, gently grasp the tick as close to the skin as possible and pull straight back slowly and steadily to reduce the risk of squeezing more bacteria into the bite.
- Third, wipe the area with alcohol or an antiseptic.
- Lastly, place the tick in a jar of rubbing alcohol to kill it.

Tick-borne Illnesses

Other diseases that can be transmitted through tick bites include:

- babesiosis
- ehrlichiosis
- Rocky Mountain spotted fever
- tularemia

Organizations

American Lyme Disease Foundation, Inc., Mill Pond Offices, 293 Route 100, Somers, NY 10589. The American Lyme Disease Foundation provides information on Lyme disease and other tick-borne illnesses on its website.
Telephone 914-277-6970
http://www.aldf.com

Lyme Disease Foundation, Inc., One Financial Plaza 18th Floor, Hartford, CT 06103. The Lyme Disease Foundation offers information on tick-borne illnesses and avoiding tick bites on its website.
Telephone 800-886-5963
http://www.lyme.org

National Center for Infectious Diseases, U.S. Centers for Disease Control and Prevention, Mailstop C-14, 1600 Clifton Road, Atlanta, GA 30333. The website for this U.S. government agency provides information about Lyme disease.
Telephone 800-311-3435
http://www.cdc.gov/ncidod

Website

KidsHealth.org. KidsHealth is a website created by the medical experts of the Nemours Foundation and is devoted to issues of children's health. It contains articles on a variety of health topics, including Lyme disease.
http://www.KidsHealth.org

▶ *See also*

Ehrlichiosis

Meningitis

Rocky Mountain Spotted Fever

Tick-borne Infections

Tularemia

M

Malaria

Malaria (mah-LAIR-e-uh) is a disease caused by a parasite that is spread to humans by the bite of an infected mosquito.

What Is Malaria?

Malaria, which literally means bad air, was once thought to be spread in the air around stagnant marshes. It is now known that mosquitoes, particularly female *Anopheles* (a-NOH-fel-eez) mosquitoes, spread the parasites that cause malaria. Four different species of a parasite in the genus *Plasmodium* (plaz-MO-dee-um) cause malaria. They are *falciparum* (fal-SIP-ar-um), *malariae* (ma-LAIR-e-eye), *ovale* (o-VAL-e), and *vivax* (VI-vax). Of the four, *P. falciparum* is the most common and the most deadly. *Plasmodium* requires time in both the mosquito vector* and human host* to complete its life cycle.

How Common Is Malaria?

Forty percent of the world's population is at risk for contracting malaria from infected mosquitoes, primarily in tropical and subtropical regions. Worldwide, there are 300 to 500 million cases of malaria and more than one million deaths from malaria each year. More than 90 percent of all malaria deaths occur in sub-Saharan Africa, a vast area south of the Sahara Desert, and 75 percent of deaths occur in children. *Plasmodium falciparum* causes malaria in this region, and poverty, poor nutrition, and poor access to health care all contribute to the high death rate. Malaria is increasingly common in Central and South America, Asia, the Middle East, and the Pacific Islands. About 1,200 cases of malaria are diagnosed in the United States each year, mostly in recent immigrants or travelers from countries where malaria is found.

Mosquito control has virtually eliminated malaria in areas with temperate climates. However, the disease is making a comeback as mosquitoes become resistant to insecticides and *Plasmodium* becomes resistant to medications used to treat malaria.

Is Malaria Contagious?

Malaria is not passed directly from one person to another. Mosquitoes spread the disease. When a mosquito bites an infected person, it ingests

KEYWORDS
for searching the Internet
and other reference sources

Anopheles mosquito

Chloroquine

Mosquito-borne illness

Plasmodium

Quinine

* **vector** (VEK-tor) is an animal or insect that carries a disease-causing organism and transfers it from one host to another.

* **host** is an organism that provides another organism (such as a parasite or virus) with a place to live and grow.

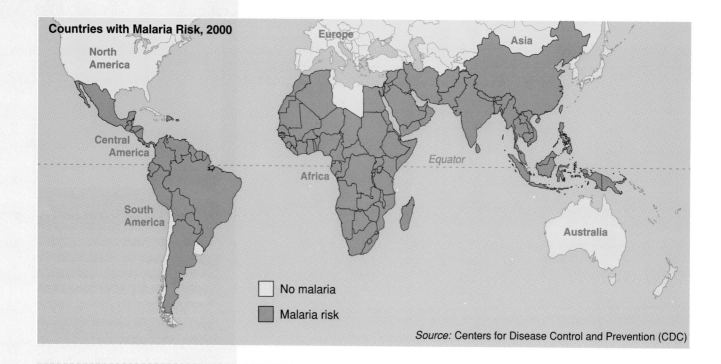

Countries with Malaria Risk, 2000

North America

Central America

South America

Europe

Asia

Africa

Equator

Australia

☐ No malaria

■ Malaria risk

Source: Centers for Disease Control and Prevention (CDC)

In most of Latin America, Africa, the Middle East, and Asia, people are at a higher risk of getting malaria. Drug-resistant malaria has caused the disease to be on the rise in these parts of the world.

* **incubation** (ing-kyoo-BAY-shun) **period** is the time between infection by a germ and when symptoms first appear. Depending on the germ, this period can be from hours to months.

* **anemia** (uh-NEE-me-uh) is a blood condition in which there is a decreased amount of oxygen-carrying hemoglobin in the blood and, usually, fewer than normal numbers of red blood cells.

* **jaundice** (JON-dis) is a yellowing of the skin, and sometimes the whites of the eyes, caused by a buildup in the body of bilirubin, a chemical produced in and released by the liver. An increase in bilirubin may indicate disease of the liver or certain blood disorders.

malaria parasites contained in that person's blood. The parasites need an incubation period* of about 1 week in the mosquito before the mosquito can spread the disease when it bites another person. Once in a person's body, the parasites travel to the liver where they can remain dormant, or inactive, for months or even years. In the liver, the parasites grow and multiply and are then ready to move into the body's red blood cells, where they continue to grow until the red blood cells burst, freeing more parasites to attack more blood cells. The parasite can be ingested by a mosquito and spread to another person only during the time that *Plasmodium* is in the blood.

What Are the Signs and Symptoms of Malaria?

Malaria causes fever and symptoms similar to those of the flu. In the early stages of the disease when the parasite is in the liver, the infected person does not feel sick. When the parasites invade the red blood cells and cause them to burst, toxins (poisons that harm the body) are released into the blood and the person experiences fever, chills, sweating, headache, muscle aches, and tiredness. Symptoms typically begin 9 to 16 days after infection with the parasite, but the time may vary depending on the infecting species. Episodes of these symptoms reoccur every 48 to 72 hours. Other symptoms may include nausea (NAW-zee-uh), vomiting, and diarrhea (dye-uh-REE-uh).

How Is Malaria Diagnosed and Treated?

Under the microscope, a blood sample from a person who has malaria will show one of the four species of *Plasmodium* parasites within the red blood cells. Malaria is treated with antimalarial drugs, many of them derived from quinine, which is found naturally in the bark of the cinchona tree from Peru. Which drug is chosen to treat a patient depends on the parasite causing the infection, the severity of symptoms, the age of the patient, and whether the parasite is resistant to certain drugs. Some patients may need intensive hospital care.

Treatment can last several weeks or months. In some infections, the parasite can remain dormant in the liver for months or years and the disease may return even after treatment. Destruction of red blood cells in cases of malaria can result in anemia* and jaundice*. Severe and untreated infection may cause liver and kidney* problems, seizures*, mental confusion, coma*, and death; malaria is fatal in 1 in 500 cases. Children and pregnant women are particularly vulnerable to complications. Infected pregnant women are at risk for miscarriage*, premature delivery*, and stillbirth*, and anemia in children can have long-term effects on growth and development.

Can Malaria Be Prevented?

In areas where malaria is endemic*, people can avoid being bitten by mosquitoes by wearing long-sleeved shirts and long pants, using insect

* **kidney** is one of the pair of organs that filter blood and remove waste products and excess water from the body in the form of urine.

* **seizures** (SEE-zhurs) are sudden bursts of disorganized electrical activity that interrupt the normal functioning of the brain, often leading to uncontrolled movements in the body and sometimes a temporary change in consciousness.

* **coma** (KO-ma) is an unconscious state in which a person cannot be awakened and cannot move, see, speak, or hear.

* **miscarriage** is the ending of a pregnancy through the death of the embryo or fetus before birth.

* **premature delivery** is when a baby is born before it has reached full term.

* **stillbirth** is the birth of a dead fetus.

* **endemic** (en-DEH-mik) describes a disease or condition that is present in a population or geographic area at all times.

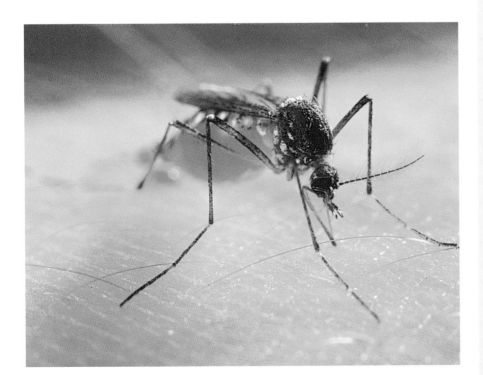

◄

Scientists, in searching for alternative means of malaria control, have recently been able to genetically modify mosquitoes carrying a form of malaria that affects rodents. The genetically modified mosquitoes were less susceptible to infection after feeding on a malaria-infected mouse and were far less likely than normal mosquitoes to transmit the malaria parasite to other mice. *Phototake*

repellent, and staying in a screened or air-conditioned room from dusk to dawn when mosquitoes are most active. Bed nets treated with certain insecticides repel mosquitoes for 6 to 12 months. Travelers to foreign countries where malaria is found should take preventive drugs prescribed by a doctor before leaving.

Scientists are working to develop a vaccine that will prevent malaria. However, the different species of *Plasmodium* and the complicated life cycle of these parasites have made developing a vaccine difficult.

Resources

Book

Jones, Ann. *Looking for Lovedu: Days and Nights in Africa*. Knopf: New York, 2001. The author's account of her journey across Africa in search of the legendary Lovedu tribe is full of adventure and complications such as malaria.

Organization

World Health Organization (WHO), Avenue Appia 20, 1211 Geneva 27, Switzerland. WHO provides information about malaria at its website.
Telephone 011-41-22-791-2111
http://www.who.int

Measles (Rubeola)

Measles (ME-zuls) is a viral respiratory system* infection that is best known for the rash of large, flat, red blotches that appear on the arms, face, neck, and body.

What Is Measles?

Measles, also known as rubeola (roo-be-O-luh), is a highly contagious viral infection caused by the measles virus. Most people are familiar with its most recognized feature: a near full-body rash of red blotches. In fact, measles is primarily an infection of the respiratory system. The disease has been diagnosed throughout the world, and before a vaccine* was available it commonly appeared in the United States in springtime epidemics* every few years. In the United States, 1 to 2 deaths occur for every 1,000 cases of measles. In developing countries, the fatality rate can be as high as 1 in every 4 people who contract the disease. Most deaths from measles in the United States are caused by pneumonia (nu-MO-nyah, inflammation of the lung), either from the measles virus itself or from a bacterial infection that arises as a complication of measles.

▶ *See also*
West Nile Fever
Yellow Fever

KEYWORDS
for searching the Internet and other reference sources

Koplik spots

MMR vaccine

Rubeola

* **respiratory system**, or respiratory tract, includes the nose, mouth, throat, and lungs. It is the pathway through which air and gases are transported down into the lungs and back out of the body.

* **vaccine** (vak-SEEN) is a preparation of killed or weakened germs, or a part of a germ or product it produces, given to prevent or lessen the severity of the disease that can result if a person is exposed to the germ itself. Use of vaccines for this purpose is called immunization.

How Common Is Measles?

Before the introduction of the measles vaccine in 1963, approximately 500,000 reported cases of measles and 500 deaths occurred in the United States each year. Since the start of measles vaccination programs, though, infection rates have dropped by more than 98 percent, and epidemics have all but disappeared. According to the U.S. Centers for Disease Control and Prevention, between 1993 and 2001 there were fewer than 500 cases of measles diagnosed each year (in 2000 there was an all-time low of 86 cases). However, an earlier resurgence of measles between 1989 and 1991 led to more than 55,000 diagnosed cases and 123 deaths. This epidemic arose because many children were not being vaccinated.

By contrast, the effect of measles in the developing world remains staggering. The disease accounted for about 777,000 deaths in 2001. Limited access to the vaccine is the primary reason that developing countries continue to see huge numbers of measles cases. Immigrants to the United States who have not received the vaccine in their native countries account for many of the cases of the disease that occur in the United States.

How Does Measles Spread?

Measles is highly contagious and can spread quickly among people who have not been immunized against it. The measles virus spreads by direct contact with an infected person or by breathing in tiny drops of fluid sent into the air when the person sneezes, coughs, or laughs. A cough or sneeze releases thousands of microscopic particles that contain the virus. They can stay in the air, able to infect people, for up to 2

Measles Redux

Cases of measles infection rose dramatically during the years 1989 to 1991 in the United States and other countries. Nearly half of the U.S. patients were unvaccinated preschool children living in urban areas. The epidemic began because of a lapse in measles vaccinations and public education. Many people were unaware that measles was still a threat, because years of public vaccinations had controlled the infection; some were afraid of adverse reactions to the vaccine itself. Emergency vaccinations eventually contained the epidemic, but the outbreak revealed the persistence of a virus that many believed was no longer a cause for concern.

* **epidemics** (eh-pih-DEH-miks) are outbreaks of disease, especially infectious disease, in which the number of cases suddenly becomes far greater than usual. Usually, epidemics are outbreaks of diseases in specific regions, whereas worldwide epidemics are called pandemics.

THE SPREAD OF MEASLES

Historically, infectious diseases have been powerful players on the world stage. They have toppled kingdoms, swept through countries with devastating results, and altered world economies and religions. Measles traveled around the globe with European adventurers and explorers. The disease cut a swath through the inhabitants of the Pacific Islands and the Americas (North America, South America, and Central America). When the Spanish conquistadors Hernán Cortés (1485–1547) and Francisco Pizarro (ca. 1475–1541) arrived in the Americas, they unknowingly carried with them measles and smallpox, which resulted in the death of an estimated one-third of the native populations.

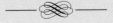

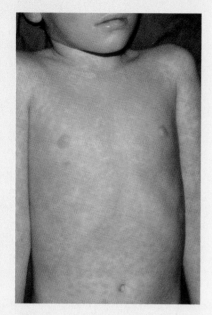

Measles poses a serious health treat to children, especially in developing countries where adequate medical treatment is difficult to obtain. *Custom Medical Stock Photo, Inc.*

* **seizures** (SEE-zhurs) are sudden bursts of disorganized electrical activity that interrupt the normal functioning of the brain, often leading to uncontrolled movements in the body and sometimes a temporary change in consciousness.

* **delirium** (dih-LEER-e-um) is a condition in which a person is confused, is unable to think clearly, and has a reduced level of consciousness.

* **antibodies** (AN-tih-bah-deez) are protein molecules produced by the body's immune system to help fight specific infections caused by microorganisms, such as bacteria and viruses.

* **dehydration** (dee-hi-DRAY-shun) is a condition in which the body is depleted of water.

* **intravenous** (in-tra-VEE-nus) **fluids** are fluids injected directly into a vein.

hours. In some cases, people have caught measles after entering a room that an infected person has already left. A person with measles is contagious from 1 to 2 days before the symptoms begin until 4 or 5 days after the rash appears.

What Are the Signs and Symptoms?

After a person has been exposed to the virus, there is an incubation period that averages 10 to 12 days. The first symptoms include fever, runny nose, cough, and reddened eyes that are sensitive to light. Koplik spots, a unique sign of measles, break out 1 to 2 days before the rash begins and usually are gone by the time it appears; they are bluish-white dots found on the inside of the cheeks and other places on the mucous membranes (moist linings) in the mouth.

The measles rash typically begins on the forehead and extends down across the face, neck, and body. It generally takes several days for the rash to travel from head to toes. The red blotches often spread out and join, completely covering the skin, especially on the face and shoulders. Once the rash appears, 2 to 4 days after the onset of illness, the fever rises and may peak at 104 to 105 degrees Fahrenheit. During this time, the patient looks and feels very ill. Symptoms improve soon after the rash has traveled down to the legs and feet, usually accompanied by a rapid drop in temperature. The rash fades along the same path that it appeared, beginning at the forehead and working its way down. As the rash disappears, the skin may temporarily look brown, dry, and flaky. Other symptoms of measles include loss of appetite, vomiting, and diarrhea (dye-uh-REE-uh), especially in young children. Hemorrhagic (heh-muh-RAH-jik) measles is a rare and serious form of the disease characterized by hemorrhaging (uncontrolled or abnormal bleeding), high fever, seizures*, and delirium*.

How Do Doctors Make the Diagnosis?

Measles can be diagnosed by asking a patient about symptoms and performing a physical examination. If there is a question about the diagnosis or if it is necessary to confirm a suspected case of measles, blood tests can determine whether antibodies* to the virus have developed in the body.

What Is the Treatment for Measles?

Because measles is caused by a virus, treatment generally is aimed at keeping the patient comfortable until the infection runs its course. The high fever and sweating that accompany measles raise the risk of dehydration*, so patients should have plenty of rest and fluids. Taking vitamin A may aid recovery in some cases, especially among children with poor nutrition. Serious cases may require a hospital stay and intravenous fluids*. Antibiotics are given when bacterial infections (such as ear infections or pneumonia) develop as complications of the disease.

What to Expect

Measles generally lasts between 10 and 14 days from the onset of symptoms through the fading of the rash. Ear infections, croup*, and pneumonia sometimes accompany measles. Less commonly, inflammation of the brain (known as encephalitis, en-seh-fuh-LYE-tis) or inflammation of the heart muscle (known as myocarditis, my-oh-kar-DYE-tis) can occur. Subacute sclerosing panencephalitis* (SSPE), a type of encephalitis, is an extremely rare late complication of lasting measles virus infection that can cause gradual loss of brain function. SSPE may occur months, years, or even decades after measles infection, but it is almost never seen in the United States, as a result of widespread use of the measles vaccine. If a pregnant woman contracts measles, the infection can harm her developing baby, leading to miscarriage*, premature labor*, or low birth weight.

How Can Measles Be Prevented?

The best protection against measles is immunization. The vaccine usually is given as part of a combined measles-mumps-rubella (MMR) vaccine that children typically receive twice in their lives. The first round is given when an infant is 12 to 15 months old and the second when the child is ready to start school, at 4 to 5 years old. Children also may receive the second vaccine when they are 11 or 12 years old, if they do not receive it earlier. Because about 5 percent of people do not develop protective antibodies after the first MMR vaccine, the second dose offers better protection against infection. If someone comes into contact with a person who has measles and then is vaccinated within 3 days of that exposure, the vaccine may prevent or lessen the severity of a case of measles. Immune globulin* can have the same result if it is given within 6 days of exposure to the virus.

Resources

Organization

U.S. Centers for Disease Control and Prevention (CDC), 1600 Clifton Road, Atlanta, GA 30333. Through the website of the National Center for Infectious Diseases, the CDC provides a fact sheet and other information on measles.
Telephone 800-311-3435
http://www.cdc.gov/ncidod/

Website

KidsHealth.org. KidsHealth is a website created by the medical experts of the Nemours Foundation and is devoted to issues of children's health. It contains articles on a variety of health topics, including measles.
http://www.KidsHealth.org

* **croup** (KROOP) is an infection involving the trachea (windpipe) and larynx (voice box) that typically occurs in childhood. It causes inflammation and narrowing of the upper airway, sometimes making it difficult to breathe. The characteristic symptom is a barking cough.

* **subacute sclerosing panencephalitis** (sub-uh-KYOOT skluh-RO-sing pan-en-seh-fuh-LYE-tis), or SSPE, is a chronic brain disease of children and adolescents that occurs months or years after having had measles; it causes convulsions, movement problems, and mental retardation and is usually fatal.

* **miscarriage** is the ending of a pregnancy through the death of the embryo or fetus before birth.

* **premature labor** is labor (the birth process) that begins too early, before the fetus has developed fully in the womb.

* **immune globulin** (ih-MYOON GLAH-byoo-lin), also called gamma globulin, is the protein material that contains antibodies.

▶ *See also*

227

Meningitis

Meningitis (meh-nin-JY-tis) is an inflammation of the membranes that surround the brain and the spinal cord (the meninges, meh-NIN-jeez). Meningitis is most often caused by infection with a virus or a bacterium.

What Is Meningitis?

Meningitis is an inflammation of the meninges, the membranes that enclose and protect the brain and the spinal cord. It is usually caused by infection, most often with viruses or bacteria. Meningitis caused by bacteria is known as septic meningitis. Meningitis caused by other organisms, including viruses, fungi, and parasites, is called aseptic (a-SEP-tik) meningitis. Viral meningitis is the most common and mildest form of the disease, and most people fully recover from it without complications. Bacterial meningitis, if not diagnosed early, can cause serious and sometimes fatal complications.

Enteroviruses, a group of viruses that includes several strains of coxsackieviruses (kok-SAH-kee-vy-ruh-sez) and echoviruses, cause about 90 percent of cases of aseptic meningitis. Two types of bacteria that are most likely to cause septic meningitis are *Streptococcus pneumoniae* (strep-tuh-KAH-kus nu-MO-nye) and *Neisseria meningitidis* (nye-SEER-e-uh meh-nin-JIH-tih-dis), also called meningococcus (meh-NIN-guh-kah-kus). Before the introduction of a vaccine* in the 1980s to prevent infection with *Haemophilus influenzae* type b (Hib), the bacterium was a common cause of septic meningitis in young children. Meningitis can be caused by other pathogens* as well, such as some species of parasites and fungi and the bacteria that cause Lyme disease*, tuberculosis*, and syphilis*. Meningitis from these organisms is usually a complication of widespread infection throughout the body and is more likely to be seen in people who have immune problems or other diseases, such as those with AIDS* or cancer. Sometimes, chemical irritations, severe drug allergies, or tumors can lead to inflammation in the central nervous system*, resulting in meningitis.

How Common Is Meningitis?

Bacterial meningitis, especially meningococcal meningitis, sometimes occurs in epidemics* in underdeveloped parts of the world, but epidemics are less common in the United States. Because of vaccinations (vak-sih-NAY-shunz) against some of the bacteria that can cause meningitis, the overall number of cases of septic meningitis has steadily declined since 1990. Vaccinated infants and young children are much less likely to contract bacterial meningitis. However, since the late 1990s there has been an increase in the number of cases of meningococcus in-

KEYWORDS

for searching the Internet and other reference sources

Coxsackieviruses

Echoviruses

Enteroviruses

Meninges

Neisseria meningitidis

Streptococcus pneumoniae

Vaccinations

* **vaccine** (vak-SEEN) is a preparation of killed or weakened germs, or a part of a germ or product it produces, given to prevent or lessen the severity of the disease that can result if a person is exposed to the germ itself. Use of vaccines for this purpose is called immunization.

* **pathogens** (PAH-tho-jens) are microorganisms that can cause disease in another living organism.

* **Lyme** (LIME) **disease** is a bacterial infection that is spread to humans by the bite of an infected tick. It begins with a distinctive rash and/or flulike symptoms and, in some cases, can progress to a more serious disease with complications affecting other body organs.

* **tuberculosis** (too-ber-kyoo-LO-sis) is a bacterial infection that primarily attacks the lungs but can spread to other parts of the body.

* **syphilis** (SIH-fih-lis) is a sexually transmitted disease that, if untreated, can lead to serious lifelong problems throughout the body, including blindness and paralysis.

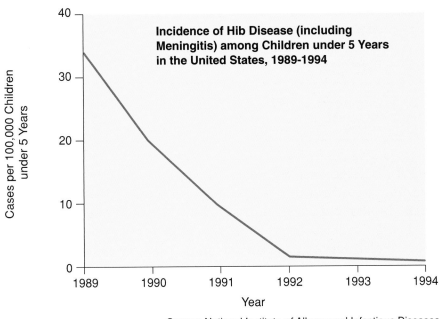

Incidence of Hib Disease (including Meningitis) among Children under 5 Years in the United States, 1989-1994

Source: National Institute of Allergy and Infectious Diseases

The rate of incidence of Hib-related disease, such as meningitis, decreased dramatically since Hib vaccination programs were started in 1989.

fection seen in young adults, particularly in college students who live in dormitories.

How Does Meningitis Spread?

Some forms of bacterial meningitis are contagious, but these are not easily spread (compared to germs that cause colds and the flu). Bacterial meningitis almost never results from simply being in the same room or building with someone who has meningitis. Only a small fraction of people who come in contact with these bacteria and viruses will actually develop meningitis.

Bacteria that can cause meningitis are sometimes found in the throats and noses of healthy people. They are spread through direct contact with respiratory secretions (drops of fluid from the mouth, nose, or lungs). This means they can be passed to someone who kisses an infected person or to someone who touches the secretions from someone who is sneezing or coughing and then touches his or her own nose or mouth. Meningococcus can spread in this way through households, daycare centers, and college dormitories.

Enteroviruses commonly are passed from person to person through contact with respiratory secretions, by breathing in drops from someone who is coughing or sneezing, and from contact with an infected person's feces (FEE-seez, or bowel movements).

* **AIDS**, or acquired immunodeficiency (ih-myoo-no-dih-FIH-shen-see) syndrome, is an infection that severely weakens the immune system; it is caused by the human immunodeficiency virus (HIV).

* **central nervous system** is the part of the nervous system that includes the brain and spinal cord.

* **epidemics** (eh-pih-DEH-miks) are outbreaks of diseases, especially infectious diseases, in which the number of cases suddenly becomes far greater than usual. Usually, epidemics are outbreaks of diseases in specific regions, whereas worldwide epidemics are called pandemics.

* **seizures** (SEE-zhurs) are sudden bursts of disorganized electrical activity that interrupt the normal functioning of the brain, often leading to uncontrolled movements in the body and sometimes a temporary change in consciousness.

* **computerized tomography** (kom-PYOO-ter-ized toe-MAH-gruh-fee) or CT, also called computerized axial tomography (CAT), is a technique in which a machine takes many X rays of the body to create a three-dimensional picture.

* **abscess** (AB-ses) is a localized or walled off accumulation of pus caused by infection that can occur anywhere in the body.

* **sepsis** is a potentially serious spreading of infection, usually bacterial, through the bloodstream and body.

* **shock** is a serious condition in which blood pressure is very low and not enough blood flows to the body's organs and tissues. Untreated, shock may result in death.

What Are the Signs and Symptoms of Meningitis?

Symptoms of meningitis often include fever, headache, stiff neck and back, photophobia (painful sensitivity of the eyes to light), abnormal sleepiness, and confusion. Vomiting may also be seen. Infants' symptoms are not as specific as those in older children and adults but usually include irritability, lethargy, poor feeding, crying when moved, and vomiting. Infants may not have neck or back stiffness while ill with meningitis. Meningococcus can cause a reddish-purple rash (from bleeding under the skin) that rapidly spreads over the body. Seizures* can occur in anyone with meningitis, regardless of age.

How Is Meningitis Diagnosed and Treated?

A doctor will first ask questions about the illness, do a physical examination, and then perform some tests. The brain is sometimes viewed with a computerized tomography* (CT) scan to rule out other reasons for severe headache and illness, such as an abscess*, tumor, or other problems within the brain. A lumbar puncture (also called a spinal tap) is usually done to take a sample of the cerebrospinal (seh-ree-bro-SPY-nuhl) fluid (CSF), the fluid that surrounds the brain and spinal cord. The CSF will be examined under a microscope to look for bacteria or other infectious agents, and increased numbers of white blood cells indicating inflammation.

Antibiotics are not used to treat viral meningitis because it is caused by a virus, not bacteria. Once a case of meningitis is known to be viral, rest and pain medication for body aches and headache can help the person feel better until the infection resolves on its own.

Bacterial meningitis requires prompt medical treatment, usually in the hospital. Antibiotics are given to fight the invading organism for at least 2 weeks. Treatment of complications may require intensive care and other medications.

Meningitis that results from other types of infection or other causes is treated with medications, such as antifungal or antiparasitic drugs, and may require hospitalization, especially during the early stages of medical care.

Most cases of viral meningitis last 1 to 2 weeks, and most people recover completely. Symptoms from bacterial meningitis can last weeks, and people may have severe complications from the disease, especially if it is not diagnosed and treated promptly.

What Complications Can Meningitis Cause?

Complications from viral meningitis are not as common as those from bacterial meningitis, but they can include inflammation and swelling of the brain. Sometimes, permanent learning disability and other brain damage can result.

Complications from bacterial meningitis can occur rapidly and be severe, even with quick diagnosis and treatment of the disease. Complications include sepsis*, brain swelling, seizures, shock*, organ failure (such as of the kidneys*), and death. Up to 15 percent of cases of meningitis caused by meningococcus are fatal. Long-term effects are seen in about 10 percent of those who survive bacterial meningitis and can include hearing loss, seizure disorder, learning disabilities, and other problems resulting from brain injury. Meningitis caused by the bacteria that cause tuberculosis is particularly likely to damage the nervous system.

Can Meningitis Be Prevented?

Vaccinations against *Haemophilus influenzae* type b and *Streptococcus pneumoniae* are now given routinely to American children before the age of 2. A vaccine against meningococcus is also available, although it is not regularly used in the United States and is not effective in young children. Young people going off to college, especially those who plan to live in a dormitory, should consider getting the vaccine, as recommended by the U.S. Centers for Disease Control and Prevention and the American Academy of Pediatrics. It also is recommended for people traveling outside the United States, people living in certain institutional settings, the elderly, and people with some chronic* medical conditions.

During outbreaks of bacterial meningitis, especially those caused by meningococcus, in schools, dormitories, or daycare people may be given prophylactic* antibiotics to keep the disease from occurring in those who were in close contact with the infected person.

It is difficult to keep viruses such as enteroviruses from spreading from person to person. Risk of viral infection can be decreased by washing hands regularly, especially after using the toilet, and avoiding close contact with anyone who is ill, including not sharing food, eating or serving utensils, razors, or other personal items.

Resources

Organizations

Meningitis Foundation of America Inc., 6610 North Shadeland Avenue, Suite 200, Indianapolis, IN 46220. The Meningitis Foundation of America offers information about the disease, including prevention and treatment, at its website.
Telephone 800-668-1129
http://www.musa.org

U.S. Centers for Disease Control and Prevention (CDC), 1600 Clifton Road, Atlanta, GA 30333. The CDC is the U.S. government authority for information about infectious and other diseases. It provides fact sheets about meningitis at its website.
Telephone 800-311-3435
http://www.cdc.gov

* **kidneys** are the pair of organs that filter blood and remove waste products and excess water from the body in the form of urine.

* **chronic** (KRAH-nik) means continuing for a long period of time.

* **prophylactic** (pro-fih-LAK-tik) refers to something that is used to prevent an illness or other condition, such as an infection or pregnancy.

▶ *See also*
AIDS and HIV Infection
Coxsackievirus and Other Enteroviruses
Fungal Infections
Lyme Disease
Syphilis
Tuberculosis

Mononucleosis, Infectious

Infectious mononucleosis (mah-no-nu-klee-O-sis), also known as mono, is an infectious illness usually caused by the Epstein-Barr (EP-steen BAR) virus (EBV). It often leads to fever, sore throat, swollen lymph nodes*, and tiredness.

KEYWORDS
for searching the Internet
and other reference sources

Burkitt's lymphoma

Cytomegalovirus

Epstein-Barr virus (EBV)

Mono

* **lymph** (LIMF) **nodes** are small, bean-shaped masses of tissue that contain immune system cells that fight harmful microorganisms. Lymph nodes may swell during infections.

* **acute** describes an infection or other illness that comes on suddenly.

* **cytomegalovirus** (sy-tuh-MEH-guh-lo-vy-rus), or CMV, infection is very common and usually causes no symptoms. It poses little risk for healthy people, but it can lead to serious illness in people with weak immune systems.

* **HIV**, or the human immunodeficiency (HYOO-mun ih-myoo-no-dih-FIH-shen-see) virus, is the virus that causes AIDS (acquired immunodeficiency syndrome).

* **immune** (ih-MYOON) means resistant to or not susceptible to a disease.

* **respiratory tract** includes the nose, mouth, throat, and lungs. It is the pathway through which air and gases are transported down into the lungs and back out of the body.

What Is Mononucleosis?

By the time they are 40, as many as 95 percent of adults in the United States have evidence in their blood of a previous EBV infection. Many of these infections are never recognized, especially if they occur in early childhood, because the symptoms look like those of other childhood viral illnesses. Some people infected with EBV have no symptoms. This occurs in many parts of the world where most people are infected early in life. In the United States, EBV infection is most common during adolescence and early adulthood (ages 15 to 25). One-third to one-half of teens who come into contact with the virus for the first time will develop symptoms of classic infectious mono: sore throat, swollen lymph nodes, fever, and extreme tiredness.

Mono most often is associated with acute* infection by EBV, but it is sometimes seen with acute cytomegalovirus* (CMV) infection, acute HIV* infection, and, rarely, other viruses.

Although the symptoms may be unpleasant, mono is generally a mild disease. After a person recovers, the virus remains dormant (inactive) in the body for life. It occasionally may reactivate but it rarely causes symptoms again. When people have been infected with the virus, whether or not they had symptoms, they usually will be immune* to future EBV-related illness.

How Common Is Mononucleosis?

EBV is one of the most common human viruses in the world. In the United States, cases of mono with symptoms most often are found in teens between the ages of 15 and 17. The illness occurs in 2 out of every 1,000 adolescents and young adults and is less common in other age groups.

How Is Mononucleosis Spread?

Mono is contagious, although less so than the common cold. EBV passes from person to person primarily through contact with saliva. Kissing and sharing food, drinks, or utensils commonly spread the virus. Although EBV is present in the respiratory tract*, it usually is not transmitted by coughing or sneezing. Some people will become sick and be able to spread the virus for weeks, especially those who are infected but do not feel sick and pass the virus to others without realizing it. The virus usually remains inactive after the first infection, but some people may spread it from time to time throughout their life.

How Do People Know They Have Mononucleosis?

Symptoms of mono develop between 4 and 6 weeks after infection and generally last 2 to 4 weeks. These include swollen lymph nodes, extreme tiredness, fever, sore muscles, and sore throat. Up to 50 percent of people with classic infectious mononucleosis will have a swollen spleen, and some will have an enlarged liver. Other symptoms may include loss of appetite, weakness, nausea (NAW-zee-uh), stiffness, headache, chest pain, and, rarely, jaundice*.

How Is Mononucleosis Diagnosed and Treated?

Symptoms of mono usually show up 1 to 4 weeks before the diagnosis is made. A physical exam, the patient's age, and sometimes a history of contact with an infected person help the doctor make the diagnosis. An adolescent patient with a lasting fever, sore throat, and swollen lymph nodes, with or without an enlarged spleen, is likely to have mono.

Blood tests will confirm the diagnosis. A blood count will show an increased number of lymphocytes*, and many of them will look unusual. A positive rapid screening test may confirm the diagnosis by revealing EBV in the blood, but this test can be negative, especially early in the illness. More accurate antibody* testing may be done to rule out other viruses that can cause mono-like illnesses. Antibody testing checks several antibodies to determine if there is a current infection or evidence of past infection.

There is no specific treatment for mono. Because it is a viral illness, antibiotics are not prescribed unless a secondary bacterial illness is present, such as strep throat. The best treatment for mono is rest. Over-the-counter medications such as acetaminophen (uh-see-teh-MIH-noh-fen) or ibuprofen may be taken to relieve fever and pain.

Steroids, medications that reduce inflammation, may be given to decrease swelling in the tonsils* and lymph nodes in the neck if a patient is experiencing difficulty swallowing or breathing. Playing contact sports is prohibited for someone who has mono because when the spleen and liver enlarge, they are more vulnerable to injury. Patients with mono are advised not to play contact sports for at least 1 month and to be examined and get a doctor's permission before they start again.

Symptoms of mono usually clear up 1 to 2 months after they appear, but they can last as long as 4 months.

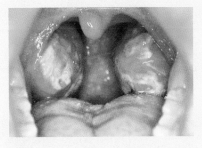

A person with mononucleosis typically has inflamed, pus-covered tonsils and may also have high fever and swollen lymph nodes. *Dr. P. Marazzi/Science Photo Library*

* **jaundice** (JON-dis) is a yellowing of the skin, and sometimes the whites of the eyes, caused by a buildup in the body of bilirubin, a chemical produced in and released by the liver. An increase in bilirubin may indicate disease of the liver or certain blood disorders.

* **lymphocytes** (LIM-fo-sites) are white blood cells, which play a part in the body's immune system, particularly the production of antibodies and other substances to fight infection.

* **antibody** (AN-tih-bah-dee) is a protein molecule produced by the body's immune system to help fight a specific infection caused by a microorganism, such as a bacterium or virus.

* **tonsils** are paired clusters of lymphatic tissue in the throat that help protect the body from bacteria and viruses that enter through a person's nose or mouth.

Kiss and Tell

Mono often is referred to as the "kissing disease" because the infection is spread primarily through direct contact with infected saliva.

EBV and Cancer

EBV has been linked to the development later in life of Burkitt's lymphoma (a rare blood disease of the lymph nodes seen mainly in Africa) and nasopharyngeal carcinoma (nay-zo-fair-in-JEE-ul kar-sih-NO-muh, a cancer in the throat area seen mainly in China). EBV also is linked to lymphoma in the United States, most notably in people with weakened immune systems, such as people who have HIV.

* **anemia** (uh-NEE-me-uh) is a blood condition in which there is a decreased amount of oxygen-carrying hemoglobin in the blood and, usually, fewer than normal numbers of red blood cells.

* **paralysis** (pah-RAH-luh-sis) is the loss or impairment of the ability to move some part of the body.

* **lymphoma** (lim-FO-muh) refers to a cancerous tumor of lymphocytes, cells that normally help the body fight infection.

What Are Some Complications of Mononucleosis?

Recovery from mono is usually uneventful, but sometimes complications occur. An enlarged spleen may rupture, which is an emergency that needs surgery. Fifty percent of patients with infectious mononucleosis will have some liver inflammation, but only a small number will have significant inflammation, or hepatitis (heh-puh-TIE-tis). Blood problems that can result from the infection include anemia*, decreased white cells (cells that fight infection), and low numbers of platelets (cells that help the blood clot). Mononucleosis also can lead to encephalitis (en-seh-fuh-LYE-tis, inflammation of the brain), Guillain-Barre (GEE-yan bah-RAY) syndrome (an inflammation of the nerves, which causes muscle weakness and paralysis*), and Bell's palsy (PAWL-zee, a temporary weakness or paralysis of the muscles on one side of the face). Myocarditis (my-oh-kar-DYE-tis, an inflammation of the muscular walls of the heart) is a rare complication.

EBV also has been associated with cancers, such as lymphoma*, especially in patients with weak immune systems, such as people who have had organ transplants or who have HIV.

Can Mononucleosis Be Prevented?

There is nothing specific that a person can do to avoid contracting mono because EBV often is spread in the saliva of healthy people who have been infected in the past and who can still transmit the virus. Normal human behavior makes it practically impossible to prevent the spread of the disease.

Resources

Organizations

U.S. Centers for Disease Control and Prevention (CDC), 1600 Clifton Road, Atlanta, GA 30333. The CDC is the U.S. government authority for information about infectious and other diseases. It posts information about mononucleosis at its website.
Telephone 800-311-3435
http://www.cdc.gov

U.S. National Library of Medicine, 8600 Rockville Pike, Bethesda, MD 20894. The National Library of Medicine has a website packed with information on diseases such as mononucleosis, consumer resources, dictionaries and encyclopedias of medical terms, and directories of doctors and helpful organizations.
Telephone 888-346-3656
http://www.nlm.nih.gov

Website

KidsHealth.org. KidsHealth is a website created by the medical experts of the Nemours Foundation and is devoted to issues of children's health. It contains articles on a variety of health topics, including mononucleosis.

http://www.KidsHealth.org

Mumps

Mumps is a contagious viral infection that causes inflammation and swelling in the glands of the mouth that produce saliva.

What Is Mumps?

Mumps is an infection caused by a virus. The mumps virus can infect various parts of the human body but typically attacks the salivary glands. The mouth has three pairs of salivary glands: one pair under the mouth and lower jaw; a second pair under the tongue; and a third pair in the back of both cheeks between the ear and the jaw. In most cases, mumps affects the third pair, called the parotid glands*, causing them to swell painfully.

In some patients, the virus spreads to the central nervous system* and causes a condition called aseptic meningitis*. Up to 15 percent of patients who have mumps, most commonly adults, will develop cases of meningitis with symptoms (such as headache and stiff neck).

Before the introduction of the mumps vaccine in 1967, the infection was also a major cause of acquired (not present at birth) deafness in childhood. Deafness occurs in about 1 out of 20,000 cases of mumps, often in only one ear.

Is Mumps Common?

Mumps was a common childhood illness in the United States until 1967, when a vaccine was made available to the public. Before the vaccine, most mumps infections occurred in children under the age of 15, and 5- to 9-year-olds were the most frequently affected age group. In the twenty-first century, many cases are diagnosed in young adults who have not been immunized.

Since 1967, cases of mumps have declined steadily. Statistics indicate the dramatic impact that the vaccine has had. In 1964, approximately 212,000 cases of mumps were diagnosed in the United States. By 2001, that number had dropped to 231 cases, according to the U.S. Centers for Disease Control and Prevention.

Epidemics* of mumps are rare and usually break out among people who have not been vaccinated and who live in close quarters, such as

▶ *See also*

AIDS and HIV Infection

Cytomegalovirus (CMV) Infection

Encephalitis

Hepatitis, Infectious

Myocarditis/Pericarditis

KEYWORDS
for searching the Internet and other reference sources

MMR vaccination

Orchitis

Parotitis

Salivary glands

* **parotid** (puh-RAH-tid) **gland** is the salivary gland located in the jaw just beneath and in front of each ear.

* **central nervous** (SEN-trul NER-vus) **system** is the part of the nervous system that includes the brain and spinal cord.

* **aseptic meningitis** (a-SEP-tik meh-nin-JY-tis) is a milder, non-bacterial form of meningitis that is usually caused by a virus. Meningitis is an inflammation of the meninges, or the membranes that surround the brain and the spinal cord.

* **epidemics** (eh-pih-DEH-miks) are outbreaks of diseases, especially infectious diseases, in which the number of cases suddenly becomes far greater than usual. Usually, epidemics that involve worldwide outbreaks are called pandemics.

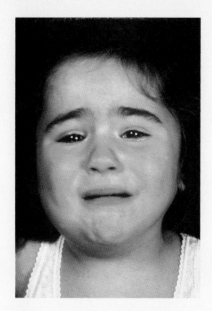

▲

Although swollen salivary glands are typically associated with mumps, approximately one-fifth of people infected with the virus show no symptoms. *Photo Researchers, Inc.*

* **antibodies** (AN-tih-bah-deez) are protein molecules produced by the body's immune system to help fight specific infections caused by microorganisms, such as bacteria and viruses.

* **culturing** (KUL-chur-ing) means being subjected to a test in which a sample of fluid or tissue from the body is placed in a dish containing material that supports the growth of certain organisms. Typically, within days the organisms will grow and can be identified.

army camps and college dormitories. For example, a small outbreak of the disease occurred between 1986 and 1987, mostly in older children and college-age students, because of insufficient immunization during a period from 1967 to 1977.

How Do People Contract Mumps?

Mumps is highly contagious. People infected with the mumps virus can spread it when they laugh, cough, or sneeze. Direct contact with saliva or fluid from an infected person's nose also can spread mumps. Patients are contagious from about 1 day before their glands become swollen to up to 3 days after the swelling has improved.

What Happens When People Have Mumps?

Signs and symptoms   About 1 in 5 people who develop mumps have no symptoms. Many patients who do show signs of infection have only general symptoms such as a low fever, extreme tiredness, loss of appetite, muscle pain, and headache. Symptoms usually appear within 14 to 25 days after exposure to the virus.

Only 30 to 40 percent of people who become infected with the mumps virus have the swelling in the jaw area that most people associate with mumps. Earache and tenderness in the jaw are often the first signs of inflamed parotid glands. In 2 out of 3 cases of mumps, both parotid glands become swollen and painful, with one side swelling a few days before the other. Some patients also experience swelling in the other salivary glands. Talking, chewing, and swallowing can be painful, especially if the person eats or drinks acidic or sour food and beverages (such as lemonade and orange juice), which make the salivary glands squeeze out more saliva and increase discomfort.

Diagnosis and treatment   A doctor typically diagnoses mumps by examining a person who has symptoms of the infection. Other infections can cause swelling in the salivary glands, too, so a doctor may take a sample of blood to look for antibodies* to the virus. Other tests that can be used to diagnose mumps include culturing* samples of saliva or urine to find the mumps virus.

Most cases of mumps can be treated at home. Over-the-counter pain medication, such as acetaminophen (uh-see-teh-MIH-noh-fen), can ease pain and fever, and warm or cold packs can soothe the pain of swollen, inflamed parotid glands. Resting and drinking plenty of non-acidic fluids help the body recover. The symptoms of mumps begin to clear up after 1 week and are usually gone within 10 days.

Complications   Complications of mumps are rare but can be serious and may require additional treatment under a doctor's care or even hospitalization. The infection can lead to inflammation and swelling of the brain (encephalitis, en-seh-fuh-LYE-tis), as well as inflammation of the pancreas* (pancreatitis, pan-kree-uh-TIE-tis), other organs, or the membranes covering the brain and the spinal cord (meningitis). If symptoms of encephalitis or meningitis occur, it usually is within 3 to 7 days after the swelling of the parotid glands begins. These symptoms include high fever, stiff neck, and headache. In some patients with mumps, an electrocardiogram* (EKG) will show signs of myocarditis*, but the condition rarely is severe enough to produce symptoms with mumps.

Up to half of all males who become infected with the mumps virus after puberty experience painful swelling of the testicles* as a complication of the disease. Usually one testicle becomes swollen, but in some cases both do. High fever, chills, headache, nausea (NAW-zee-uh), and vomiting accompany the swelling, which generally goes away within a week after it appears, along with the fever and other symptoms. In rare cases, this swelling can permanently damage the testicle leading to infertility* because of reduced ability to produce sperm cells. Only 5 percent of females who contract mumps after puberty will develop inflammation of the ovaries*, which causes abdominal* pain and other symptoms similar to those of appendicitis*.

Can Mumps Be Prevented?

Immunization is the best way to prevent mumps, and the vaccine usually is administered during early childhood. The vaccine requires two doses and generally is given in the same shot with the vaccines for measles and rubella. It is known as the MMR (measles-mumps-rubella) vaccine. The first dose typically is given when an infant is between 12 and 15 months old and the second when the child is between 4 and 5 years old. Avoiding close contact with someone who has been diagnosed with mumps also reduces the risk of contracting the virus, particularly if the uninfected person has not been vaccinated.

Resources

Organizations

U.S. Centers for Disease Control and Prevention (CDC), 1600 Clifton Road, Atlanta, GA 30333. The CDC posts information about mumps at its website.
Telephone 800-311-3435
http://www.cdc.gov

U.S. National Library of Medicine, 8600 Rockville Pike, Bethesda, MD 20894. The National Library of Medicine has a website packed with information on diseases such as mumps, consumer resources, dictionaries and encyclopedias of medical terms, and directories of doctors and helpful organizations.
Telephone 888-346-3656
http://www.nlm.nih.gov

* **pancreas** (PAN-kree-us) is a gland located behind the stomach that produces hormones and enzymes necessary for metabolism and digestion.

* **electrocardiogram** (e-lek-tro-KAR-dee-o-gram), also known as an EKG, is a test that records and displays the electrical activity of the heart.

* **myocarditis** (my-oh-kar-DYE-tis) is an inflammation of the muscular walls of the heart.

* **testicles** (TES-tih-kulz) are the paired male reproductive glands that produce sperm.

* **infertility** (in-fer-TIH-lih-tee) is the inability of females to become pregnant or of males to cause pregnancy.

* **ovaries** (O-vuh-reez) are the sexual glands from which ova, or eggs, are released in women.

* **abdominal** (ab-DAH-mih-nul) refers to the area of the body below the ribs and above the hips that contains the stomach, intestines, and other organs.

* **appendicitis** (ah-pen-dih-SY-tis) is an inflammation of the appendix, the narrow, finger-shaped organ that branches off the part of the large intestine in the lower right side of the abdomen.

World Health Organization (WHO), Avenue Appia 20, 1211 Geneva 27, Switzerland. WHO provides information about mumps at its website.
Telephone 011-41-22-791-2111
http://www.who.int

Website

KidsHealth.org. KidsHealth is a website created by the medical experts of the Nemours Foundation and is devoted to issues of children's health. It contains articles on a variety of health topics, including mumps.
http://www.KidsHealth.org

Mycobacterial Infections, Atypical

Atypical mycobacterial (my-ko-bak-TEER-e-ul) infections are infections caused by mycobacteria* other than those that cause tuberculosis*.

What Are Atypical Mycobacterial Infections?

Atypical mycobacteria are commonly found in the environment, like in soil and water, and in food. Most of the time they do not cause infection or illness in healthy people. When a person's immune system is weakened, however, as in people who have HIV or AIDS, several strains of mycobacteria can cause opportunistic infections*. Atypical mycobacteria are related to the bacterium that causes tuberculosis (TB), but they often are resistant to the drugs used to treat TB. These strains are called mycobacteria other than tuberculosis, or MOTT.

Although some mycobacteria can live on human skin or in the nose, atypical mycobacterial infections are not known to spread from person to person. Rather, infection comes from direct contact with the bacteria in the environment.

Are Atypical Mycobacterial Infections Common?

Mycobacterial infections other than tuberculosis are uncommon, and they most frequently affect people with HIV or AIDS. As cases of HIV and AIDS have increased, so have cases of mycobacterium infections. In the United States, these infections are more common than tuberculosis. People with seriously weakened immune systems or chronic lung disease are at greatest risk.

How Do People Know They Have an Atypical Mycobacterial Infection?

Signs and symptoms of atypical mycobacterial infections include fever, swollen lymph nodes, extreme tiredness, night sweats, weight loss, diar-

▶ See also
Encephalitis
Measles (Rubeola)
Meningitis
Rubella (German Measles)
Vaccination (Immunization)

KEYWORDS
for searching the Internet and other reference sources

Mycobacteria other than tuberculosis (MOTT)

Mycobacterium avium complex (MAC)

Mycobacterium intracellulare

Mycobacterium kansasii

Mycobacterium marinum

Mycobacterium ulcerans

Opportunistic infections

* **mycobacteria** (my-ko-bak-TEER-e-uh) belong to a family of bacteria called "fungus bacteria" because they are found in wet environments.

* **tuberculosis** (too-ber-kyoo-LO-sis) is a bacterial infection that primarily attacks the lungs but can spread to other parts of the body.

* **opportunistic infections** are infections caused by infectious agents that usually do not produce disease in people with healthy immune systems but can cause widespread illness in patients with weak or faulty immune systems.

rhea (dye-uh-REE-uh), joint and bone pain, cough, shortness of breath, skin lesions*, general discomfort, and paleness. Many of these symptoms can be signs of less serious conditions, but in a person with a weakened immune system a combination of such symptoms suggests a MOTT infection. In children, lymphadenitis* is the most common type of MOTT infection, whereas lung infections, which occur less often in children, are the most common in adults.

What Are Some Specific Infections?

Mycobacterium avium complex (MAC) MAC includes the species *Mycobacterium avium* (A-vee-um) and *Mycobacterium intracellulare* (in-truh-sel-yoo-LAR-e) and most commonly causes lymphadenitis and lung disease in otherwise healthy people. Patients who have AIDS are particularly susceptible to MAC, and it often spreads to the blood, lungs, spleen, liver, bone marrow*, and intestines in people with HIV. MAC infection in an HIV-positive person can signal the start of full-blown AIDS. Disseminated disease* rarely occurs in people with healthy immune systems.

Mycobacterium marinum This infection causes skin lesions, sometimes known as swimming pool granuloma* or fish tank granuloma. Infection with *M. marinum* (MAR-ih-num) is very rare, occurring in less than 1 in 100,000 people. Those who are most at risk include people with weakened immune systems and people who handle fish, are exposed to contaminated water in aquariums, or swim in fresh or salt water that contains the mycobacterium. Several weeks after a person has contact with contaminated water, a bump appears on a hand, arm, or foot where there was a break in the skin. The lesion grows and drains over several weeks, leaving an ulcer*. Occasionally, a deep infection will cause tenderness and swelling in the nearby bone or joints.

Mycobacterium ulcerans *Mycobacterium ulcerans* (UL-sir-ans) is found in tropical and subtropical regions in Asia, the Western Pacific, and Latin America, although it is most common in West Africa. The infection causes skin lesions known as Buruli (boo-REH-lee) ulcers, named for a region in Uganda in Africa. The ulcers develop mainly on the limbs, grow slowly, and release a toxin (or poison) that damages the skin and underlying tissue. The infection is relatively painless, but if left untreated it can destroy massive amounts of skin and bone, leading to permanent deformities.

Mycobacterium kansasii Infection with *Mycobacterium kansasii* (kan-ZAS-e-eye) causes a lung disease similar to tuberculosis, although not as severe. Patients may experience fever and cough, and a doctor often hears wheezing and "crackling" when listening to the patient's lungs. It also can involve the lymph nodes and cause skin lesions. In people

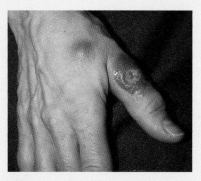

▲

Exposure to *Mycobacterium marinum* can lead to a rare infection known as "swimming pool granuloma" or "aquarium granuloma." About 3 weeks after the bacteria enters through a break in the skin, usually on the hands, reddish bumps appear. This infection can be prevented by avoiding contact with contaminated water and wearing gloves or washing thoroughly when cleaning aquariums. *Custom Medical Stock Photo, Inc.*

* **lesions** (LEE-zhuns) is a general term referring to a sore or a damaged or irregular area of tissue.

* **lymphadenitis** (lim-fah-den-EYE-tis) is inflammation of the lymph nodes and channels of the lymphatic system.

* **bone marrow** is the soft tissue inside bones where blood cells are made.

* **disseminated disease** describes a disease that has spread widely in the body.

* **granuloma** (gran-yoo-LO-muh) is chronically inflamed and swollen tissue that often develops as the result of an infection.

* **ulcer** is an open sore on the skin or the lining of a hollow body organ, such as the stomach or intestine. It may or may not be painful.

with weak immune systems, the infection can erupt into widespread disease. This infection is rare in the United States, but people with chronic lung disease are especially susceptible. If left untreated, the disease frequently worsens and can be fatal.

How Do Doctors Diagnose and Treat Atypical Mycobacterial Infections?

A doctor can perform several tests to detect mycobacteria, including examination and culture* of samples of blood, sputum*, bowel movement, or bone marrow. Chest X rays or computerized tomography* (CT) scans can show disease in the lungs. Some cases may require endoscopy* to collect a sample of lung or stomach tissue or biopsies* of skin or lymph node tissue. Quickly diagnosing mycobacterial infections is crucial, as treatment needs to begin as soon as possible.

The PPD (purified protein derivative) skin test for tuberculosis will often be positive, although not as strongly so, in people who have an atypical mycobacterial infection, because atypical mycobacteria are so similar to the bacterium that causes TB.

Treatment for mycobacterial infections depends on the type of bacterium, the location and severity of the infection, and the status of the person's immune system. Resistant and severe infections usually need to be treated with a combination of antibiotics, and up to six medications may be used at once. Surgery, sometimes along with medications, is the most effective way to treat lymph node infections and skin lesions.

Treatment for MOTT infections can take as long as 6 months to 2 years. Antibiotics work during the growth stage of bacteria, and mycobacteria are slow growing. If left untreated, MOTT infections can spread throughout the body, especially in people with weak immune systems. They can cause abscesses*, bone and joint infections, and infections of the lymph nodes, lungs, or soft tissue. Widespread infections can lead to serious illness and even death.

Can People Prevent Atypical Mycobacterial Infections?

Because mycobacteria are common in the environment, these infections are difficult to prevent, especially in people with weakened immune systems. Preventive medications are prescribed for people at risk, such as those with HIV or AIDS. Getting enough sleep and eating a healthy diet also can help these patients cope with and fight these infections.

Resources

Organizations

U.S. Centers for Disease Control and Prevention (CDC), 1600 Clifton Road, Atlanta, GA 30333. The CDC is the U.S. government

* **culture** (KUL-chur) is a test in which a sample of fluid or tissue from the body is placed in a dish containing material that supports the growth of certain organisms. Within days or weeks the organisms will grow and can be identified.

* **sputum** (SPYOO-tum) is a substance that contains mucus and other matter coughed out from the lungs, bronchi, and trachea.

* **computerized tomography** (kom-PYOO-ter-ized toe-MAH-gruh-fee) or CT, also called computerized axial tomography (CAT), is a technique in which a machine takes many X rays of the body to create a three-dimensional picture.

* **endoscopy** (en-DOS-ko-pee) is a type of diagnostic test in which a lighted tube-like instrument is inserted into a part of the body.

* **biopsies** (BI-op-seez) are tests in which small samples of skin or other body tissue are removed and examined for signs of disease.

* **abscesses** (AB-seh-sez) are localized or walled off accumulations of pus caused by infection that can occur anywhere in the body.

authority for information about infectious and other diseases. It provides information about *Mycobacterium avium* complex at its website. Telephone 800-311-3435
http://www.cdc.gov

U.S. National Library of Medicine, 8600 Rockville Pike, Bethesda, MD 20894. The National Library of Medicine has a website packed with information on diseases (including atypical mycobacterial infections) and drugs, consumer resources, dictionaries and encyclopedias of medical terms, and directories of doctors and helpful organizations. Telephone 888-346-3656
http://www.nlm.nih.gov

Mycoplasma Infections

Mycoplasma (my-ko-PLAZ-muh) infections are caused by a type of very small bacteria. These infections usually involve the lungs or the urinary and genital tracts.

What Are Mycoplasma Infections?

Scientists have identified at least 16 species of these tiny bacteria; three have been linked to disease in humans, and researchers are looking at possible relationships between other species and a variety of diseases.

Mycoplasma pneumoniae (my-ko-PLAZ-muh nu-MO-nye) is the cause of atypical or "walking" pneumonia (nu-MO-nyah, inflammation in the lungs), a form of pneumonia that is characterized by symptoms similar to those of the flu and is generally less serious than other types of pneumonia. Widespread outbreaks of mycoplasma pneumonia occur every 4 to 8 years. Most people recover without lasting effects, but elderly patients and people with weak immune systems may experience complications from the infection.

Commonly found in the genital and urinary tracts of adults, *Mycoplasma hominis* (HAH-mih-nis) and *Ureaplasma urealyticum* (yoo-REE-uh-plaz-muh yoo-ree-uh-LIH-tih-kum) are known as the genital mycoplasmas. These organisms can cause urethritis* and contribute to vaginitis* in women. They have been associated with sexually transmitted diseases (STDs) and with chronic infections in people with weakened immune systems. Up to 50 percent of sexually active women are colonized* with *U. urealyticum*, which can spread to newborn babies during delivery. In premature infants, *U. urealyticum* may contribute to pneumonia and other infections, as well as to chronic lung disease.

Because these organisms are also found in healthy people and infants, their presence in someone who is sick does not necessarily mean mycoplasma

► *See also*
AIDS and HIV Infection
Tuberculosis

KEYWORDS
for searching the Internet and other reference sources

Atypical pneumonia

Mycoplasma hominis

Mycoplasma pneumoniae

Ureaplasma urealyticum

Urethritis

Walking pneumonia

* **urethritis** (yoo-ree-THRY-tis) is inflammation of the urethra (yoo-REE-thra), which is the tube through which urine passes from the bladder out of the body.

* **vaginitis** (vah-jih-NYE-tis) is inflammation of the vagina (vah-JY-nah), which is the canal in a woman that leads from the uterus to the outside of the body.

* **colonized** means that a group of organisms, particularly bacteria, are living on or inside the body without causing symptoms of infection.

241

is the culprit behind that particular infection. Although mycoplasma species such as *U. urealyticum* or *M. hominis* may be responsible for some infections, in many cases it appears that they help start or worsen an illness that is actually caused by another infectious organism.

Mycoplasma Pneumonia

The U.S. Centers for Disease Control and Prevention estimates that 2 million people contract mycoplasma pneumonia in the United States each year. Of these, 100,000 require hospitalization. Fatal cases are rare and usually occur in the elderly and in people with sickle-cell disease*.

Mycoplasma pneumonia most frequently affects people between the ages of 5 and 40; it is rarely seen in children under 5. Outbreaks are common in groups of young adults, often in places where people are crowded together, such as in military facilities and college dormitories.

Mycoplasma is contagious, spreading through tiny drops of moisture from the nose and throats of infected people when they cough, sneeze, laugh, or talk. Sharing drinking glasses or eating utensils can spread the bacteria as well. To become infected, someone must have close contact with the sick person.

The time between exposure and the appearance of symptoms is relatively long (1 to 4 weeks), so the disease can spread for months within a home without family members realizing they are passing along the same infection. After a bout of *Mycoplasma pneumoniae* infection, antibodies* will protect a person from re-infection, but this immunity* does not last for life.

Signs and symptoms Symptoms of mycoplasma pneumonia infection come on gradually. Many people have symptoms similar to those of the flu, such as sore throat, headache, weakness, fever, cough, and chills. Less common symptoms include earaches, eye pain, muscle aches, joint stiffness, skin rash, swollen lymph nodes* in the neck, and difficulty breathing. Some people have only a mild illness, whereas others will develop the more full-blown classic walking pneumonia.

Diagnosis The physical exam is an important part of diagnosing mycoplasma pneumonia. A school-age child with fever, a cough, and wheezing or crackling sounds in the lungs may have mycoplasma. A chest X ray will help confirm the diagnosis. Doctors do not usually order cultures* on samples of fluid from the nose or throat because the mycoplasma bacteria do not grow easily in cultures.

Although blood tests are not helpful in making a diagnosis early on, after about a week of illness, a blood test known as cold agglutinins (uh-GLOO-tuh-nins) is positive in half to three-fourths of all patients. This test is not specific for *M. pneumoniae* (other infections also can give a positive test result), but information from it can help support a diagnosis of suspected walking pneumonia. Tests for specific antibodies pro-

* **sickle-cell disease** is a hereditary condition in which the red blood cells, which are usually round, take on an abnormal crescent shape and have a decreased ability to carry oxygen throughout the body.

* **antibodies** (AN-tih-bah-deez) are protein molecules produced by the body's immune system to help fight specific infections caused by microorganisms, such as bacteria and viruses.

* **immunity** (ih-MYOON-uh-tee) is the condition of being protected against an infectious disease. Immunity often develops after a germ is introduced to the body. One type of immunity occurs when the body makes special protein molecules called antibodies to fight the disease-causing germ. The next time that germ enters the body, the antibodies quickly attack it, usually preventing the germ from causing disease.

* **lymph** (LIMF) **nodes** are small, bean-shaped masses of tissue that contain immune system cells that fight harmful microorganisms. Lymph nodes may swell during infections.

* **cultures** (KUL-churs) are tests in which samples of fluid or tissue from the body are placed in dishes containing material that supports the growth of certain organisms. Typically, within days the organisms will grow and can be identified.

duced by the body to mycoplasma require at least two blood samples over time to show the body's response to the infection.

Treatment   Antibiotics, along with rest and fluids, will help most patients recover. Some people get better without medicine, especially those who have only a mild illness. In severe cases, patients may need to be hospitalized so they can receive oxygen and other breathing support.

Symptoms usually last from 1 to 4 weeks, although the dry cough and extreme tiredness may linger for several more weeks.

Complications   Few people die from mycoplasma pneumonia, but the elderly are most at risk. Complications are not common but can include acute respiratory distress (extreme difficulty in breathing) and respiratory failure.

Other complications are even rarer: pericarditis (per-ih-kar-DYE-tis, inflammation of the sac around the heart); anemia (uh-NEE-me-uh, a deficiency of red blood cells); and diseases of the central nervous system*, including Guillain-Barré syndrome (GEE-yan bah-RAY SIN-drome, a temporary inflammation of the nerves that causes muscle weakness and paralysis*), encephalitis (en-seh-fuh-LYE-tis, inflammation of the brain), and meningitis (meh-nin-JY-tis, inflammation of the membranes lining the brain and spinal cord).

* **central nervous system** is the part of the nervous system that includes the brain and spinal cord.

* **paralysis** (pah-RAH-luh-sis) is the loss or impairment of the ability to move some part of the body.

Prevention   The best defenses against mycoplasma pneumonia are frequent, thorough hand washing and not sharing food, drinks, or eating utensils.

Genital Mycoplasma Infection

Mycoplasma hominis infects up to 30 to 50 percent of sexually active men and women. *Ureaplasma urealyticum* may infect more than half of sexually active women and 5 to 20 percent of sexually active men.

Twenty percent of newborns are colonized with these bacteria, but colonization rates drop significantly by 3 months of age. Premature infants have the greatest risk of colonization; up to half of all premature infants less than 34 weeks' gestational age* whose mothers are colonized may pick up the bacteria during birth. Genital mycoplasmas spread through direct contact during all forms of sexual intercourse. Mothers also can pass the bacteria to their babies during pregnancy and delivery.

* **gestational** (jes-TAY-shuh-nul) **age** is the length of time a fetus has remained developing within the womb.

Signs and symptoms   Most people with genital mycoplasma infection have no symptoms. Those who do may have a discharge (flow of fluid) from the urethra and pain or difficulty urinating. In rare cases, symptoms can include respiratory problems and joint pain, usually in people with weak immune systems.

Occasionally, women develop urethritis from mycoplasma infection, and although genital mycoplasma does not cause vaginitis, it may contribute to infections caused by other vaginal organisms, resulting in

* **pelvic inflammatory disease** refers to an infection of a woman's internal reproductive organs, including the fallopian tubes, uterus, cervix, and ovaries.

* **stillbirth** is the birth of a dead fetus.

* **premature delivery** is when a baby is born before it has reached full term.

* **infertility** (in-fer-TIH-lih-tee) is the inability of females to become pregnant or of males to cause pregnancy.

vaginal discharge. Pelvic (lower belly) pain may be a symptom of pelvic inflammatory disease* brought on by mycoplasma, alone or with other STDs. In pregnant women, *U. urealyticum* can cause inflammation of the membranes and fluid surrounding the unborn baby called asymptomatic chorioamnionitis (a-simp-toh-MAH-tik kor-e-o-am-nee-ahn-EYE-tis), which has been linked to a greater risk of stillbirth* and premature delivery*.

The symptoms of infection in newborns can be subtle. Fever, changes in blood pressure and heart rate, and difficulty breathing may be the first signs of a problem.

Diagnosis Samples are taken from the areas of suspected infection (such as a swab of discharge from the vagina), and the organism is grown with special culture techniques.

Treatment Antibiotics are prescribed to treat genital mycoplasma infections in people who have symptoms. In cases where mycoplasma is found along with other disease-causing organisms, these other infections must be treated as well.

Genital mycoplasma infections generally respond to treatment within 1 to 2 weeks, although these infections commonly return.

Complications Complications are rare in healthy adults but may include inflammation of other parts of the genital tract. Some adults, especially those with weakened immune systems, may have bone and joint infections, skin infections, and lung disease. The bacteria also have been linked to infertility* in women. Infected newborns, especially premature babies, may develop pneumonia or chronic lung disease and are at risk for meningitis and for spread of the disease throughout their bodies.

Prevention Because many people carry genital mycoplasma bacteria but do not know they are infected, preventing their spread is difficult. Abstaining from all forms of sex (not having sex) is the only sure way to prevent infection.

Resources

Organization

U.S. Centers for Disease Control and Prevention (CDC), 1600 Clifton Road, Atlanta, GA 30333. The CDC is the U.S. government authority for information about infectious and other diseases. It provides information about mycoplasma infections at its website. Telephone 800-311-3435
http://www.cdc.gov

Website

KidsHealth.org. KidsHealth is a website created by the medical experts of the Nemours Foundation and is devoted to issues of children's health. It contains articles on a variety of health topics, including mycoplasma pneumonia.
http://www.KidsHealth.org

Myocarditis/Pericarditis

Myocarditis (my-oh-kar-DYE-tis) is inflammation of the heart muscle, and pericarditis (per-ih-kar-DYE-tis) is inflammation of the smooth sac surrounding the heart.

What Are Myocarditis and Pericarditis?

Myocarditis, or inflammation of the muscular walls of the heart, is most commonly caused by viruses, however, it can also be caused by bacteria, parasites, and fungi. Other causes of the condition include radiation, chemicals, cocaine use, and prescription medications. Conditions that affect several parts of the body, such as autoimmune diseases*, also can be associated with both myocarditis and pericarditis.

When the pericardium (per-ih-KAR-dee-um), the smooth, double-layered sac-like covering that surrounds the heart, becomes inflamed—known as pericarditis—fluid usually accumulates in the space between its layers. As the amount of fluid increases, the buildup puts pressure on the beating heart and can limit its ability to function. Many of the same infections that cause myocarditis can cause pericarditis as well, and the two often appear together. In addition to the infectious causes of pericarditis, heart surgery or a heart attack* can lead to an inflamed pericardium and accumulation of fluid around the heart.

How Common Are Myocarditis and Pericarditis?

Myocarditis and pericarditis are uncommon complications of many infectious diseases. Many cases of myocarditis are mild and go undetected when the person is sick. In fact, it is difficult to determine exactly how many people develop myocarditis or pericarditis. However, some evidence of myocarditis is found in 1 to 4 percent of autopsies*. In almost all of these cases, there were no symptoms of the disease while the person was alive.

Are Myocarditis and Pericarditis Contagious?

Neither condition is directly contagious. However, many of the organisms that cause infections that can lead to myocarditis or pericarditis are

 See also
Pneumonia
Sexually Transmitted Diseases
Urinary Tract Infections

KEYWORDS
for searching the Internet and other reference sources

Cardiomyopathy

Heart disease

Heart transplant

Pericardium

*autoimmune (aw-toh-ih-MY-OON) diseases are diseases in which the body's immune system attacks some of the body's own normal tissues and cells.

*heart attack is a general term that usually refers to a sudden, intense episode of heart injury. It is usually caused by a blockage of a coronary artery, which stops blood from supplying the heart muscle with oxygen.

*autopsies (AW-top-seez) are examinations of bodies after death to look for causes of death or the effects of diseases.

* **genes** (JEENZ) are chemical structures composed of deoxyribonucleic acid (DNA) that help determine a person's body structure and physical characteristics. Inherited from a person's parents, genes are contained in the chromosomes found in the body's cells.

* **congestive** (kon-JES-tiv) **heart failure**, or heart failure, is a condition in which a damaged or overworked heart cannot pump enough blood to meet the oxygen and nutrient needs of the body. People with heart failure may find it hard to exercise due to the insufficient blood flow, but many people live a long time with this condition.

* **electrocardiogram** (e-lek-tro-KAR-dee-o-gram), also known as an EKG, is a test that records and displays the electrical activity of the heart.

* **echocardiogram** (eh-ko-KAR-dee-uh-gram) is a diagnostic test that uses sound waves to produce images of the heart's chambers and valves and blood flow through the heart.

* **biopsy** (BI-op-see) is a test in which a small sample of skin or other body tissue is removed and examined for signs of disease.

* **computerized tomography** (kom-PYOO-ter-ized toe-MAH-gruh-fee) or CT, also called computerized axial tomography (CAT), is a technique in which a machine takes many X rays of the body to create a three-dimensional picture.

* **magnetic resonance imaging**, or MRI, uses magnetic waves, instead of X rays, to scan the body and produce detailed pictures of the body's structures.

spread from person to person by coughing or sneezing. It is not clear why myocarditis or pericarditis develops in some people but not in others. A combination of the infection, a person's genes*, and an individual's immune response probably determines who will develop these conditions.

What Are the Signs and Symptoms of Myocarditis and Pericarditis?

Because both conditions can seriously affect the heart's function, they may lead to signs and symptoms of heart failure. Patients with myocarditis may experience fever, rapid heartbeat, extreme tiredness, difficulty breathing, and chest pain that can range from mild to severe, sometimes with heart attack-like intensity. In serious cases, congestive heart failure*, fainting, and, sometimes, sudden death can occur.

Pericarditis often is accompanied by sharp chest pains, trouble breathing, and pain when taking a deep breath. These conditions usually improve when the patient is sitting or standing rather than lying down. Other symptoms may include dry cough, extreme tiredness, fever, rapid heartbeat, and chills.

How Are Myocarditis and Pericarditis Diagnosed?

A doctor will suspect myocarditis based on symptoms and a physical exam. For instance, a rapid heartbeat, fluid in the lungs, and swollen ankles and feet may point to heart failure, which can occur with myocarditis. The history of the patient's illness is another important clue, as the patient often has had symptoms of a viral infection within the previous 2 weeks to 6 months.

To assess the heart's condition, the doctor may order any of a variety of tests. Although a chest X ray often appears normal in the early stages of the illness, it may show an enlarged heart or fluid-filled lungs. An electrocardiogram* (EKG) may show evidence of heart inflammation and can help identify a heart attack as the possible cause of the symptoms. An echocardiogram* may show the decreased heart function seen in myocarditis. Blood tests that reveal inflammation of the heart muscle are often abnormal in people with myocarditis and can help in making the diagnosis. A biopsy* of a piece of heart muscle can provide a definitive diagnosis. Other tests may be done to identify a specific virus or other infectious organism, but in many cases the exact cause of the inflammation is never found.

To diagnose pericarditis, doctors look for signs of fluid around the heart. During a physical exam, physicians also listen for a rubbing sound that can be heard when the pericardial sac is inflamed. If enough fluid is present, the heart may appear enlarged on a chest X ray. The fluid itself can be seen on an echocardiogram, a computerized tomography* (CT) scan, or a magnetic resonance imaging* (MRI) scan. An EKG can be helpful in making the diagnosis as well.

How Are Myocarditis and Pericarditis Treated?

Myocarditis and pericarditis may be difficult or impossible to prevent, but prompt recognition and treatment of these conditions will improve the chances of recovery. With both myocarditis and pericarditis, doctors strive to identify and treat the underlying cause, reduce the inflammation, and improve the heart's function. These are serious conditions that usually require hospitalization once the patient has developed detectable symptoms.

Anti-inflammatory medicines such as aspirin, nonsteroidal anti-inflammatory medications, or corticosteroids* may be prescribed to reduce inflammation. Patients also may receive medicine to ease pain and diuretics* to remove excess fluid from the body. Depending on the cause and the complications of the inflammation, other treatments may be necessary as well, including antibiotics and medications that control heart rhythm problems and improve heart function.

Some cases of pericarditis may require pericardiocentesis (per-ih-KAR-dee-o-sen-tee-sis), or the removal of fluid from the pericardial sac with a needle. This relieves pressure on the heart and collects fluid for tests. In chronic or recurrent cases, the doctor may recommend surgery to cut or remove part of the pericardium. During recovery, the patient's activity usually is restricted, and doctors typically recommend diet changes such as eating less salt. Cases of myocarditis and pericarditis may last from 2 weeks to 3 months, although some people never fully recover their prior heart function.

What Are Some Complications of Myocarditis and Pericarditis?

Complications of these conditions can be very serious. The heart muscle may become damaged and unable to pump effectively. Heart failure, irregular heartbeat, and death may occur. In some cases, if the heart muscle has been severely and permanently damaged, a heart transplant may be considered.

Resource

Organization

American Heart Association, National Center, 7272 Greenville Avenue, Dallas, TX 75231. The American Heart Association posts fact sheets about myocarditis and pericarditis, as well as general information about the heart and how it works, at its website.
Telephone 800-242-8721
http://www.americanheart.org

* **corticosteroids** (kor-tih-ko-STIR-oyds) are chemical substances made by the adrenal glands that have several functions in the body, including maintaining blood pressure during stress and controlling inflammation. They can also be given to people as medication to treat certain illnesses.

* **diuretics** (dye-yoor-EH-tiks) are medications that increase the body's output of urine.

▶ *See also*
Endocarditis, Infectious

O

Oncogenic Infections

Oncogenic (on-ko-JEH-nik) infections are infections that may increase a person's risk of developing a certain type or types of cancer.

KEYWORDS
for searching the Internet and other reference sources

Burkitt's lymphoma

Epstein-Barr virus

Helicobacter pylori

Hepatitis

Human lymphotrophic virus

Human papillomavirus

What Are Oncogenic Infections?

Cancer often is linked to lifestyle choices (such as smoking), a person's genetic* makeup, and environmental influences. Researchers now have begun to make connections between the development of certain types of cancer and specific viral, bacterial, and parasitic infections. These infections are referred to as oncogenic, or tumor-producing, infections.

Oncogenic viruses transfer their genetic material to other cells and then remain in the body for a long time as a latent infection (meaning that they are dormant, or inactive, but not dead) or as a chronic (KRAH-nik) infection (meaning that the infection continues for a long time). For example, Epstein-Barr (EP-steen BAR) virus remains in the body for life, occasionally flaring up and being subdued by the body's immune system. Chronic infections such as hepatitis (heh-puh-TIE-tis) B or C often damage the body slowly, over many years.

Another characteristic of oncogenic infections is that they seem to encourage cells to reproduce at an unusually fast rate, which may damage the genetic material in those cells. Additional factors, such as smoking or exposure to other carcinogens*, may be needed to trigger the final change of a normal cell into a cancer cell. These exposures, along with each person's individual genetic makeup, may explain why cancer develops in some people who have had oncogenic infections but not others.

Specific Oncogenic Infections

There are several infections that have been linked to the development of cancer. Human papillomavirus (pah-pih-LO-muh-vy-rus), or HPV, is a family of more than 70 different types of viruses that can produce warts* on various parts of the body. Some strains* of HPV are spread sexually and cause genital* warts. Sexually transmitted HPVs are linked to the development of cervical*, penile*, and anal* cancer. (Anal and penile cancers are rare in the United States.)

According to the American Cancer Society, the most important risk factor for a woman in the development of cervical cancer is HPV infection. HPV is found in 90 percent of cervical cancer cases. Its presence

* **genetic** (juh-NEH-tik) refers to heredity and the ways in which genes control the development and maintenance of organisms.

* **carcinogens** (kar-SIH-no-jenz) are substances or agents that can cause cancer.

* **warts** are small, hard growths on the skin or inner linings of the body that are caused by a type of virus.

* **strains** are various subtypes of organisms, such as viruses or bacteria.

* **genital** (JEH-nih-tul) refers to the external sexual organs.

* **cervical** refers to the cervix (SIR-viks), the lower, narrow end of the uterus that opens into the vagina.

* **penile** (PEE-nile) refers to the penis, the external male sexual organ.

* **anal** refers to the anus, the opening at the end of the digestive system through which waste leaves the body.

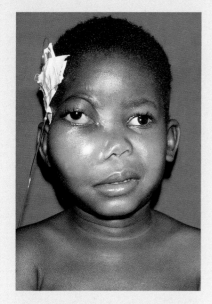

▲

A child with Burkitt's lymphoma, a type of tumor first discovered in Africa. The African form of Burkitt's lymphoma is strongly associated with early childhood infection by the Epstein-Barr virus. *Custom Medical Stock Photo, Inc.*

* **Pap smear** is a common diagnostic test used to look for cancerous cells in the tissue of the cervix.

* **mononucleosis** (mah-no-nu-klee-O-sis) is an infectious illness caused by a virus that often leads to fever, sore throat, swollen glands, and tiredness.

* **lymphocytes** (LIM-fo-sites) are white blood cells, which play a part in the body's immune system, particularly the production of antibodies and other substances to fight infection.

* **lymphoma** (lim-FO-muh) refers to a cancerous tumor of lymphocytes, cells that normally help the body fight infection.

may make a woman more likely to have cervical dysplasia (SIR-vih-kul dis-PLAY-zhuh), or precancerous cells in the cervix. This condition can lead to cancer if it is left untreated. Early discovery and treatment can lessen a woman's risk of cervical cancer, and doctors advise women diagnosed with HPV to have frequent Pap smears*. HPV is the most common sexually transmitted disease in the United States, with 5 million new infections diagnosed each year. There is no cure for HPV, and treatment is aimed at controlling the infection.

Epstein-Barr virus (EBV) is commonly known as the virus that causes infectious mononucleosis*. Up to 95 percent of adults in the United States have been infected with the virus by the time they are 40 years old. EBV is transmitted through contact with fluid from the mouth and nose of someone who is infected. Children who contract EBV rarely have symptoms, and when they do, the symptoms typically are the same as those of common viral infections. When adolescents or adults are infected with EBV, they can have infectious mononucleosis.

EBV remains in the body, primarily in the lymphocytes*, for the rest of a person's life. It is dormant for much of the time, although it occasionally flares up without causing any real harm. People with weakened immune systems are at particular risk that EBV will flare up and cause illness. EBV is associated primarily with the development of Hodgkin's disease and non-Hodgkin's lymphoma* (both cancers of the lymphatic system*), nasopharyngeal* carcinoma*, and Burkitt's lymphoma, a rare cancer arising in the lymph nodes* that is a common type of childhood tumor in some parts of the world, primarily central Africa.

Hepatitis B and C virus (HBV and HCV) infections primarily affect the liver. They are spread through contact with infected blood, such as through the sharing of needles (including needles for tattooing, body piercing, and drug use). HBV also can spread through contact with the body fluids of an infected person during sexual intercourse. Some people with hepatitis have no symptoms at all, but in others the infection eventually can result in liver cancer or liver damage from cirrhosis (sir-O-sis), a condition in which liver cells die and are replaced with scar tissue. Because HBV and HCV infections generally are chronic, the viruses are present in the body for a long time and can do significant damage. As the body tries to overcome this damage, new cells are created at a faster rate, increasing the risk of cell mutation* and liver cancer. Hepatitis is treated with injections of interferon (in-ter-FEER-on) alpha-2b, a drug that strengthens the immune system to fight the virus. HBV infection can be prevented by vaccination against the infection.

It is now known that the *Helicobacter pylori** bacterium causes most cases of gastric (stomach) and duodenal* ulcers*. The infection can be treated with antibiotics. People infected with *H. pylori* are at higher risk of stomach cancers, such as gastric lymphoma and adenocarcinoma (ah-deh-no-kar-sin-O-muh). Gastric cancer has been diagnosed more often

Oncogenic Infections	Associated Cancers
Human papilloma virus (HPV) infection	Cervical and penile cancers
Epstein-Barr virus (EBV) infection	Lymphomas and nasopharyngeal cancer
Hepatitis B and C virus (HBV or HCV) infection	Liver cancer
Helicobacter pylori infection	Stomach cancer
Human lymphotrophic virus type 1 (HLTV-1) infection	Lymphomas

in countries where *H. pylori* infection is common, such as China and Colombia, and it is believed that the combination of infection, diet, and other factors contributes to these cancers. The bacteria may spread through contact with feces (FEE-seez), or bowel movements, found in contaminated water sources or on hands that have not been washed thoroughly.

Human lymphotrophic (lim-fo-TRO-fik) virus type 1 is a virus that has been linked to the development of certain types of leukemia* and lymphoma primarily in people from Japan, the southern Pacific islands, the Caribbean, parts of central Asia, and central and western Africa. Infection with the virus often occurs at birth, but it can remain inactive for years and sometimes decades before cancer develops. The virus usually is spread through contact with contaminated blood, from prolonged exposure to an infected sexual partner, or from mother to child through breast milk. The earlier a person contracts the infection, the higher the risk of lymphoma. This virus is related to the human immunodeficiency (ih-myoo-no-dih-FIH-shen-see) virus (HIV), the cause of acquired immunodeficiency syndrome (AIDS). HIV itself is an oncogenic virus that has been linked to several types of cancer.

How Can People Protect Themselves from Oncogenic Infections?

Exposure to oncogenic infections does not mean that a person will get cancer. Many people contract such infections and never get cancer. Scientists believe that many factors play a role in the development of cancer

* **lymphatic** (lim-FAH-tik) **system** is a system that contains lymph nodes and a network of channels that carry fluid and cells of the immune system through the body.

* **nasopharyngeal** (nay-zo-fair-in-JEE-ul) refers to the nose and pharynx (FAIR-inks), or throat.

* **carcinoma** (kar-sih-NO-muh) is a cancerous tumor that arises in the epithelium (eh-puh-THEE-lee-um), the sheets of cells that line body surfaces, such as the insides of hollow organs and cavities.

* **lymph** (LIMF) **nodes** are small, bean-shaped masses of tissue that contain immune system cells that fight harmful microorganisms. Lymph nodes may swell during infections.

* **mutation** (myoo-TAY-shun) is a change in an organism's gene or genes.

* **Helicobacter pylori** (HEEL-ih-ko-bak-ter pie-LOR-eye) is a bacterium that causes inflammation and ulcers, or sores, in the lining of the stomach and the upper part of the small intestine, also known as peptic ulcer disease.

* **duodenal** (do-uh-DEE-nul) refers to the upper part of the small intestine.

* **ulcer** is an open sore on the skin or the lining of a hollow body organ, such as the stomach or intestine. It may or may not be painful.

* **leukemia** (loo-KEE-me-uh) is a form of cancer characterized by the body's uncontrolled production of abnormal white blood cells.

and think that these infectious agents increase the risk only for some people. Avoiding exposure to these infections can lower the risk of certain types of cancer. People can avoid HPV infection, as well as human lymphotrophic virus type 1 and HIV infection, by limiting the number of their sexual partners and practicing abstinence (not having sex) or safe sex. To prevent hepatitis B and C, it is wise to avoid poorly sanitized needles for tattoos, piercing, or intravenous* drug use. Thorough hand washing, particularly after using a bathroom or changing a diaper, can lessen the risk of infection with *H. pylori*. It is almost impossible to avoid exposure to Epstein-Barr virus.

Resources

Organization

U.S. Centers for Disease Control and Prevention (CDC), 1600 Clifton Road, Atlanta, GA 30333. The CDC offers information about many infectious diseases, including *H. pylori* and HPV infections, at its website.
Telephone 800-311-3435
http://www.cdc.gov

Website

KidsHealth.org. KidsHealth is a website created by the medical experts of the Nemours Foundation and is devoted to issues of children's health. It contains articles on a variety of health topics, including Epstein-Barr virus, HPV, and hepatitis.
http://www.KidsHealth.org

Oral Infections

Oral infections are infections that occur in or around the mouth.

What Are Oral Infections?

Bacteria and viruses usually cause oral infections. They can affect the teeth, gums, palate (PAL-it, the roof of the mouth), tongue, lips, and inside of the cheeks. Simple oral infections are limited to the mouth and are different from oral lesions*, which are non-infectious and may be a sign of an illness that involves other parts of the body.

Oral infections are very common. Tooth decay is the second most common infectious condition, after the common cold.

Many oral infections are not contagious because bacteria that exist naturally in every person's mouth cause them. However, herpangina (her-

intravenous (in-tra-VEE-nus) means within or through a vein. For example, medications, fluid, or other substances can be given through a needle or soft tube inserted through the skin's surface directly into a vein.

▶ *See also*
AIDS and HIV Infection
Helicobacter Pylori Infection (Peptic Ulcer Disease)
Hepatitis, Infectious
Mononucleosis, Infectious
Sexually Transmitted Diseases
Warts

lesions (LEE-zhuns) is a general term referring to sores or damaged or irregular areas of tissue.

pan-JY-na) and recurrent herpes labialis (HER-peez lay-be-AL-us) are contagious and spread through contact with fluid from an infected person's mouth and nose.

What Are Some Common Oral Infections?

Canker sores Canker sores, also called aphthous (AF-thus) ulcers, are painful but benign* sores that occur on the tongue, inside of the lips and cheeks, gums, and palate. There is no evidence that canker sores are caused by an infectious organism. However, they are very common and can be confused with the sores that appear with some mouth infections. The ulcers may appear one at a time or in groups. They are small, pale, shallow, gray-white, and usually surrounded by bright red tissue.

These sores most frequently affect children and young adults. Sometimes they erupt when people accidentally bite the inside of their mouth or where braces rub the inside of the cheek. Stress, sensitivity to a particular food, not getting enough iron or B vitamins, and changes in hormones*, like those that occur during women's normal menstrual cycles, also may trigger canker sores. Often there is no apparent reason why a person develops a canker sore, although some people may be more likely to have them, especially if other people in their family have had canker sores. It previously was thought that canker sores were the result of an infection, but no infectious agent has been found. Now it is believed that something triggers the immune system, and the cells that normally fight infection "attack" the body's own tissue, leading to a canker sore.

Someone who has a canker sore may feel a tingling or burning sensation before a sore, reddish spot appears. The pain from a canker sore lasts up to 10 days, and the sore heals completely in 1 to 3 weeks. Canker sores usually come and go throughout a person's life. Occasionally, a person who develops a severe outbreak of canker sores may have a fever or a generally ill feeling.

A doctor (or dentist) usually diagnoses canker sores simply by examining the sore. Rarely, a biopsy* may be taken if the sore is unusually large or is not healing as expected, to distinguish it from other types of mouth ulcers. These sores heal without treatment, but over-the-counter medicines for canker sores can ease pain. People with more serious sores may be prescribed medication to apply to them. Experts advise anyone with a canker sore to avoid acidic, hot, or spicy foods and to rinse the mouth and gargle with warm saltwater to relieve pain. There is no known way to prevent the sores.

Cavities Dental caries (KARE-eez), also known as tooth decay and cavities, are areas where the hard enamel of a tooth has been destroyed, leaving small holes that are susceptible to further decay. Tooth decay occurs most frequently in children and teens and is the leading cause of tooth loss in younger people. Up to 80 percent of teens have had cavities by the time they finish high school, although tooth decay is much

KEYWORDS
for searching the Internet
and other reference sources

Aphthous ulcer

Candidiasis

Canker sore

Cavity

Cold sore

Dental caries

Gingivitis

Gingivostomatitis

Gum disease

Herpangina

Herpes labialis

Periodontal disease

Thrush

Tooth care

Tooth decay

* **benign** (beh-NINE) means a condition is not cancerous.

* **hormones** are chemical substances that are produced by various glands and sent into the bloodstream carrying messages that have certain effects on other parts of the body.

* **biopsy** (BI-op-see) is a test in which a small sample of skin or other body tissue is removed and examined for signs of disease.

less common today than it was before fluoride supplements and regular dental care were available to most people.

Bacteria that live in the mouth, especially certain kinds of streptococcus (strep-tuh-KAH-kus), cause tooth decay. The bacteria change food, particularly sweet and starchy foods, into acid, which eats away at the enamel of teeth. The acid, bacteria, and bits of food in the mouth combine into a thin film known as plaque (PLAK), which coats the teeth and collects in their grooves. A person with dental caries may experience pain or sensitivity in the affected tooth, usually when eating cold, hot, or sweet foods. Some people may not feel anything at all until the cavity extends into the middle part of the tooth, which houses the tooth's blood vessels and nerves. If left untreated, caries can lead to long-term tooth sensitivity, abscesses*, weakened teeth that can break easily, and even tooth loss.

Sugary foods and drinks and other foods contain carbohydrates* that increase the risk of tooth decay. Frequent meals and snacks also give the bacteria more chances to produce acid. Infants and young children who sip milk or juice throughout the day or go to bed with a bottle may develop bottle caries, a pattern of tooth decay that can damage baby teeth extensively.

Tooth decay usually is diagnosed during regular dental visits, and, depending on how badly the tooth has decayed, it may be treated with a filling, crown, or root canal (surgery to remove the pulp of the tooth). A dentist can apply a protective sealant to the molars or use fluoride to help prevent caries. Limiting sweets and frequent snacks; good dental hygiene (brushing and flossing); getting fluoride from drinking water, toothpaste, or other supplements; and regular dental visits are the best ways to prevent tooth decay.

Gingivitis Gingivitis (jin-juh-VY-tis) is inflammation of the gums, also known as the gingiva. It is caused by plaque that coats the teeth along the gum line. The bacteria and acid inflame and irritate the gums, making them red, swollen, and tender. If the plaque is not removed by brushing, flossing, and regular dental visits, it hardens into tartar at the base of the teeth and at the gum line, which further irritates the gums. As gingivitis progresses, the buildup of plaque and tartar causes the gums to recede and affects the ligaments* and bones supporting the teeth. Gingivitis often appears during puberty or early adulthood, and it is the first stage of periodontal* disease.

Some causes of gum irritation, which can lead to gingivitis, include:

- poor dental care and habits
- dental devices or appliances (such as bridges or braces) that have rough, irritating edges
- extremely vigorous tooth brushing or flossing
- teeth that are not aligned properly

*abscesses (AB-seh-sez) are localized or walled off accumulations of pus caused by infection that can occur anywhere within the body.

*carbohydrates are nutrients in food that help provide energy to the body.

*ligaments are bands of fibrous tissue that connect bones or cartilage, supporting and strengthening the joints. Ligaments in the mouth hold the roots of teeth in the tooth sockets.

*periodontal (pare-e-o-DON-tul) means located around a tooth.

- pregnancy
- poorly controlled diabetes* or certain other long-lasting illnesses

Swollen, bright red, tender gums that bleed easily and mouth sores are signs of gingivitis. It is diagnosed by examining the gums during a dental visit, and dental X rays may be taken to determine how much damage has been done to underlying structures in the mouth. People with gingivitis are treated with a thorough dental cleaning, followed by careful and regular at-home cleaning of the teeth and gums. Antibacterial mouthwash also may be prescribed. Gingivitis will not clear up on its own and can progress to serious periodontal disease that eventually affects the ligaments that hold the teeth in the gums and the tooth sockets, leading to tooth loss. Untreated gingivitis also may cause abscesses or a condition known as trench mouth, which is a severe and painful form of gum disease.

__Herpangina__ Herpangina is an infection marked by painful sores on the roof of the mouth, the tonsils*, and sometimes the inside of the cheeks. The lesions start as small bumps but become whitish sores with a red border. Herpangina usually is caused by coxsackievirus (kok-SAH-kee-vy-rus), which also causes hand, foot, and mouth disease; in hand, foot, and mouth disease, small blisters are found on the palms and the soles as well as the mouth. A day or two before the sores of herpangina appear, a person may have a fever, sore throat, and headache. Symptoms last less than a week.

Herpangina tends to affect young children and occurs most frequently in summer and fall. Like many other infections from common viruses, it is difficult to prevent. A doctor diagnoses herpangina by examining the appearance and location of the patient's lesions. Treatment includes drinking enough fluid and using over-the-counter medication such as acetaminophen (uh-see-teh-MIH-noh-fen) for pain and fever relief. A person also may apply numbing cream to the lesions to ease discomfort.

__Gingivostomatitis__ Gingivostomatitis (jin-juh-vo-sto-muh-TY-tis) is an infection of the gums and mouth caused by herpes simplex virus type 1 (genital* herpes is caused by herpes simplex virus type 2) and other common childhood viruses. As with herpangina, fever and illness appear before the mouth sores do. The lesions begin as blisters that pop soon after they form, leaving the base of the blister. When this covering peels off, a tender ulcer is formed. It will look grayish or yellowish with a red border. These painful sores often make it difficult to eat.

The diagnosis of gingivostomatitis is based on the presence of mouth sores, usually accompanied by other symptoms of a viral illness. Gingivostomatitis caused by herpes virus has a distinctive appearance and usually does not require more tests. Cultures* or biopsies rarely are done. Treatment for gingivostomatitis includes easing pain and preventing

* **diabetes** (dye-uh-BEE-teez) is a condition in which the body's pancreas does not produce enough insulin or the body cannot use the insulin it makes effectively, resulting in increased levels of sugar in the blood. This can lead to increased urination, dehydration, weight loss, weakness, and a number of other symptoms and complications related to chemical imbalances within the body.

* **tonsils** are paired clusters of lymph tissues in the throat that help protect the body from bacteria and viruses that enter through a person's nose or mouth.

* **genital** (JEN-nih-tul) refers to the external sexual organs.

* **cultures** (KUL-churs) are tests in which a sample of fluid or tissue from the body is placed in a dish containing material that supports the growth of certain organisms. Typically, within days the organisms will grow and can be identified.

*** dehydration** (dee-hi-DRAY-shun) is a condition in which the body is depleted of water, usually caused by excessive and unreplaced loss of body fluids, such as through sweating, vomiting, or diarrhea.

*** vaginal** (VAH-jih-nul) refers to the vagina, the canal in a woman that leads from the uterus to the outside of the body.

*** AIDS**, or acquired immunodeficiency (ih-myoo-no-dih-FIH-shensee) syndrome, is an infection that severely weakens the immune system; it is caused by the human immunodeficiency virus (HIV).

dehydration*. Over-the-counter pain medicine, medicated mouthwash or saltwater gargles, or numbing cream may provide some relief. Brushing teeth and gums gently will help prevent bacterial infection of the sores. Fluids and a bland diet are recommended as well.

Herpes Recurrent herpes labialis, also known as cold sores or fever blisters, is a condition caused by herpes simplex virus type 1. Cold sores are extremely common. Most Americans are infected with the virus by age 20. The virus stays in the body for life, although it usually causes no disease or only an occasional cold sore in most people. Many things can trigger a reactivation of the herpes virus to cause recurrent cold sores, such as fever, sun exposure, and stress.

Burning, tingling, or itching may occur a day or two before a small, sometimes painful blister appears on the gums, lips, inside of the mouth, or around the mouth. The blister is filled with clear or yellowish fluid. Shortly after it forms, the sore crusts over, and the crust eventually falls off. Sometimes a person also develops a mild fever or feels ill.

A doctor diagnoses herpes labialis based on the appearance of the cold sores, although fluid from a blister may be examined or cultured to confirm the diagnosis. Patients with cold sores often report having had them before. The blisters usually disappear on their own after 1 to 2 weeks, but if a person has frequent or severe cold sores, a doctor may prescribe antiviral medication to shorten the outbreak. However, the medicine does not get rid of the virus. When cold sores appear, ice or warm compresses may ease any discomfort or pain.

Cold sores are contagious. Kissing spreads the virus by direct contact, but the virus may spread indirectly by sharing food, drinks, lipstick, or utensils. It is difficult to prevent this infection because it can spread when no sores are visible.

Thrush Thrush, or candidiasis (kan-dih-DYE-uh-sis), is an overgrowth of *Candida*, a yeast-like fungus that can thrive in moist areas around body openings such as the mouth. Candidiasis can cause cracks in the corners of the mouth, and the lips, tongue, palate, and inside of the cheeks can have crusty whitish or yellowish patches. *Candida* also can cause other conditions, such as diaper rash and vaginal* yeast infections.

Thrush generally is not contagious, but newborns may come in contact with the fungus during birth if the mother has a vaginal yeast infection. People with weakened immune systems, such as those with AIDS* or cancer, may be more susceptible to thrush.

How Can People Prevent Oral Infections?

Frequent hand washing and avoiding exposure to people who are sick whenever possible helps prevent the spread of viral infections. Taking care of the teeth and mouth also goes a long way toward preventing oral infections. Tips for good oral hygiene include:

- Visiting a dentist regularly (every 6 months) for teeth cleanings and check-ups, and brushing teeth twice daily. Fluoride toothpaste is recommended for children; anti-tartar toothpaste is recommended for adults.
- Brushing the gums and tongue gently.
- Flossing daily.
- Brushing teeth after eating sugary or starchy foods.
- Wearing a helmet, and possibly a mouth guard, when playing certain sports, such as football or hockey, to protect teeth from injury.
- Not using tobacco products.

Resources

Organizations

U.S. Centers for Disease Control and Prevention (CDC), 1600 Clifton Road, Atlanta, GA 30333. The CDC's Division of Oral Health offers information about children's and adults' oral health at its website.
Telephone 800-311-3435
http://www.cdc.gov/OralHealth/index.htm

U.S. National Institute of Dental and Craniofacial Research, 45 Center Drive, MSC 6400, Bethesda, MD 20892. The National Institutes of Health's National Institute of Dental and Craniofacial Research provides information about oral and dental health at its website.
Telephone 301-496-4261
http://www.nidcr.nih.gov

Osteomyelitis

Osteomyelitis (ah-stee-o-my-uh-LYE-tis) is a bone infection that is usually caused by bacteria. It can involve any bone in the body, but it most commonly affects the long bones of the arms and legs.

What Is Osteomyelitis?

Osteomyelitis usually is caused by infection with bacteria. *Staphylococcus aureus* (stah-fih-lo-KAH-kus ARE-ree-us), streptococcal (strep-tuh-KAH-kul) species of bacteria, and *Pseudomonas aeruginosa* (su-doe-MO-nas air-ew-jih-NO-suh) are the major organisms associated with osteomyelitis. These bacterial intruders can travel from other parts of the body, such as the ear, throat, or intestines*, through the bloodstream and to a bone,

► See also
Abscesses
Coxsackieviruses and Other Enteroviruses
Herpes Simplex Virus Infections

KEYWORDS
for searching the Internet and other reference sources
Orthopedics
Staphylococcus aureus
Streptococcus bacteria

* **intestines** are the muscular tubes that food passes through during digestion after it exits the stomach.

257

* **trauma** is severe injury to the body.

* **vertebrae** (VER-tuh-bray) are the bones that form a column surrounding the spinal cord; there are 39 vertebrae in the spine.

* **diabetes** (dye-uh-BEE-teez) is a condition in which the body's pancreas does not produce enough insulin or the body cannot use the insulin it makes effectively, resulting in increased levels of sugar in the blood. This can lead to increased urination, dehydration, weight loss, weakness, and a number of other symptoms and complications related to chemical imbalances within the body.

* **ulcerations** are open sores on the skin or tissue lining a body part.

* **acute** describes an infection or other illness that comes on suddenly and usually does not last very long.

* **chronic** (KRAH-nik) means continuing for a long period of time.

* **intravenous** (in-tra-VEE-nus) means within or through a vein. For example, medications, fluid, or other substances can be given through a needle or soft tube inserted through the skin's surface directly into a vein.

where they can start an infection. Bones that have been weakened or damaged, such as one that has been injured recently, are more susceptible to bacterial invasion. When there is trauma* to the bone, like a puncture wound from stepping on a nail, bacteria can infect the bone directly. Rarely, fungi may cause osteomyelitis, and the spread of tuberculosis (too-ber-kyoo-LO-sis), a contagious disease that typically affects the lungs, through the body also can lead to bone infection, usually in the spine.

In children, osteomyelitis occurs most often in the long bones of the leg, such as the femur (FEE-mur) and tibia (TIH-be-uh). Adults tend to have the infection in the hipbones and vertebrae*, where it may occur following surgery on a bone or from an infection that has spread from the skin. People with diabetes* can have osteomyelitis in the foot bones from ulcerations* on their feet. Osteomyelitis that evolves rapidly is called acute* osteomyelitis. If a bone infection persists because it is not treated or it does not respond to treatment, it is known as chronic* osteomyelitis. Over time, the infection may interfere with the blood supply to the bone, causing the bone tissue to die.

How Common Is Osteomyelitis?

Chronic osteomyelitis occurs in about 2 in 10,000 adults. Children have the acute form of the disease more often than adults do, at a rate of about 1 in 5,000. People who have diabetes, who have had a traumatic injury recently, or who use intravenous* drugs are at greatest risk for chronic infection.

AN HISTORIC INFECTION

Some cases of osteomyelitis last for years, even a lifetime. Joshua Lawrence Chamberlain rose to the rank of general in the U.S. Civil War and was a hero in the Battle of Gettysburg. General Ulysses S. Grant selected Chamberlain to receive the official surrender of the Confederate Army's weapons at Appomatox, Virginia, in 1865. He later served as governor of Maine and president of Bowdoin College. Before he reached that lofty standing, Confederate soldiers had shot him in the groin in a battle at Petersburg, Virginia, in 1864. The ball pierced both hipbones, but despite the crude battlefield surgery of the time he survived his injury. His wound never healed completely, though, and Chamberlain lived another 50 years with chronic osteomyelitis. He died in 1914, at the age of 85, from complications of that long-lasting wound.

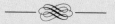

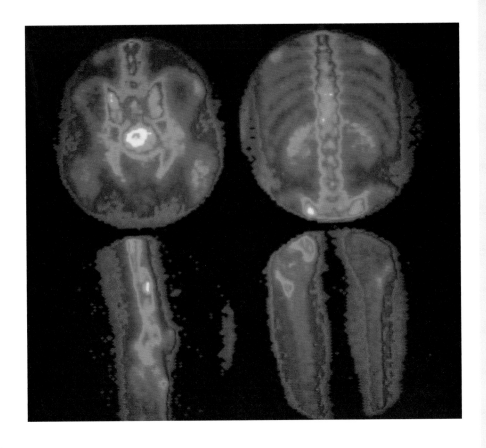

Special bone scans are used to diagnose osteomyelitis. The affected areas of bone "light up" on these scans. *Custom Medical Stock Photo, Inc.*

Is It Contagious?

Bone infections are not contagious. However, some types of bacteria that cause the infections that can progress to osteomyelitis are passed from person to person.

What Are the Signs and Symptoms of Osteomyelitis?

The first sign of acute infection may be a fever that begins suddenly. The area over the infected bone may become warm, red, and swollen, and the joints next to the bone may swell as well. As the infection progresses, it can cause pain in the affected bone and may limit the person's movement in that area. Some people with osteomyelitis feel irritable, nauseated, and generally sick. Patients with long-term bone infection may experience drainage of pus* through the skin covering the affected bone.

How Is the Disease Diagnosed?

To help make the diagnosis, a doctor may order an X ray of the suspect area to look for signs of bone inflammation or damage, but changes in the bone may not show up for weeks after the infection begins. Magnetic resonance imaging* (MRI) or a computerized tomography* (CT) scan

* **pus** is a thick, creamy fluid, usually yellow or greenish in color, that forms at the site of an infection. Pus contains infection-fighting white blood cells and other substances.

* **magnetic resonance imaging (MRI)** uses magnetic waves, instead of X rays, to scan the body and produce detailed pictures of the body's structures.

* **computerized tomography** (kom-PYOO-ter-ized toe-MAH-gruh-fee) or CT, also called computerized axial tomography (CAT), is a technique in which a machine takes many X rays of the body to create a three-dimensional picture.

* **radionuclide** (ray-dee-o-NU-klide) **scans** are tests that begin by giving a patient a small amount of a radioactive substance. The radioactive substance shows up on a scan, producing a view of the structure or function of the part of the body being studied.

* **cultures** (KUL-churz) are tests in which a sample of fluid or tissue from the body is placed in a dish containing material that supports the growth of certain organisms. Typically, within days the organisms will grow and can be identified.

* **biopsy** (BI-op-see) is a test in which a small sample of skin or other body tissue is removed and examined for signs of disease.

may show changes that reflect osteomyelitis sooner than X rays will. Radionuclide scans* may help pinpoint the location of the infection early in the course of the disease. Blood cultures* or, less commonly, a bone biopsy* may identify the infectious agent.

What Is the Treatment for Osteomyelitis?

Patients with osteomyelitis usually need to be hospitalized. They typically receive antibiotics for 4 to 6 weeks to combat the infection. At first, the medication is given intravenously, but patients may be switched to oral (by mouth) medicine as the treatment continues and their condition improves. In more serious and chronic cases, patients may need an operation to remove bits of bone that have died. To help new bone grow, surgeons may perform a bone graft, in which bone from another part of the body is placed in the spot where dead bone has been removed; doctors may use packing material to fill in the open area temporarily.

How Long Does the Disease Last?

Patients with osteomyelitis often need several weeks or months of treatment before the infection clears up. Acute cases may resolve after as little as 1 month of antibiotic therapy, but chronic cases can linger much longer.

What Are the Complications?

In children, osteomyelitis can damage growing bones permanently, especially if it is not promptly and adequately treated. Infection may spread to the blood, overlying skin, or nearby joints. Bones may be weakened and break more easily. Movement of nearby joints or limbs may become limited. Occasionally in chronic cases, severe infection or damage to the bone may result in the need to amputate, or remove, part or all of a limb.

How Can Osteomyelitis Be Prevented?

Quick, thorough treatment of any infection, particularly those from deep wounds, can lower the risk of osteomyelitis. It is recommended that patients who are more susceptible to osteomyelitis, such as those with diabetes, contact a doctor promptly if they notice signs of infection.

Resource

Website

KidsHealth.org. KidsHealth is a website created by the medical experts of the Nemours Foundation and is devoted to issues of children's health. It contains articles on a variety of health topics, including osteomyelitis.
http://www.KidsHealth.org

▶ *See also*
Arthritis, Infectious
Staphylococcal Infections
Streptococcal Infections
Tuberculosis

Otitis (Ear Infections)

Otitis (o-TIE-tis) is an inflammation of the internal or external parts of the ear, usually caused by infection.

Ears have three main parts: outer, middle, and inner. The eardrum is between the outer and middle ear and is the part of the ear that responds to sound waves by vibrating. The pea-size middle ear normally is filled with air, and when the eardrum vibrates, the tiny bones of the middle ear are set into motion to send sound signals to the inner ear, which is filled with fluid. The eustachian (yoo-STAY-she-un) tube connects the middle ear with the throat and nose, normally allowing air and fluid to move in and out of the middle ear.

When parts of the ear become infected, an earache may occur. There are two basic types of ear infection: otitis media and otitis externa.

Otitis Media

Middle ear infections If a person has a cold or allergies, the eustachian tube may not function properly and fluid can become trapped in the middle ear, which can lead to infection if bacteria or viruses get in. In acute* otitis media, the middle ear becomes inflamed and fills with fluid or pus*.

Chronic* otitis media results if the infection does not go away (with or without treatment) within a few weeks. In more severe or long-lasting cases of chronic otitis media, the eardrum may become permanently damaged or the infection may spread to surrounding structures. More often in chronic otitis media, the infection may be gone but fluid remains and the eardrum cannot move freely to transmit sound waves. This condition is known as chronic otitis media with effusion* and can cause a temporary hearing loss in the affected ear. Recurrent otitis media occurs when a person has repeated ear infections but gets better between infections.

Otitis media is not contagious, but common colds and other infections of the respiratory tract* that can lead to it are. When people cough, sneeze, laugh, or talk, they can spread the viruses or bacteria that cause colds and respiratory illnesses to their hands, to the surfaces around them, and into the air. Other people can breathe in these germs or touch contaminated surfaces with their hands and spread the germs to their noses and mouths. If the conditions are right, the germs enter the middle ear through the eustachian tube or cause a blockage in the eustachian tube, setting the stage for an ear infection to develop.

Adults can get otitis media, but it is more common in children, especially those under age 3. The eustachian tubes of children are narrower, shorter, and more horizontal than those in adults, making it

KEYWORDS
for searching the Internet and other reference sources

Earaches

Eardrum

Ear infections

Eustachian tube

Otitis externa

Otitis media

Otolaryngology

Swimmer's ear

* **acute** describes an infection or other illness that comes on suddenly and usually does not last very long.

* **pus** is a thick, creamy fluid, usually yellow or greenish in color, that forms at the site of an infection. Pus contains infection-fighting white cells and other substances.

* **chronic** (KRAH-nik) means continuing for a long period of time.

* **effusion** (ih-FYOO-zhun) is an excessive accumulation of body fluid in a body space or cavity, such as the middle ear.

* **respiratory tract** includes the nose, mouth, throat, and lungs. It is the pathway through which air and gases are transported down into the lungs and back out of the body.

Three by Three

A third of all children experience three or more ear infections by the time they turn 3 years old. Otitis media is the number-one diagnosis among children for sick visits to the doctor, and it is the leading cause of hearing loss in children.

Source: *American Academy of Otolaryngology*

** **mastoiditis** (mas-toy-DYE-tis) is an infection of the mastoid bone, located behind the ear.

** **diabetes** (dye-uh-BEE-teez) is a condition in which the body's pancreas does not produce enough insulin or the body cannot use the insulin it makes effectively, resulting in increased levels of sugar in the blood. This can lead to increased urination, dehydration, weight loss, weakness, and a number of other symptoms and complications related to chemical imbalances within the body.

** **cellulitis** (sel-yoo-LYE-tis) is an infection of the skin and the tissues beneath it.

easier for germs to enter and fluid to build up. Young children also have frequent respiratory infections, which are often accompanied by ear infections in children this age.

Signs and symptoms Signs and symptoms of otitis media include:
- in babies, irritability, fussiness, or tugging on the ear
- ear pain or a feeling of pressure
- buzzing or ringing sounds in the ear
- pus draining or bleeding from the ear (if the eardrum has ruptured)
- mild hearing loss
- fever
- vomiting or diarrhea (dye-uh-REE-uh)

Complications of otitis media include a ruptured ear drum due to high-pressure fluid buildup in the middle ear, mastoiditis*, and, rarely, spread of infection to the brain. Hearing loss also can occur; it is typically temporary, except in long-standing chronic disease.

Otitis Externa

Swimmer's ear Otitis externa, often called swimmer's ear, is an inflammation or infection of the outer ear canal. It is not contagious but occurs when bacteria or fungi enter through a break in the skin inside the ear.

Otitis externa often occurs after swimming or diving, when moisture can break down the protective wax and skin in the ear canal. Although it is called swimmer's ear, it can occur whenever these barriers are broken down in other ways, such as by frequent cleaning with cotton swabs or scratching inside the ear too roughly. Once the skin is broken, bacteria or fungi can enter and cause an infection. The ear will become red, swollen, and painful to the touch.

Otitis externa is fairly common and affects mostly teens and young adults. People who spend a long time swimming or diving are most susceptible.

Occasionally otitis externa can have complications. In about 1 percent of cases, the infection persists and results in chronic otitis externa. Rarely, this can lead to malignant otitis externa, a serious condition in which the infection spreads to the bones and nerves of the ear, skull, and brain; this occurs almost exclusively among people with diabetes*. Cellulitis* is another possible complication.

Signs and symptoms Signs and symptoms of otitis externa include:
- ear pain that usually worsens if the ear is touched or pulled
- red, swollen outer ear canal

- green or yellow pus draining from the ear
- mild loss of hearing

How Are Ear Infections Diagnosed?

A doctor will examine a person's ears, inside and out, checking for redness, swelling, and abnormal collections of fluid. The doctor will take a close look at the eardrum by using a lighted instrument called an otoscope (O-toh-skope). An audiogram may be performed to test the person's hearing and a tympanogram (tim-PAH-no-gram) may be done to check for normal vibration of the eardrum and pressure levels in the middle ear.

Samples of fluid, pus, and blood from inside the ear may be tested to discover whether a bacterium, virus, or fungus is causing the infection. If the doctor thinks the infection has spread to surrounding bone or cartilage, an X ray or computerized tomography* (CT) scan of the head may be performed.

How Do Doctors Treat Ear Infections?

Over-the-counter, non-aspirin painkillers such as acetaminophen (uh-see-teh-MIH-noh-fen) and warm heating pads can be used to ease the throbbing pain of earaches. Antibiotic eardrops are used to treat otitis externa. Oral (by mouth) antibiotics are used to treat otitis media and may be prescribed in more severe cases of otitis externa. However, antibiotics are not always necessary to treat otitis media because the condition is not always caused by bacteria. Many cases of otitis media are caused by viruses, which do not respond to antibiotic treatment, but it is often difficult to tell the difference. Even if bacteria are the cause of an ear infection, many cases will get better on their own, although antibiotic treatment lowers the risk of the infection spreading and clears up symptoms sooner. Typically, the symptoms of acute otitis media improve within the first 2 to 3 days of antibiotic treatment. Chronic infections, however, can last several weeks or months. In children with chronic otitis media, it may be helpful to surgically insert a small plastic tube in the eardrum that allows air to flow into the middle ear and prevent fluid buildup that can interfere with hearing.

In cases of external otitis, doctors recommend that water be kept out of the ear canal during recovery; earplugs or shower caps can help keep out water while bathing, and swimming should be avoided.

How Can Ear Infections Be Prevented?

Frequent hand washing can help prevent spread of the germs that cause colds and other respiratory illnesses, which often lead to ear infections, especially in young children. Toys should be washed often to keep infections from spreading among babies and young children in daycare settings.

To prevent fluid from pooling in eustachian tubes, experts recommend that babies be bottle-fed in an upright position and not sleep with

* **computerized tomography** (kom-PYOO-ter-ized toe-MAH-gruh-fee) or CT, also called computerized axial tomography (CAT), is a technique in which a machine takes many X rays of the body to create a three-dimensional picture.

▶ *See also*
Common Cold
Influenza
Streptococcal Infections

a bottle. Breastfeeding also can help prevent otitis media in babies, as can avoiding exposure to cigarette smoke.

Vaccinations* against *Streptococcus pneumoniae* (strep-tuh-KAH-kus nu-MO-nye), a common cause of otitis media, and influenza* can reduce the likelihood of contracting otitis media. Treating allergies or removing enlarged adenoids* that block the eustachian tubes may decrease the chances of having recurrent or chronic ear infection in some patients.

After swimming or bathing, thoroughly drying ears with a towel can help get rid of water and lower the risk of contracting otitis externa. For avid swimmers, preventive eardrops can be used after swimming. Nothing should be inserted into the ears because of the risk of injuring the skin of the ear canal or damaging the eardrum.

Resources

Organization

American Academy of Otolaryngology—Head and Neck Surgery, 1 Prince Street, Alexandria, VA 22314. This group of doctors who specialize in treating ear, nose, and throat disorders has information about ear infections on their website.
Telephone 703-836-4444
http://www.entnet.org

Website

KidsHealth.org. KidsHealth is a website created by the medical experts of the Nemours Foundation and is devoted to issues of children's health. It contains articles on a variety of health topics, including otitis.
http://www.KidsHealth.org

P

Peptic Ulcer Disease *See* Helicobacter Pylori Infection (Peptic Ulcer Disease)

Pertussis (Whooping Cough)

Pertussis (per-TUH-sis) is a bacterial infection of the respiratory tract* that causes severe coughing.

What Is Pertussis?

Pertussis is a respiratory disease found only in humans that is caused by the bacterium *Bordetella pertussis.* The first account of the infection was recorded in the sixteenth century, but it was not until the early twentieth century that *B. pertussis* was identified as the cause.

The infection causes a violent series of coughing fits ending in a high-pitched intake of breath that sounds like a "whoop," giving the disease its other name: whooping cough. These coughing fits can be so severe that patients may vomit, lose consciousness, or turn blue from lack of oxygen.

Do Many People Contract Pertussis?

Pertussis occurs throughout the world in all age groups. In the early twentieth century, it was a common childhood disease and a leading cause of infant death. Since the widespread use of a vaccine* starting in the mid-1940s, however, infection rates in children in the United States have declined. Teens and adults account for the majority of infections in the twenty-first century, which may indicate that childhood immunization with the vaccine does not offer lifelong immunity*.

Before the introduction of the vaccine, more than 200,000 cases of pertussis were diagnosed each year in the United States. Since the 1980s, the U.S. Centers for Disease Control and Prevention (CDC) has reported yearly U.S. averages ranging from about 3,000 to 8,000 cases. In many developing countries in Asia, Africa, and Latin America, however, pertussis is still a major cause of childhood deaths; the CDC attributes 300,000 deaths worldwide every year to the disease.

Is Pertussis Contagious?

Pertussis is an extremely contagious infection. The bacteria can spread through the air in drops of fluid released from the mouth and nose of a

KEYWORDS
for searching the Internet
and other reference sources

DTaP

Immunization

Respiratory system

Whooping cough

* **respiratory tract** includes the nose, mouth, throat, and lungs. It is the pathway through which air and gases are transported down into the lungs and back out of the body.

* **vaccine** (vak-SEEN) is a preparation of killed or weakened germs, or a part of a germ or product it produces, given to prevent or lessen the severity of the disease that can result if a person is exposed to the germ itself. Use of vaccines for this purpose is called immunization.

* **immunity** (ih-MYOON-uh-tee) is the condition of being protected against an infectious disease. Immunity often develops after a germ is introduced to the body. One type of immunity occurs when the body makes special protein molecules called antibodies to fight the disease-causing germ. The next time that germ enters the body, the antibodies quickly attack it, usually preventing the germ from causing disease.

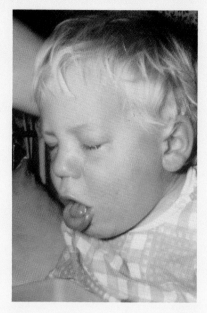

▲

Pertussis, or whooping cough, affected many children in the United States until a vaccine was developed in the 1940s. The name whooping cough comes from the high-pitched sound made during the deep breath taken following the characteristic severe coughing spells. *Custom Medical Stock Photo, Inc.*

* **incubation** (ing-kyoo-BAY-shun) is the period of time between infection by a germ and when symptoms first appear. Depending on the germ, this period can be from hours to months.

* **toxins** are poisons that harm the body.

* **mucus** (MYOO-kus) is a thick, slippery substance that lines the insides of many body parts.

* **lymphocytes** (LIM-fo-sites) are white blood cells, which play a part in the body's immune system, particularly the production of antibodies and other substances to fight infection.

coughing or sneezing person who is infected. Inhaling those airborne drops can lead to disease, as can direct contact with the drops, such as touching them and transferring bacteria from a hand to the mouth or nose. Up to 90 percent of susceptible (non-immune) people living in the same house with someone who has whooping cough will become infected as well.

Pertussis is different from most other contagious respiratory illnesses because children generally do not infect adults. Instead, adults usually have a mild case of the disease first and unknowingly pass the bacteria to their children, who develop a more serious form of the illness.

What Happens to People Who Have Pertussis?

Signs and Symptoms   Following exposure to the bacteria, an incubation* period begins and generally lasts 7 to 10 days but occasionally stretches to as long as a month. During this time, the bacteria settle in the lungs where they produce toxins* that cause inflammation and make it difficult to clear out the mucus* that forms in the respiratory tract.

After the incubation period, there are three distinct stages of pertussis infection: the catarrhal (kah-TAR-hul), paroxysmal (PAIR-ok-siz-mul), and convalescent (kon-vuh-LEH-sent) stages. In the catarrhal stage, the first symptoms of the disease appear and often are mistaken for those of a common cold or the flu. They include runny nose, sneezing, mild fever, and a cough that gradually worsens. This stage typically lasts 1 to 2 weeks.

In the paroxysmal stage, the characteristic symptoms of whooping cough take center stage. The occasional cough develops into sudden violent attacks, or paroxysms, of rapid coughing ending with the whooping noise. The coughing is due to the buildup of mucus in the respiratory tract and occurs frequently at night. Babies under 6 months of age may not have the strength to make the whooping sound that older children, teens, and adults typically do, but they do have bursts of coughing. It is difficult to breathe during these fits, and many patients turn blue from lack of oxygen. The severe coughing also can lead to vomiting and extreme tiredness. Between these bouts, patients look normal. The paroxysmal stage generally lasts from 1 to 6 weeks but can linger for up to 10 weeks.

In the final, convalescent stage, coughing slowly subsides over 2 or 3 weeks.

Diagnosis   In some cases, the doctor can make the diagnosis of whooping cough based solely on hearing the cough, but a definitive diagnosis requires an examination of fluid from the nose or throat. Samples of this fluid are checked for bacteria. Blood tests can look for the increased number of lymphocytes* commonly seen with this disease and for antibodies* to the bacterium.

Treatment   Doctors commonly prescribe a 2-week course of antibiotics to keep the disease from spreading to others. Antibiotics also can be prescribed for other people living in the same household with the patient to prevent them from contracting the infection. However, antibiotics can do little to improve the illness if they are not prescribed until after the characteristic whooping cough symptoms appear. Cough medicines do not ease the cough significantly, but using a cool-mist vaporizer and avoiding irritants such as smoke or fumes can help.

Children 18 months old and younger who contract whooping cough need to be watched carefully because they may choke or stop breathing during a coughing spasm. Infants less than 6 months old usually are hospitalized and given oxygen and intravenous* fluids, and their mouth and nose may need to be suctioned to keep their breathing passages clear of mucus.

Whooping cough usually lasts between 6 weeks and 2 months, but it can take even longer for a patient to recover completely. The coughing spasms may continue on and off for several months.

Complications Complications of whooping cough include bacterial infections such as ear infections or pneumonia*; dehydration* due to poor fluid intake and vomiting after coughing; broken blood vessels in the eyes, nose, and brain from forceful coughing; problems associated with lack of oxygen such as seizures* or, rarely, brain damage; and, particularly among young infants, death.

Can Pertussis Be Prevented?

Vaccination (vak-sih-NAY-shun) is the best way to prevent pertussis in children. The vaccine for pertussis is given in a combined vaccine including those for diphtheria* and tetanus*. The DTaP vaccine (made with acellular pertussis, which contains only parts of the pertussis bacterium and does not cause as many side effects as the vaccine made with the whole bacterium) is given in multiple doses, starting at 2 months of age.

Adults can lower their chances of becoming infected or spreading the disease by practicing good hygiene, such as regularly washing their hands; not sharing food, silverware, or drinking glasses; and covering their mouth when they sneeze or cough.

Resources

Organization

U.S. Centers for Disease Control and Prevention (CDC), 1600 Clifton Road, Atlanta, GA 30333. The CDC is the U.S. government authority for information about infectious and other diseases. It offers information on pertussis and vaccinations at its website.
Telephone 800-311-3435
http://www.cdc.gov

*** antibodies** (AN-tih-bah-deez) are protein molecules produced by the body's immune system to help fight specific infections caused by microorganisms, such as bacteria and viruses.

*** intravenous** (in-tra-VEE-nus), or IV, means within or through a vein. For example, medications, fluid, or other substances can be given through a needle or soft tube inserted through the skin's surface directly into a vein.

*** pneumonia** (nu-MO-nyah) is inflammation of the lungs.

*** dehydration** (dee-hi-DRAY-shun) is a condition in which the body is depleted of water, usually caused by excessive and unreplaced loss of body fluids, such as through sweating, vomiting, or diarrhea.

*** seizures** (SEE-zhurs) are sudden bursts of disorganized electrical activity that interrupt the normal functioning of the brain, often leading to uncontrolled movements in the body and sometimes a temporary change in consciousness.

*** diphtheria** (dif-THEER-e-uh) is an infection of the lining of the upper respiratory tract (the nose and throat). It is a disease that can cause breathing difficulty and other complications, including death.

*** tetanus** (TET-nus) is a serious bacterial infection that affects the body's central nervous system.

▶ *See also*

Croup

Diphtheria

Pneumonia

Tetanus (Lockjaw)

Vaccination (Immunization)

KEYWORDS
*for searching the Internet
and other reference sources*

Gastrointestinal tract

Intestinal parasites

Nematodes

Roundworms

* **intestines** are the system of muscular tubes that food passes through during digestion after it exits the stomach.

* **roundworm** is one of several types of cylinder-shaped worms that live in people. Roundworms are also known as nematodes (NEE-muh-todes).

* **small intestine** is the part of the intestine—the system of muscular tubes that food passes through during digestion—that directly receives the food after it passes through the stomach.

* **larvae** (LAR-vee) are the immature forms of an insect or worm that hatches from an egg.

* **colon** (KO-lin), also called the large intestine, is a muscular tube through which food passes as it is digested, just before it moves into the rectum and out of the body through the anus.

* **anus** (A-nus) is the opening at the end of the digestive system, through which waste leaves the body.

Website

KidsHealth.org. KidsHealth is a website created by the medical experts of the Nemours Foundation and is devoted to issues of children's health. It contains articles on a variety of health topics, including pertussis.
http://www.KidsHealth.org

Pinworm Infestation

In cases of pinworm infestation, or enterobiasis (en-tuh-roh-BY-uh-sis), a species of small worm lives and reproduces in the human intestines*.

What Is Pinworm Infestation?

Human pinworms, *Enterobius vermicularis (en-tuh-ROH-be-us ver-MIH-kyoo-lar-is)*, are a species of roundworm* about the size of a staple. People become infested when they swallow tiny pinworm eggs, usually after touching something that a person with pinworms has touched. The eggs travel to the small intestine* and hatch into larvae*. The larvae then migrate to the colon*, where they grow into adult worms. Female adult pinworms emerge from a person's anus* at night to lay their eggs on the skin of the perianal region*. The worms return to the colon, where they usually die, but the eggs can survive for up to 2 weeks outside the human body. If the person scratches around the anus and later touches the lips, it is possible to transfer the eggs from the hands to the mouth, where they are swallowed and begin a new cycle of infestation.

How Common Is It?

The U.S. Centers for Disease Control and Prevention estimates that about 40 million people, or 1 person in 7, in the United States have pinworms, making it the most common worm infestation in the country. Children in school and preschool are most frequently infested, and pinworms are also common in people living in crowded conditions. When one person in a household becomes infested, other family members often wind up with the worms as well.

Is Pinworm Infestation Contagious?

Pinworms can spread directly from person to person. Someone with an infestation may unknowingly leave the parasite's eggs in their clothes or bed or anywhere that they put their hands after scratching the anal area. When another person picks up the clothes or makes the bed, he or she may get the eggs on the fingers. By touching the mouth, this person can swallow the eggs and start an infestation. Young children have the greatest chance of becoming infested, because they often put their hands in their mouths. The parasites spread easily in preschools, schools, and childcare settings.

What Are the Signs and Symptoms of Infestation?

Many people with pinworms have no symptoms at all. In others, symptoms are generally mild. The most common symptom is itching around the anus. The sensation becomes strongest at night, when the female worms are active on the skin; this may lead to restless sleep or even trouble sleeping. Children with infestations may become irritable from lack of peaceful sleep, and they occasionally lose their appetites. If a child constantly scratches around the anus, the skin there can become raw and infected. In girls, adult worms sometimes enter the vagina* instead of returning to the anus, which may cause vaginal itching.

How Is the Diagnosis of Pinworm Infestation Made?

Doctors usually use the "tape" test to diagnose a suspected pinworm infestation: a piece of transparent tape is applied briefly over the anus and then removed. If a person has pinworms, the worms or their eggs may stick to the tape. The tape then is taken to the doctor's office for examination, because the evidence is visible only under a microscope. The doctor may provide a special adhesive "pinworm paddle" to conduct this test. The tape is applied at home as soon as the person wakes up, because bathing or having a bowel movement can dislodge the eggs. The patient may need to take several tape tests if the first one or two do not show the presence of worms. The doctor also might examine scrapings from under the fingernails, where pinworm eggs can become stuck after the patient scratches the anal area. In some cases, the worms, which look like fine threads, can be spotted at night around the anus or in the bed sheets.

What Is the Treatment?

Once an infestation is confirmed, the doctor generally prescribes medication to get rid of the worms. The patient takes the first dose, often in the form of a chewable pill, right away and a second dose 2 weeks later. Sometimes doctors recommend that all people who live in the same house with the infested person take the medicine as well. Patients may need more than one round of treatment to get rid of the worms entirely, if they become infested a second time.

Are There Complications of Pinworm Infestation?

Complications of pinworm infestation are uncommon and generally minor, such as the development of a bacterial infection of the perianal skin from scratching.

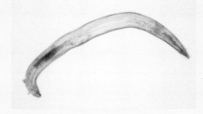

Pinworms are about one-third of an inch long and live in the human intestine. Female pinworms deposit eggs on the skin surrounding a person's anus. The eggs can then be spread to other family members through contact with sheets or clothing. *Custom Medical Stock Photo, Inc.*

* **perianal** (pair-e-A-nul) **region** is the area of skin surrounding the anus.

* **vagina** (vah-JY-nah) is the canal, or passageway, in a woman that leads from the uterus to the outside of the body.

What Are the Preventive Measures?

Practicing good personal hygiene is the best way to avoid infestation. For example, it is a good idea to wash the hands after going to the bathroom and before eating and to avoid scratching the anal area and biting the nails. To limit the spread of pinworms, people with the parasites are advised to change into clean underwear every day and frequently change their nightclothes. Taking a bath or shower after waking up in the morning can help get rid of pinworm eggs, and trimming fingernails short can prevent eggs from lodging there and later being deposited somewhere else. Doctors advise that after each course of treatment for pinworms, sheets and sleeping clothes be washed, to lower the risk of re-infestation.

Resources

Organizations

American Academy of Family Physicians, 11400 Tomahawk Creek Parkway, Leawood, KS 66211. The American Academy of Family Physicians publishes fact sheets about pinworms at its website. Telephone 800-274-2237
http://familydoctor.org

U.S. Centers for Disease Control and Prevention (CDC), 1600 Clifton Road, Atlanta, GA 30333. The CDC is the U.S. government authority for information about infectious and other diseases. It provides a fact sheet and other information on pinworm infestation through the website of the National Center for Infectious Diseases. Telephone 800-311-3435
http://www.cdc.gov/ncidod/

▶ *See also*
Ascariasis

Plague

Plague (PLAYG) is a potentially serious bacterial infection that is spread to humans by infected rodents and their fleas.

What Is Plague?

Plague is a disease caused by the bacterium *Yersinia pestis* (yer-SIN-e-uh PES-tis). It has been in existence for at least 2,000 years and in the twenty-first century is still found in Africa, Asia, South America, and North America.

There are three types of plague. Pneumonic (nu-MOH-nik) involves the lungs; bubonic (byoo-BAH-nik), the most common form, involves the body's lymphatic system*; and septicemic (sep-tih-SEE-mik) involves the bloodstream and spreads throughout the body. Septicemic plague can occur by itself or along with pneumonic or bubonic plague.

Wild rats and fleas often are associated with plague, because they were the primary carriers of the disease during history's most devastating outbreaks. Other types of rodents (and their fleas) can carry plague as well, such as prairie dogs, chipmunks, wood rats, and ground squirrels.

How Common Is Plague?

The World Health Organization reports 1,000 to 3,000 cases of plague worldwide annually. In the United States, 10 to 20 cases are reported every year, usually in rural areas in northern New Mexico, northern Arizona, southern Colorado, California, western Nevada, and southern Oregon. The last outbreak in the United States was in 1924–25 in Los Angeles. Plague has not been seen in Europe since World War II.

How Is Plague Spread?

Plague is transmitted in several ways. The most common is from animal to human through the bite of infected fleas. Fleas living on infected animals ingest the animals' blood and the bacteria in it. They then spread the disease to other animals and humans through their bite, which can result in the bubonic or septicemic form of plague. Bacteria also can

* **lymphatic** (lim-FAH-tik) **system** is a system that contains lymph nodes and a network of channels that carry fluid and cells of the immune system through the body.

Bioweapons

Plague bacteria are considered to be one of several deadly organisms that could be used in biological warfare*. It is feared that the bacteria could be aerosolized (AIR-o-suh-lized), or processed into tiny particles that could be released into the air.

A plague vaccine* was available to the general public but was discontinued by its manufacturers in 1999. Even if the vaccine were made available today, it would not be able to prevent the pneumonic form of plague, which is resistant to treatment as well.

The plague has been used as a weapon before. In 1346 the Tartar army tried to capture the port city of Caffa on the Black Sea in the Crimea. The army catapulted bodies of plague victims over the city wall; an epidemic of plague ensued and the city surrendered.

* **biological warfare** is a method of waging war by using harmful microorganisms to purposely spread disease to many people.

* **vaccine** (vak-SEEN) is a preparation of killed or weakened germs, or a part of a germ or product it produces, given to prevent or lessen the severity of the disease that can result if a person is exposed to the germ itself. Use of vaccines for this purpose is called immunization.

THE BLACK DEATH

The first pandemic (an outbreak of disease over a large geographical area, often worldwide) of plague chronicled by historians occurred between 542 and 546 A.D., during the Roman emperor Justinian's reign. The plague followed trade routes to other countries, and the Roman army itself carried plague during war campaigns throughout Asia Minor, Western Europe, Italy, and Africa. Outbreaks continued for the next 300 years before the disease finally subsided.

An equally devastating second pandemic erupted nearly 800 years later, as plague once again traveled across trade routes and infected population pockets throughout Europe. Known as the Black Death, this fourteenth century outbreak killed more than one third of Europe's population.

During these first two pandemics, the source of plague (rats and, more importantly, their infected fleas) was unknown. The spread of disease went unexplained, and many people feared it was a punishment sent by God.

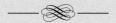

* **lymph** (LIMF) **nodes** are small, bean-shaped masses of tissue that contain immune system cells that fight harmful microorganisms. Lymph nodes may swell during infections.

* **sepsis** is a potentially serious spreading of infection, usually bacterial, through the bloodstream and body.

* **pneumonia** (nu-MO-nyah) is inflammation of the lung.

* **meningitis** (meh-nin-JY-tis) is an inflammation of the meninges, the membranes that surround the brain and the spinal cord. Meningitis is most often caused by infection with a virus or a bacterium.

* **abdominal** (ab-DAH-mih-nul) refers to the area of the body below the ribs and above the hips that contains the stomach, intestines, and other organs.

* **clot** is the process by which the body forms a thickened mass of blood cells and protein to stop bleeding.

* **sputum** (SPYOO-tum) is a substance that contains mucus and other matter coughed out from the lungs, bronchi, and trachea.

* **respiratory failure** is a condition in which breathing and oxygen delivery to the body is dangerously altered. This may result from infection, nerve or muscle damage, poisoning, or other causes.

* **shock** is a serious condition in which blood pressure is very low and not enough blood flows to the body's organs and tissues. Untreated, shock may result in death.

enter the body through an open cut or wound after direct contact with infected people or animals.

In addition, humans and animals (such as cats) with plague can spread the disease by releasing tiny drops containing the bacteria from their mouth and nose; in humans, this happens when a person coughs, sneezes, or talks. As these drops enter the air, the smaller ones can float for up to 1 hour, whereas the larger drops settle on nearby objects. A sneeze or cough can send thousands of infected particles into the air. If inhaled, these drops can cause the pneumonic form of plague. This way of spreading the disease requires relatively close contact with an infected person or animal.

What Are the Signs and Symptoms of Plague?

Symptoms typically appear 2 to 6 days after infection. Sudden fever, chills, and headache, followed by swollen, painful, hot-to-the-touch lymph nodes*, known as buboes (BYOO-boze), are the hallmarks of bubonic plague. Lymph nodes in the groin are most commonly affected. If left untreated, the infection eventually spreads to the bloodstream, causing sepsis*, pneumonia*, or meningitis*.

In septicemic plague, the bacteria multiply in the blood, causing symptoms such as fever, chills, weakness, abdominal* pain, nausea (NAW-zee-uh), and vomiting. As the infection progresses, the blood pressure drops and the blood is unable to clot* normally. The skin looks bruised from uncontrolled bleeding, which is why historically the disease was called the Black Death.

The pneumonic form of plague takes hold rapidly, with symptoms such as fever, cough, chills, chest pain, bloody sputum*, and headache. It can progress to respiratory failure* and shock* within 2 to 4 days.

How Do Doctors Diagnose and Treat Plague?

Determining whether a person was in close contact with animals that can carry plague or has traveled to an area where the plague is known to occur can be key in making the diagnosis. Bubonic plague can be identified by the characteristic swollen lymph nodes. A blood culture* and a lymph node biopsy* may be done, as well as a culture of a sputum sample to look for *Yersinia pestis* bacteria.

Getting timely treatment for plague is critical. Without treatment, bubonic plague is fatal in 50 to 60 percent of cases. Septicemic plague and pneumonic plague are fatal in almost all cases if not treated within 24 to 48 hours.

Suspected plague patients are isolated and hospitalized, where they are treated with antibiotics, intravenous* (IV) fluids, and oxygen. Anyone who has come in close contact with someone diagnosed with plague is treated with antibiotics to prevent contracting the infection. All suspected cases of plague must be reported to state and local health departments. Treatment and full recovery from plague can take several weeks or longer. Complications of plague include damage to vital organs

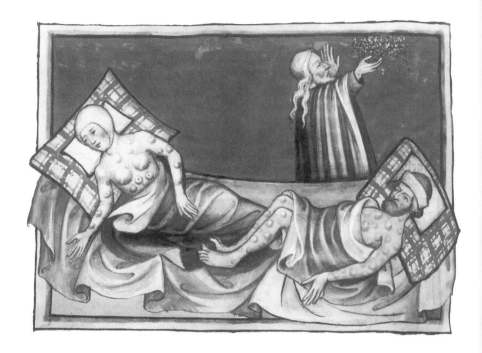

This fifteenth-century painting depicts the characteristic "buboes," or swollen lymph nodes, of bubonic plague. The buboes are red at first, but then turn a dark purple or black, which lead the disease to be called the Black Death. A fourteenth-century plague epidemic killed 25 million people in Europe. *Corbis Corporation (Bellevue)*

◀

due to lack of blood flow associated with sepsis, brain damage from lack of oxygen, lung damage, and death.

How Can People Prevent Becoming Infected?

Some people are at a higher risk for developing plague than others, such as lab technicians who handle the bacterium or blood samples taken from people who are infected, people who work in areas where plague occurs, and people who work with animals that carry the disease.

A person's risk of developing plague can be lowered by limiting contact with wild animals that might carry the disease, removing potential food sources and shelter for rodents near the home, treating pet dogs and cats weekly for fleas, and using insecticides to kill fleas around the home during outbreaks of plague in wild animals. Rat management in rural and urban areas also can minimize the potential for disease.

Antibiotics sometimes are prescribed to prevent infection if a person has been exposed to plague.

Resources

Organizations

U.S. Centers for Disease Control and Prevention (CDC), 1600 Clifton Road, Atlanta, GA 30333. The CDC is the U.S. government authority for information about infectious and other diseases, including plague.
Telephone 800-311-3435
http://www.cdc.gov

* **culture** (KUL-chur) is a test in which a sample of fluid or tissue from the body is placed in a dish containing material that supports the growth of certain organisms. Typically, within days the organisms will grow and can be identified.

* **biopsy** (BI-op-see) is a test in which a small sample of skin or other body tissue is removed and examined for signs of disease.

* **intravenous** (in-tra-VEE-nus) means within or through a vein. For example, medications, fluid, or other substances can be given through a needle or soft tube inserted through the skin's surface directly into a vein.

U.S. National Library of Medicine, 8600 Rockville Pike, Bethesda, MD 20894. The National Library of Medicine has a website packed with information on diseases (such as plague) and drugs, consumer resources, dictionaries and encyclopedias of medical terms, and directories of doctors and helpful organizations.
Telephone 888-346-3656
http://www.nlm.nih.gov

World Health Organization (WHO), Avenue Appia 20, 1211 Geneva 27, Switzerland. WHO provides information about plague at its website.
Telephone 011-41-22-791-2111
http://www.who.int

Pneumonia

Pneumonia (nu-MO-nyah) is an inflammation of the lungs, usually caused by infection, that can result in breathing difficulty.

What Is Pneumonia?

When a person breathes, air enters the lungs and travels through millions of tiny sacs. These sacs, known as alveoli (al-VEE-o-lye), are where oxygen is transferred to the blood, which carries it to all parts of the body. When someone has pneumonia, the lung tissue becomes inflamed and the alveoli fill with mucus* and other debris, making it difficult for oxygen to be transferred. When normal amounts of oxygen cannot reach the body's cells, many symptoms may develop.

Bacteria or viruses usually cause pneumonia. In some cases, a virus may directly cause the disease. Also, viral infections that lead to respiratory symptoms (such as those of a common cold) often produce inflammation and mucus buildup that makes it easier for bacteria to take hold and infect the lungs. Fungi or parasites are less common causes of pneumonia. Chemicals, drugs, or radiation also can cause lung inflammation. Aspiration (as-puh-RAY-shun) pneumonia occurs when someone accidentally inhales food or vomited material into the lungs.

Pneumonia is a common infection among people who are hospitalized for something else. Such hospital-acquired infections are especially widespread among people recovering from surgery and those who are placed on breathing machines (ventilators). Hospital-acquired pneumonia is almost always bacterial and is often caused by strains* of bacteria that are resistant to many antibiotics. For this reason, and because it affects people who are already sick, hospital-acquired pneumonia is more frequently serious or fatal compared to cases of pneumonia acquired outside the hospital.

► *See also*

Bioterrorism

Pneumonia

Sepsis

Travel-related Infections

Zoonoses

KEYWORDS
for searching the Internet and other reference sources

Atypical pneumonia

Mycoplasma pneumonia

Pneumococcal vaccine

Pneumococcus

Streptococcal pneumonia

Walking pneumonia

* **mucus** (MYOO-kus) is a thick, slippery substance that lines the insides of many body parts.

* **strains** are various subtypes of organisms, such as viruses or bacteria.

What Are Some Different Types of Pneumonia?

Bacterial pneumonia Bacterial pneumonia can attack anyone, from infants to adults, and it is most frequently fatal among the elderly. The most common cause of bacterial pneumonia is *Streptococcus pneumoniae* (strep-tuh-KAH-kus nu-MO-nye), also called pneumococcus (nu-moh-KAH-kus). If the infection is not properly treated with antibiotics, the bacteria can multiply and cause infection not only in the lungs but also in the bloodstream, brain, and other parts of the body. Other bacterial causes include:

- *Mycoplasma pneumoniae* (my-ko-PLAZ-muh nu-MO-nye), which leads to an infection known as "walking pneumonia" because it is often mild enough to go undiagnosed for a long period of time
- *Staphylococcus* (stah-fih-lo-KAH-kus), which usually affects patients in hospitals
- *Chlamydia trachomatis* (kla-MIH-dee-uh truh-KO-mah-tis), often seen in infants; two other species of chlamydia also can cause pneumonia, usually in adults: *Chlamydia pneumoniae* (kla-MIH-dee-uh nu-MO-nye) and *Chlamydia psittaci* (kla-MIH-dee-uh sih-TAH-see)
- Species of the bacteria *Klebsiella* (kleb-zee-EH-luh), *Pseudomonas* (su-doh-MO-nus), and *Legionella pneumophila* (lee-juh-NEL-uh nu-MO-fee-luh, the bacterium that causes Legionnaire's, lee-juh-NAIRS, disease)

Viral pneumonia Viral pneumonia, usually seen in children, makes up nearly half of all pneumonia cases. This type of pneumonia is usually not severe or long lasting. Causes of viral pneumonia include:

- respiratory syncytial (RES-puh-ruh-tor-e sin-SIH-she-ul) virus, or RSV, which typically causes more severe illness in infants and very young children
- adenoviruses (ah-deh-no-VY-ruh-sez), which affect the tissue lining the respiratory tract* and sometimes the eyes, intestines*, and bladder*
- influenza (in-floo-EN-zuh) viruses, which cause flu; pneumonia arising from influenza viruses is an important cause of serious illness among the elderly and people with other health problems
- parainfluenza (pair-uh-in-floo-EN-zuh) viruses, which also cause croup*

Fungal pneumonia Fungal pneumonia usually targets people with weakened immune systems. For instance, pneumonia caused by *Pneumocystis carinii* (nu-mo-SIS-tis kah-RIH-nee-eye), which was recently identified as a fungus, is most common in patients with compromised

* **respiratory tract** includes the nose, mouth, throat, and lungs. It is the pathway through which air and gases are transported down into the lungs and back out of the body.

* **intestines** are the muscular tubes that food passes through during digestion after it exits the stomach.

* **bladder** is a sac-like organ that stores urine before releasing it from the body.

* **croup** (KROOP) is an infection involving the trachea (windpipe) and larynx (voicebox) that typically occurs in childhood. It causes inflammation and narrowing of the upper airway, sometimes making it difficult to breathe. The characteristic symptom is a barking cough.

275

* **AIDS**, or acquired immunodeficiency syndrome (ih-myoo-no-dih-FIH-shen-see), is an infection that severely weakens the immune system; it is caused by the human immunodeficiency virus (HIV).

immune systems, particularly those who have AIDS*. Other fungal infections that can involve the lungs include histoplasmosis (his-toh-plaz-MO-sis), blastomycosis (blas-toh-my-KO-sis), coccidioidomycosis (kok-sih-dee-oyd-o-my-KO-sis), and aspergillosis (as-per-jih-LO-sis).

How Common Is Pneumonia?

Pneumonia was a leading cause of death in the United States in the early decades of the twentieth century. With the help of antibiotics, it dropped to number five by 2000. Although that is certainly an improvement, the disease is still common enough to affect between 3 and 5 million people each year in the United States, with more than 60,000 deaths annually.

Is Pneumonia Contagious?

The bacteria and viruses that cause pneumonia can pass from person to person. When people who are infected sneeze, cough, laugh, or talk, they expel bacteria or viruses into the air in tiny drops of moisture that can be breathed in by others. The germs also can contaminate surfaces that an infected person touches, such as doorknobs, desks, and keyboards. If people do not wash their hands after touching these things, they could become infected by casually touching their eyes, mouth, or nose. An infection contracted this way can lead to pneumonia, although it usually does not.

How Do People Know They Have Pneumonia?

Depending on the cause of the pneumonia and the health of the person with the infection, its symptoms can vary. Symptoms of bacterial pneumonia may appear suddenly and include high fever, chills, rapid breathing, a deep cough that brings up greenish mucus that is sometimes mixed with blood, and severe chest pain that worsens with breathing and coughing. A persistent dry cough, sore throat, and skin rash mark mycoplasma pneumonia (walking pneumonia).

WILLIAM OSLER, 1849–1919

Sir William Osler, often called the father of modern medicine, spent much of his life studying pulmonary diseases (diseases of the lungs) and is known for dubbing pneumonia the "old man's friend." Ironically, Osler himself died of pneumonia after contracting influenza.

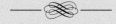

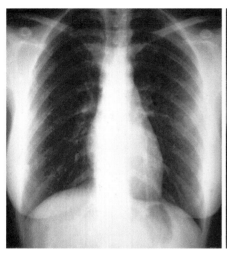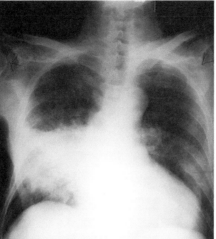

These chest X rays compare clear, healthy lungs with the cloudy, inflamed lung tissue of pneumonia. *Custom Medical Stock Photo, Inc.*

◀

Viral pneumonia can produce symptoms similar to those of the flu, including fever, muscle aches, breathlessness, rapid breathing, and a dry cough, which can worsen and eventually bring up a small amount of mucus.

Other symptoms that may accompany both bacterial and viral pneumonia include loss of appetite, nausea (NAW-zee-uh), vomiting, headache, and excessive sweating. In people with weakened immune systems, pneumonia can quickly become worse.

How Do Doctors Diagnose and Treat Pneumonia?

Diagnosis To identify the infection, the doctor first takes a history of the patient's symptoms and then will listen to a patient's chest with a stethoscope. Fluid in the lungs often produces a crackling sound when a person breathes, which can point to pneumonia. Sometimes the doctor will not be able to hear any air moving through the affected part of the lung. Chest X rays also may be taken, and a cloudy, dense-appearing area may be seen in one or both lungs, particularly in a person who has bacterial pneumonia.

Next, the doctor may take samples of blood and sputum (SPYOO-tum, coughed-up mucus) to try to find out what is causing the pneumonia. These samples can be examined under a microscope and sent to the lab for culture* and identification of the organism causing the infection. In severe cases, a bronchoscopy* or a lung biopsy* may be performed.

Treatment Antibiotics are used to treat bacterial pneumonia. Antiviral or antifungal medicines are prescribed in some cases of viral or fungal illness. In severe cases, patients may need to be hospitalized, particularly if they are in danger of dehydration*, need more oxygen, or cannot breathe well enough on their own.

* **culture** (KUL-chur) is a test in which a sample of fluid or tissue from the body is placed in a dish containing material that supports the growth of certain organisms. Typically, within days the organisms will grow and can be identified.

* **bronchoscopy** (brong-KOS-ko-pee) is a procedure used to examine the bronchi, the major air passages in the lungs, with an instrument called a bronchoscope, which is a tool for looking inside the lungs that is made up of a lighted tube with viewing lenses.

* **biopsy** (BI-op-see) is a test in which a small sample of skin or other body tissue is removed and examined for signs of disease.

* **dehydration** (dee-hi-DRAY-shun) is a condition in which the body is depleted of water, usually caused by excessive and unreplaced loss of body fluids, such as through sweating, vomiting, or diarrhea.

277

People with pneumonia get relief from symptoms and aid their recovery by:

- taking an over-the-counter, non-aspirin pain reliever such as acetaminophen (uh-see-teh-MIH-noh-fen) to ease fever and muscle aches
- resting and drinking liquids to combat dehydration
- using a humidifier to keep air cool and moist, making it easier to breathe
- staying away from cigarette smoke, which irritates the lungs

With treatment, bacterial pneumonia symptoms usually improve within a day or two and are gone in 1 to 2 weeks, but symptoms of viral pneumonia and mycoplasma pneumonia can last longer.

Medical complications   In severe cases, respiratory failure (the inability to breathe adequately) can occur, requiring the person to be hospitalized and placed on a ventilator for breathing assistance. Pus* can collect in the spaces surrounding the lungs and may need to be drained surgically. The lungs also can become scarred, leading to long-term breathing problems. These complications, particularly when they affect elderly people or patients with other health problems, can ultimately lead to death.

How Can Pneumonia Be Prevented?

The pneumococcal (nu-moh-KAH-kal) vaccine* works well against pneumococcal bacteria that cause pneumonia and is recommended for people over age 65 and children under age 2 years, those with certain other illnesses, or those with weakened immune systems. The vaccine typically needs to be given only once in a lifetime. Yearly flu vaccines can help prevent pneumonia caused by influenza viruses. Because pneumonia often is caused by contagious respiratory infections, people can protect themselves further by avoiding being near people who are sick, hand washing, not touching used tissues, and never sharing food, drinks, or eating utensils.

Resources

Organizations

The American Lung Association, 61 Broadway, 6th Floor, New York, NY 10006. The American Lung Association offers information about pneumonia on its website.
Telephone 212-315-8700
http://www.lungusa.org

U.S. Centers for Disease Control and Prevention (CDC), 1600 Clifton Road, Atlanta, GA 30333. The CDC is the U.S. government

* **pus** is a thick, creamy fluid, usually yellow or greenish in color, that forms at the site of an infection. Pus contains infection-fighting white cells and other substances.

* **vaccine** (VAK-seen) is a preparation of killed or weakened germs, or a part of a germ or product it produces, given to prevent or lessen the severity of the disease that can result if a person is exposed to the germ itself. Use of vaccines for this purpose is called immunization.

authority for information about infectious and other diseases. It provides information about pneumonia at its website.
Telephone 800-311-3435
http://www.cdc.gov

Website

KidsHealth.org. KidsHealth is a website created by the medical experts of the Nemours Foundation and is devoted to issues of children's health. It contains articles on a variety of health topics, including pneumonia.
http://www.KidsHealth.org

Polio

Poliomyelitis (po-lee-o-my-uh-LYE-tis) is a condition caused by the polio virus that involves damage of nerve cells. It may lead to weakness and deterioration of the muscles and sometimes paralysis.

What Is Polio?

Poliovirus, part of the enterovirus* group, makes its home in the gastrointestinal* tract, but when the viral infection spreads it can destroy nerve cells known as motor neurons, which make muscles work. The damaged motor neurons cannot rebuild themselves, and as a result the body's muscles no longer function correctly.

Poliovirus infections are broken down into four types: asymptomatic (a-simp-toh-MA-tik), abortive, nonparalytic (non-pair-uh-LIH-tik), and paralytic (pair-uh-LIH-tik). Most cases of polio cause no symptoms (asymptomatic) or only minor symptoms (abortive), such as sore throat, vomiting, or other symptoms resembling those of the flu. Nonparalytic polio has more severe symptoms, including stiff neck due to meningitis and muscle stiffness in the back and legs. Paralytic polio, the rarest but most severe form of the disease, attacks the central nervous system (the part of the nervous sysem that includes the brain and spinal cord) and can cause muscle weakness, spasms, and paralysis.

Types of paralytic polio include spinal, bulbar (BUL-bar), and bulbospinal (bul-boh-SPY-nul). The spinal type is most common, affecting the muscles of the legs, trunk, and neck. The bulbar form involves nerves of the brain stem* and can cause problems with breathing, talking, and swallowing. Bulbospinal polio is a combination of the first two types.

How Common Is Polio?

Polio essentially has been wiped out in the United States and many other developed countries since the introduction of a polio vaccine in 1955.

▶ *See also*
AIDS and HIV Infection
Common Cold
Croup
Influenza
Legionnaire's Disease
Mycoplasma Infections
Streptococcal Infections

KEYWORDS
*for searching the Internet
and other reference sources*

Albert Sabin

Inactivated poliovirus vaccine (IPV)

Jonas Salk

Oral polio vaccine (OPV)

Paralysis

Postpolio syndrome

Vaccine-associated paralytic polio (VAPP)

* **enterovirus** (en-tuh-ro-VY-rus) is a group of viruses that can infect the human gastrointestinal tract and spread through the body causing a number of symptoms.

* **gastrointestinal** (gas-tro-in-TES-tih-nuhl) means having to do with the organs of the digestive system, the system that processes food. It includes the mouth, esophagus, stomach, intestines, colon, and rectum and other organs involved in digestion, including the liver and pancreas.

* **brain stem** is the part of the brain that carries messages back and forth between the higher areas of the brain and the spinal cord.

279

*__epidemic__ (eh-pih-DEH-mik) is an outbreak of disease, especially infectious disease, in which the number of cases suddenly becomes far greater than usual. Usually epidemics are outbreaks of diseases in specific regions, whereas worldwide epidemics are called pandemics.

*__feces__ (FEE-seez) is the excreted waste from the gastrointestinal tract.

Before that, polio occurred in epidemic* form, with more than 21,000 paralytic cases (mostly children) in the United States in 1952 alone. The last cases of naturally occurring polio infection (known as "wild polio") acquired in the United States were reported in 1979. In the following two decades, only 152 cases of polio were reported, most of them vaccine-associated paralytic polio (VAPP), a rare complication that strikes 1 in 2 million to 3 million people who receive the oral (by mouth) polio vaccine (OPV). The last case of VAPP was recorded in 1999, and children now receive a vaccine containing an inactivated form of the virus that cannot cause polio. Although wild polio has not been found in the United States for more than two decades, it is still present in parts of Africa and Asia.

Is Polio Contagious?

Poliovirus is extremely contagious and can pass easily from person to person. The virus typically is found in feces* and can be transmitted when people come into contact with infected matter from bowel movements and unknowingly touch the mouth or nose without washing their hands first. The virus can live in feces for weeks, making the spread of infection difficult to control. It also can spread through contact with tiny drops of fluid from a sick person's mouth or nose or by drinking contaminated water. After entering the mouth or nose, the virus multiplies

ENDING POLIO: A TIMELINE

1955: Jonas Salk's vaccine containing dead, or inactive, poliovirus (IPV) is licensed, and mass numbers of school children are vaccinated, leading to an enormous decrease in the number of polio cases over the next few years and a 60 to 70 percent prevention rate.

1963: Albert Sabin's oral polio vaccine (OPV), containing a live but weakened virus, becomes the new recommended vaccination in the United States. It offers lifelong protection, can be swallowed, and is easy to administer; in very rare cases, however, it actually causes paralytic polio.

1979: The last cases of wild polio are reported in the United States.

2000: IPV becomes the exclusive polio vaccine used in the United States. Experts believe that because polio has virtually disappeared in the United States, the benefits of using OPV are no longer worth the very small risk of contracting the disease from OPV.

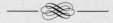

in the throat or gastrointestinal tract and eventually can invade the bloodstream. The infection is most contagious 7 to 10 days before symptoms begin and for the same period after they appear. The virus spreads more readily in areas with poor sanitation.

What Are the Signs and Symptoms?

People with abortive poliomyelitis can experience:

- fever
- headaches
- sore throat
- nausea (NAW-zee-uh) or vomiting

Nonparalytic poliomyelitis symptoms include:

- fever
- headache
- stiffness or pain in the neck, back, or legs
- muscle stiffness or spasms
- nausea and vomiting
- extreme tiredness

Paralytic poliomyelitis is marked by:

- fever
- stiffness or severe pain in the neck, back, or legs
- muscle spasms
- rapidly increasing muscle weakness leading to paralysis
- difficulty in urinating
- constipation
- difficulty in breathing, talking, and swallowing

How Do Doctors Make the Diagnosis?

Polio has been nearly wiped out worldwide. Because polio is no longer found in the United States, a doctor may ask about any recent travel to countries where the disease still occurs. A doctor may suspect polio in an ill patient with paralysis, particularly if the person has not been immunized against polio. During a physical examination, a doctor looks for evidence of muscle paralysis. Samples of blood, bowel movements, fluid from the throat, or cerebrospinal fluid* may be taken and tested for the virus.

What Is the Treatment for Polio?

There is no cure for polio. Easing a patient's symptoms is the best treatment for the disease. Controlling pain and muscle spasms and watching for progression of muscle weakness so supportive care can be given are

* **cerebrospinal** (seh-ree-bro-SPY-nuhl) **fluid** is the fluid that surrounds the brain and spinal cord.

*urinary tract infections, or UTIs, are infections that occur in any part of the urinary tract. The urinary tract is made up of the urethra, bladder, ureters, and kidneys.

*ventilator (VEN-tuh-lay-ter) is a machine used to support or control a person's breathing.

*pneumonia (nu-MO-nyah) is inflammation of the lung.

*kidney stones are hard structures that form in the urinary tract. These structures are composed of crystallized chemicals that have separated from the urine. They can obstruct the flow of urine and cause tissue damage and pain as the body attempts to pass the stones through the urinary tract and out of the body.

the main parts of treatment. Abortive cases and many nonparalytic cases of polio usually are helped by rest, fluids, and pain medication. Moist heat on muscles can ease stiffness. Antibiotics may be prescribed to treat bacterial infections that can occur in patients with polio, such as urinary tract infections*.

Patients with severe cases of polio, particularly the paralytic form, often require hospitalization. In the 1940s and 1950s, patients were placed inside metal tanks called "iron lungs" that assisted their breathing. Although medical technology has progressed since then, many people who have polio still need machines called ventilators* to assist breathing as they recover, as well as additional supportive care. Patients with paralytic polio may need physical therapy, crutches, leg braces, or surgery to help them regain their strength and movement.

What to Expect

If the disease does not damage the spinal cord and brain, patients typically make a full recovery. Symptoms in cases of abortive polio generally last less than a week, whereas in nonparalytic cases symptoms can last 1 to 2 weeks. If the polio infection causes paralysis, it can take months for muscles to begin to regain their strength and mobility. Paralysis that lingers after 12 months usually is considered permanent. Complications include:

- permanent paralysis, usually in the legs but sometimes in other muscles as well
- breathing problems due to muscle paralysis or damage to areas of the brain that control breathing
- pneumonia* due to swallowing difficulties
- fluid in the lungs
- urinary tract infections
- kidney stones*
- high blood pressure
- postpolio syndrome, which affects 25 to 50 percent of people previously infected and develops 15 to 40 years after the initial infection, causing symptoms of muscle pain, new or increased weakness, and paralysis

How Can Polio Be Prevented?

The polio vaccine is the best way to prevent the disease; its use has eliminated polio from the Western Hemisphere. Jonas Salk developed the first vaccine in 1955. It is known as inactivated poliovirus vaccine (IPV), because the poliovirus used to make the vaccine was "killed," or inactivated. Several years later, Albert Sabin developed an oral polio vaccine, which was given in the form of drops that could be swallowed. These drops contained a live, but weakened, virus.

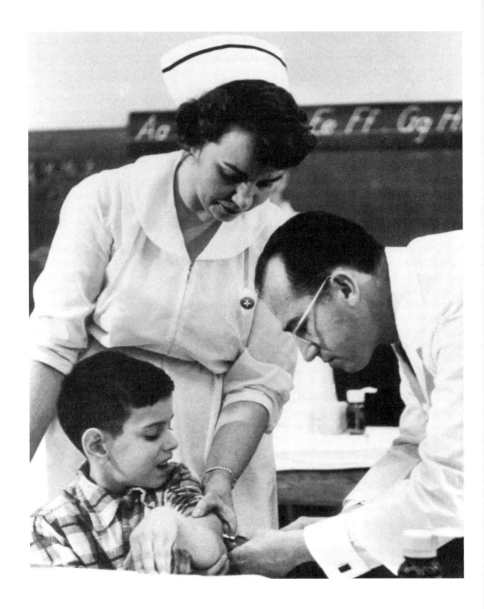

Dr. Jonas Salk started researching polio in 1949. In 1955, he announced the success of his polio vaccine, and mass immunization began. *AP/Wide World Photos*

OPV was very successful in helping rid the United States of polio. Its advantage over IPV was that once children had been immunized, they could pass the weakened virus to others who had not received the vaccine in the same way that the infectious poliovirus spread between people. This contact with the virus gave unvaccinated children immunity as if they had been vaccinated. In rare cases, however, because it contained a live virus OPV actually caused paralytic polio in the children who received the vaccine or in people who had close contact with them and had not been immunized. This is known as vaccine-associated paralytic polio. People with weakened immune systems were most at risk for VAPP.

IPV is now the only polio vaccine used in the United States, and it does not cause VAPP. Children might have a sore spot where they receive the shot, but there are rarely any side effects from the vaccine. Children receive IPV routinely as part of the childhood immunization schedule. Most adults who were vaccinated as children do not need to receive the vaccine again. People traveling to places where polio is still found (such as Africa and Asia), lab workers who handle poliovirus, and medical professionals who care for patients with polio may need to be vaccinated again. If polio is wiped out worldwide, immunization against polio may not be needed in the future.

Resources

Organization

U.S. Centers for Disease Control and Prevention (CDC), 1600 Clifton Road, Atlanta, GA 30333. Through the website of the National Immunization Program, the CDC provides information about polio and immunization schedules and vaccines.
Telephone 800-311-3435
http://www.cdc.gov/nip/

Websites

KidsHealth.org. KidsHealth is a website created by the medical experts of the Nemours Foundation and is devoted to issues of children's health. It contains articles on a variety of health topics, including polio.
http://www.KidsHealth.org

The Public Broadcasting System traces the history of polio in the United States through its companion website to the video *A Paralyzing Fear: The Story of Polio in America.*
http://www.pbs.org/storyofpolio/polio/index.html

The World Health Organization's Global Polio Eradication Initiative website offers facts, news, and immunization information about the disease.
http://www.polioeradication.org

▶ *See also*
Meningitis
Vaccination (Immunization)

Pregnancy-related and Newborn Infections
See **Congenital Infections**

R

Rabies

Rabies (RAY-beez) is a viral infection of the central nervous system that usually is transmitted to humans by the bite of an infected animal.

What Is Rabies?

Because of its devastating effects, rabies has been one of the most feared diseases in the world since it was first described in ancient times. A member of the *Rhabdoviridae* family of viruses causes rabies. In the United States, the virus lives primarily in wild bats, raccoons, skunks, and foxes; it sometimes is found in other animals as well, such as wolves, coyotes, or ferrets. Small animals such as hamsters, squirrels, mice, and rabbits typically do not carry the virus. More than 90 percent of reported rabies cases in animals occur in wild animals. The most common domestic animals that become infected, or "rabid," are cats, dogs, and cattle. Throughout the world most cases of human exposure to rabies are to rabid dogs, but in the United States cases related to dog bites are rare. Indeed, most cases are linked to bats.

When a rabid animal bites a person, the rabies virus, which lives in the animal's saliva, is transmitted through the body, where it can attack the central nervous system (the part of the nervous system that includes the brain and spinal cord), leading to encephalitis* and death. After symptoms begin, the disease can progress very quickly and can be fatal within a few days.

How Common Is Rabies?

Almost all reported cases of rabies in the United States occur in animals. In the year 2000, 7,369 cases of rabies in animals were reported to the U.S. Centers for Disease Control and Prevention; 509 of those infections were in domestic animals (pets and farm animals). Only five people were infected with rabies that year, and all of them died. On average, only one or two deaths from rabies are seen in humans each year in the United States.

Is Rabies Contagious?

Rabies has not been found to be contagious from person to person. In theory, if a person infected with rabies were to bite someone else, the virus might spread, but no such cases have been recorded. Animal bites

KEYWORDS
for searching the Internet
and other reference sources

Central nervous system infection

Encephalitis

Rhabdoviridae

Vaccination

Zoonotic diseases/Zoonoses

* encephalitis (en-seh-fuh-LYE-tis) is an inflammation of the brain, usually caused by a viral infection.

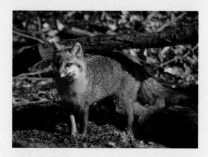

Wild foxes, along with bats, raccoons, and skunks, are among the primary carriers of rabies in the United States. *Custom Medical Stock Photo, Inc.*

* **mucous membranes** are the moist linings of the mouth, nose, eyes, and throat.

* **paralysis** (pah-RAH-luh-sis) is the loss or impairment of the ability to move some part of the body.

* **seizures** (SEE-zhurs) are sudden bursts of disorganized electrical activity that interrupt the normal functioning of the brain, often leading to uncontrolled movements in the body and sometimes a temporary change in consciousness.

* **double vision** is a vision problem in which a person sees two images of a single object.

* **coma** (KO-ma) is an unconscious state in which a person cannot be awakened and cannot move, see, speak, or hear.

* **delirium** (dih-LEER-e-um) is a condition in which a person is confused, is unable to think clearly, and has a reduced level of consciousness.

are the most common cause of rabies in people. Rarely, the virus may spread when saliva or tissue from an infected animal enters an open wound or mucous membrane*, such as when an infected animal licks a person's broken skin. In rare instances, exposure to bats, with no known bite or scratch, causes human rabies.

What Are the Signs and Symptoms of Rabies?

Once a person has been infected with the rabies virus, symptoms may appear as soon as 10 days or as long as 90 days after exposure. These symptoms typically happen in stages. The first stage may include fever, a general ill feeling, sore throat, loss of appetite, nausea (NAW-zee-uh), vomiting, depression, and headache. If the person has been bitten by an animal, there may be a tingling sensation around the area of the bite. As the disease progresses and attacks the nervous system, a person may have difficulty sleeping and experience anxiety, confusion, aggressiveness, or hallucinations (ha-loo-sin-AY-shuns, seeing or hearing things that are not really there).

Other symptoms of rabies infection include partial paralysis*, seizures* or muscle spasms, inability to speak, sensitivity to light or sound, and hydrophobia (hi-druh-FOE-bee-uh), or avoiding drinking water or other liquids due to trouble swallowing. In the final stages, the person may experience double vision* or find it difficult to swallow saliva (which can make someone appear to be "foaming at the mouth"). The disease can progress to coma* and death.

THE STRANGE FACTS IN THE CASE OF EDGAR ALLAN POE

Edgar Allan Poe, whose name is synonymous with horror and mystery, died as perplexing and shocking a death as any that he concocted in the many suspenseful and macabre tales that he wrote. Poe set out on a trip from Richmond, Virginia, to Philadelphia at the end of September 1849. The next anyone heard of him—about a week after his departure—he had collapsed outside a tavern in Baltimore and was found quivering and raving. Four days later, on October 7, he died in a nearby hospital. For many years it was thought that his symptoms of delirium*, cold sweat, confusion, memory loss, and difficulty in swallowing could be attributed to severe alcoholism. In 1996, however, R. Michael Benitez, a doctor at the University of Maryland Medical Center, concluded in a review of the historical record that Poe, in fact, might have died of rabies.

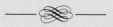

Making the Diagnosis

People who may have been exposed to rabies need immediate medical attention. If a person has symptoms of the disease, a doctor will perform a physical examination and ask questions to figure out whether the person might have been exposed to a rabid animal. To diagnose rabies in a human, doctors can perform several laboratory tests, including examination of blood and spinal fluid for antibodies* to the rabies virus. Skin biopsies* and saliva tests also may be done to search for signs of the infection. One of the best diagnostic tests is done on brain tissue from the potentially infected animal. The results can tell doctors whether the animal was rabid. Animals with less risk of being infected (such as a pet dog) can be isolated and observed by the local health department to see whether any signs of rabies develop.

How Do Doctors Treat Rabies?

It is recommended that someone who might have been exposed to rabies wash the site thoroughly with warm, soapy water. A person who has been bitten by or who has come into direct contact with an animal that may be rabid can receive immediate treatment by a doctor to prevent the disease from developing. This is called postexposure prophylaxis*. The person receives one dose of rabies immune globulin*, which provides the body with antibodies against rabies, followed by five doses of rabies vaccine* given over a period of 28 days. This treatment has proved to be very effective in preventing the development of rabies when it is started within a day of exposure. Once a person has symptoms of rabies, treatment typically is limited to life support in the hospital. Approximately 40,000 people in the United States and an estimated 10 million people throughout the world are treated as a precaution each year after having been exposed to animals suspected of being rabid.

How Long Does the Disease Last and What Are the Complications?

Once symptoms have appeared the disease can progress very quickly to coma and death, generally within 1 to 3 weeks. Rabies infection that is not treated immediately almost always causes death. In rare cases where people have survived, they often have severe and permanent brain damage.

Can Rabies Be Prevented?

Vaccinating household pets against rabies is very important in preventing the spread of the disease. This method has dramatically limited the number of rabies cases seen in domestic animals in the United States. People who are at greatest risk of exposure, such as veterinarians, travelers to areas of the world where rabid animals are common,

* **antibodies** (AN-tih-bah-deez) are protein molecules produced by the body's immune system to help fight specific infections caused by microorganisms, such as bacteria and viruses.

* **biopsies** (BI-op-seez) are tests in which small samples of skin or other body tissue are removed and examined for signs of disease.

* **prophylaxis** (pro-fih-LAK-sis) means taking specific measures, such as using medication or a device (such as a condom), to help prevent infection, illness, or pregnancy.

* **immune globulin** (ih-MYOON GLAH-byoo-lin), also called gamma globulin, is the protein material that contains antibodies.

* **vaccine** (vak-SEEN) is a preparation of killed or weakened germs, or a part of a germ or product it produces, given to prevent or lessen the severity of the disease that can result if a person is exposed to the germ itself. Use of vaccines for this purpose is called immunization.

LOUIS PASTEUR'S VACCINE BREAKTHROUGH

In 1885, Louis Pasteur (1822–1895), a French scientist known for his remarkable contributions to modern medicine, developed a vaccine that can prevent rabies in humans who have been exposed to the virus. This breakthrough led to the creation of the Pasteur Institute, a medical research organization dedicated to the understanding and prevention of infectious diseases, where Pasteur continued his important work for the last years of his life.

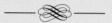

and laboratory workers who handle material that may contain the rabies virus, often are immunized (vaccinated) against the disease. Taking these safety measures also can help prevent rabies:

- avoiding contact with unfamiliar or wild animals, especially bats and raccoons
- never feeding or handling a wild or unknown animal
- keeping trash that is stored outside carefully sealed, to avoid attracting raccoons and other animals
- consulting a doctor for advice about receiving the rabies vaccine before traveling to an area where rabies is more common, such as Asia or Africa

Resources

Organization

U.S. Centers for Disease Control and Prevention (CDC), 1600 Clifton Road, Atlanta, GA 30333. The CDC tracks outbreaks of rabies in the United States and publishes information about the disease at its website.
Telephone 800-311-3435
http://www.cdc.gov

Website

KidsHealth.org. KidsHealth is a website created by the medical experts of the Nemours Foundation and is devoted to issues of children's health. It contains articles on a variety of health topics, including rabies.
http://www.KidsHealth.org

▶ See also

Encephalitis

Vaccination (Immunization)

Zoonoses

Rickettsial Infections

Rickettsial (rih-KET-see-ul) infections are a collection of diseases caused by bacteria from the Rickettsiaceae *family.*

What Are They?

The diseases caused by rickettsial infections are alike in many ways. Rocky Mountain spotted fever, typhus (TY-fis), ehrlichiosis (air-lik-e-O-sis), and Q fever all have similar symptoms, including headache, high fever, and sometimes a rash. These infections also respond to the same type of treatment, and many of them spread in the same way: through the bites of blood-sucking arthropods*, such as lice, fleas, and ticks.

How Common Are Rickettsial Infections?

These infections do not occur frequently in the United States (although typhus is relatively common in other parts of the world, especially the tropics). Rocky Mountain spotted fever is the most common rickettsial infection in the United States: up to 1,200 cases are reported yearly. Fewer than 100 typhus cases are reported annually, and a total of about 1,200 cases of ehrlichiosis have been reported during an 11-year period.

Are They Contagious?

Rickettsial infections do not spread directly from person to person. Instead, most require blood-sucking arthropods, such as lice, ticks, and fleas, to carry the organisms between animals and people or from one person to another. When a flea, for example, bites an infected animal or person, it can ingest the infectious bacteria. If the flea then bites someone else, it can spread the disease to that person. In the case of Rocky Mountain spotted fever, however, the bacterium lives and reproduces within ticks. Once a tick acquires the bacterium (from its mother when it is still an egg or through mating or feeding on an infected animal) it can infect people for the rest of its life. Q fever mainly spreads from livestock animals to people. The bacteria can pass into the animals' bowel movements, milk, urine, or fluids that accompany giving birth. People become infected by breathing in the bacteria in airborne bits of dust contaminated with one of those substances.

Specific Infections

Rocky Mountain spotted fever Rocky Mountain spotted fever first was recognized in the Rocky Mountain states (such as Idaho, Montana, and Colorado) but since then it has been found throughout the United States. It is caused by the *Rickettsia rickettsii* bacterium, which is transmitted by tick bites. The disease is most common in children, usually in tick-infested areas, where outdoor work and play create the most risk.

KEYWORDS
for searching the Internet and other reference sources

Brill-Zinsser disease

Ehrlichiosis

Murine typhus

Q fever

Rickettsiaceae

Rocky Mountain spotted fever

Typhus

* **arthropods** are members of a group of organisms that lack a spinal column and have a segmented body and jointed limbs. This group includes various insects, ticks, spiders, lice, and fleas.

*epidemic (eh-pih-DEH-mik) is an outbreak of disease, especially infectious disease, in which the number of cases suddenly becomes far greater than usual. Usually epidemics are outbreaks of diseases in specific regions, whereas worldwide epidemics are called pandemics.

Symptoms of infection include a severe headache, muscle pain, chills, fever, confusion, and a rash that appears first on the wrists and ankles before spreading. About 5 percent of Rocky Mountain spotted fever cases are fatal, usually because a person does not receive treatment quickly.

Typhus Typhus can appear in several forms, including epidemic* typhus, murine typhus, and Brill-Zinsser disease. The bacteria that cause typhus, *Rickettsia prowazekii* and *Rickettsia typhi*, spread to people through the bites of fleas or lice. People who are infected can become very sick and often have a fever that may climb as high as 105 to 107 degrees Fahrenheit. Murine typhus is the variety seen most often in the United States, usually in the southern and southeastern states. People who come into contact with fleas that feed on rats, opossums, and outdoor cats are at the greatest risk for the disease. Once someone becomes infected, that person may experience a headache, a rash, nausea (NAW-zee-uh), joint pain, belly pain, vomiting, and a dry cough. The disease is rarely fatal. Most people recover with few complications.

*stupor is a state of sluggishness or impaired consciousness.

*delirium (dih-LEER-e-um) is a condition in which a person is confused, is unable to think clearly, and has a reduced level of consciousness.

Murine typhus is a milder form of epidemic typhus, which is associated with a drop in blood pressure and stupor* or delirium*, and it can be fatal. Epidemic typhus is spread from person to person by body lice. Brill-Zinsser disease is a recurrence of epidemic typhus that appears in someone who was infected before that person's immune system was weakened by stress or illness. When the body's defenses are down, organisms left over from the earlier bout of illness may reactivate. The disease causes mild symptoms and is not fatal.

HISTORICAL IMPORTANCE OF TYPHUS

Epidemic typhus has a long history of causing death in times of war. Poor sanitation and the presence of lice and rats in crowded living quarters have contributed to high rates of illness and death among soldiers: During the Napoleonic War, the French defeat in Russia in 1812 was attributed to typhus. Conditions were no better by World War I: Thousands of soldiers had fallen victim to typhus by the war's end. It was not until the time of World War II that the disease could be controlled with vaccinations*, antibiotics, and more sanitary conditions. Typhus also has been referred to as "jail fever," because epidemics would periodically sweep through prisons, where filthy conditions made a home for rats and lice.

*vaccinations (vak-sih-NAY-shunz), also called immunizations, are the giving of doses of vaccines, which are preparations of killed or weakened germs, or a part of a germ or product it produces, to prevent or lessen the severity of a disease.

Q fever Q fever is caused by the bacterium *Coxiella burnetii*, which lives primarily in farm animals, such as sheep, goats, and cattle. People who contract the infection may have no symptoms at all or may experience symptoms similar to those of the flu, such as fever, muscle and joint aches, severe headache, and dry cough. Nausea, vomiting, diarrhea (dye-uh-REE-uh), chest and belly pain, and jaundice* also can accompany Q fever. People who work with animals, such as veterinarians, farmers, and slaughterhouse workers, are most at risk for the disease, which is contracted by breathing in the bacteria from the animals' bowel movements, milk, urine, or fluids from giving birth.

Ehrlichiosis Ehrlichiosis is caused by infection with the species of *Ehrlichia* (air-LIH-kee-uh) bacteria *E. chaffeensis* and *E. phagocytophila*. Tick bites spread the bacteria to people, where the infection produces symptoms similar to those of Rocky Mountain spotted fever. Severe cases can damage many organ systems and lead to seizures*, coma*, and death.

How Do Doctors Make the Diagnosis?

Rickettsial infections are diagnosed by finding antibodies* to the organism in the blood. These antibodies usually are not present early in the illness, so a doctor relies on the patient's history of symptoms, a physical examination, and information about where the person lives or became sick to make the diagnosis. To avoid potentially serious complications, it is important not to delay treatment of rickettsial infections while waiting for test results. In some cases, a skin biopsy* of the rash can aid in making the diagnosis.

What Is the Treatment for Rickettsial Infections?

All of these diseases are treated with antibiotics. Patients begin taking the medication as soon as possible, because a delay in treatment may increase the risk of complications. In more serious cases, often those in which the diagnosis has been delayed, it may be necessary to hospitalize patients and treat them with intravenous* (IV) antibiotics and fluids.

How Long Does a Rickettsial Infection Last?

The infections typically last from 1 week to several weeks. If they go untreated or if treatment does not begin soon after infection, the disease can linger for months.

What Are the Complications?

Untreated and severe cases of any of these diseases can be fatal. In addition, each rickettsial illness has its unique complications:

- Rocky Mountain spotted fever can cause paralysis*, hearing loss, and nerve damage.

* **jaundice** (JON-dis) is a yellowing of the skin, and sometimes the whites of the eyes, caused by a buildup in the body of bilirubin, a chemical produced in and released by the liver. An increase in bilirubin may indicate disease of the liver or certain blood disorders.

* **seizures** (SEE-zhurs) are sudden bursts of disorganized electrical activity that interrupt the normal functioning of the brain, often leading to uncontrolled movements in the body and sometimes a temporary change in consciousness.

* **coma** (KO-ma) is an unconscious state in which a person cannot be awakened and cannot move, see, speak, or hear.

* **antibodies** (AN-tih-bah-deez) are protein molecules produced by the body's immune system to help fight specific infections caused by microorganisms, such as bacteria and viruses.

* **biopsy** (BI-op-see) is a test in which a small sample of skin or other body tissue is removed and examined for signs of disease.

* **intravenous** (in-tra-VEE-nus) means within or through a vein. For example, medications, fluid, or other substances can be given through a needle or soft tube inserted through the skin's surface directly into a vein.

* **paralysis** (pah-RAH-luh-sis) is the loss or impairment of the ability to move some part of the body.

291

▶ *See also*

Ehrlichiosis

Endocarditis, Infectious

Hepatitis, Infectious

Rocky Mountain Spotted Fever

Tick-borne Infections

Zoonoses

- Typhus can lead to pneumonia*, kidney* problems, and problems with the central nervous system*.

- Chronic* Q fever in the elderly can cause endocarditis* and hepatitis*.

- Ehrlichiosis can damage various organs, including the lungs, kidneys, and brain.

How Are Rickettsial Infections Prevented?

People can take steps to protect themselves from infection by avoiding flea, tick, and louse bites. It is recommended that anyone who works or plays outdoors be particularly careful. Avoiding areas that are infested with lice, ticks, and fleas or using insecticides and repellents in those areas can help. Wearing long pants and long-sleeved shirts, especially in spots with thick bushes or tall grass, also can guard against bites. After spending time outside in areas where ticks are found, people should examine their bodies carefully, including the hair, to make sure that there are no ticks. It is wise to check pets regularly for ticks, too, because animals can carry parasites into the house.

Q fever is best prevented by regularly testing animals for infection and isolating those that are infected. Doctors recommend that people who work with animals wash hands and launder clothes carefully to lower their risk of infection.

Resources

Organization

U.S. Centers for Disease Control and Prevention (CDC), 1600 Clifton Road, Atlanta, GA 30333. Through the website of the National Center for Infectious Diseases, the CDC provides fact sheets and other information on rickettsial infections.
Telephone 800-311-3435
http://www.cdc.gov/ncidod/

Website

KidsHealth.org. KidsHealth is a website created by the medical experts of the Nemours Foundation and is devoted to issues of children's health. It contains articles on a variety of health topics, including Rocky Mountain spotted fever.
http://www.KidsHealth.org

Ringworm

Ringworm, or tinea (TIH-nee-uh), is a fungal infection of the skin, scalp, or nails. It usually causes red, dry, flaky skin.

What Is Ringworm?

Despite its name, ringworm is not caused by a worm but by mold-like fungi known as dermatophytes (dur-MAH-toh-fites) that thrive in the top layer of the skin, in the scalp, and in nails. Several different but related types of fungi, including those in the *Trichophyton* and *Microsporum* species, cause ringworm infection on different parts of the body. All of these infections are known as tinea infections.

Fungal infections take their names from the part of the body where they occur, so tinea corporis is ringworm on the body; tinea unguium is ringworm of the nails; tinea capitis is ringworm of the scalp; tinea cruris is ringworm of the groin (commonly called jock itch); and tinea pedis is ringworm of the feet (also known as athlete's foot). The same fungi that infect humans can infect cats and dogs as well, and people can contract the disease from both people and pets.

Damaged skin is more vulnerable to infection, as is skin in warm, moist areas. When the fungus takes hold, it typically causes a ring-like rash of red, flaking skin. The border of the rash may be raised, as if a worm were under the skin. The rash's shape and this raised edge led people to call the infection ringworm. When the nails are infected, they usually become yellow, thickened, and brittle.

Is Ringworm Common?

Ringworm is widespread in many countries, including the United States. Tinea corporis and tinea capitis infections most often occur in children, although they are found in people of all ages. The other types of ringworm, especially jock itch and athlete's foot, are more common in adolescents and adults.

How Do People Contract Ringworm?

Ringworm is contagious and spreads through direct contact with an infected person or pet. People also can contract the fungus from soil or from surfaces and things that an infected person has touched, such as toys, a pillow, or the locker room floor. Once someone is infected, that person is contagious until the telltale rash starts to shrink. The fading of the ring indicates that the fungus is no longer present.

How Do People Know They Have Ringworm?

As anyone who has had the infection knows, the symptoms of ringworm are annoying rather than serious. The most common signs are itching

KEYWORDS
*for searching the Internet
and other reference sources*

Athlete's foot

Dermatophyte

Jock itch

Microsporum

Tinea

Trichophyton

Latin Lesson

Capitis (KAH-pih-tis): from the Latin word for head

Corporis (KOR-poor-us): the Latin word for body

Cruris (KRU-ris): from the Latin word for leg

Pedis (PEE-dis): the Latin word for foot

Unguium (UN-gwee-um): from the Latin word for nail

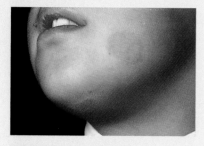

▲

This child has the red, ring-shaped rash characteristic of ringworm. Ringworm is caused by mold-like fungi, not by a worm as the name would suggest. *Custom Medical Stock Photo, Inc.*

* **pus** is a thick, creamy fluid, usually yellow or greenish in color, that forms at the site of an infection. Pus contains infection-fighting white cells and other substances.

* **cultured** (KUL-churd) means subjected to a test in which a sample of fluid or tissue from the body is placed in a dish containing material that supports the growth of certain organisms. Typically, within days the organisms will grow and can be identified.

* **ultraviolet** light is a wavelength of light beyond visible light; on the spectrum of light, it falls between the violet end of visible light and X rays.

around the infected area, dry skin, and a red, ring-shaped rash. Over time the borders of the rash spread outward and the center clears, leaving a circle of red around normal skin. Sometimes the central patch in the rash is filled with pus*, and the borders may be dry and scaly or moist and crusty.

Ringworm on the scalp can cause a temporary bald patch or areas of scaly, flaky skin, occasionally with a red, swollen spot. Infected nails become yellow, thickened, and brittle, and athlete's foot often appears as red, cracked, peeling skin between the toes.

How Do Doctors Diagnose Ringworm?

In many infected patients, doctors can identify tinea just by looking at the skin, scalp, or nails. To confirm the diagnosis, the doctor may take a scraping of the suspect area to be examined under a microscope for signs of the fungus. The scraping also can be cultured* to see if any fungi grow from it. Because some types of fungi glow under ultraviolet* (UV) light, the doctor may shine a UV lamp on the rash to see if any part of it lights up. This can help identify the fungus causing the infection.

How Is Ringworm Treated?

Doctors prescribe antifungal cream, ointment, or shampoo for most cases of infection. More advanced cases also may require oral (by mouth) medicine, including all cases of tinea capitis and tinea unguium.

Patients typically need to use the cream, ointment, or shampoo for at least 2 weeks. However, some patients may need to use medicine for several weeks or months, depending on the extent and location of the infection. Beyond that, it may take even more time for skin to heal completely or for healthy nails and hair to grow back.

Ringworm may be irritating, but it causes almost no complications. Without treatment, the infection can linger for many months, and infected nails may fall off. Sometimes areas that have been attacked by the fungus develop infection from bacteria because the damaged skin is more vulnerable.

Can Ringworm Be Prevented?

The best way to prevent ringworm is to practice good hygiene, like bathing and changing underclothes every day. Keeping the skin clean and dry will discourage the fungus from taking hold. Not sharing personal items such as brushes, towels, and clothing (especially gym shoes) will limit the spread of ringworm between people. In addition, washing an infected person's clothing and bedding frequently can help keep the infection from spreading to others. If a household pet develops ringworm, doctors advise the family to talk to a veterinarian and avoid direct contact with the animal, like cuddling and patting, until the rash heals.

Athlete's foot can flourish when the skin on the feet, especially between the toes, stays moist. Removing shoes and socks to allow moisture from sweat to dry, carefully drying feet after showering, and changing socks daily can help ward off the fungus. Wearing slip-on sandals instead of going barefoot in public places such as locker rooms and gym showers can reduce the risk of picking up tinea from surfaces an infected person has touched.

Resources

Organization

U.S. National Library of Medicine, 8600 Rockville Pike, Bethesda, MD 20894. The National Library of Medicine has a website packed with information on diseases such as ringworm, consumer resources, dictionaries and encyclopedias of medical terms, and directories of doctors and helpful organizations.
Telephone 888-346-3656
http://www.nlm.nih.gov

Website

KidsHealth.org. KidsHealth is a website created by the medical experts of the Nemours Foundation and is devoted to issues of children's health. It contains articles on a variety of health topics, including ringworm.
http://www.KidsHealth.org

▶ *See also*
Fungal Infections
Skin and Soft Tissue Infections

Rocky Mountain Spotted Fever

Rocky Mountain spotted fever is an infection transmitted by the bite of a tick*. At first its symptoms are mild, but without treatment the disease can become serious and cause organ damage and death.

What Is Rocky Mountain Spotted Fever?

Rocky Mountain spotted fever (RMSF) is the most serious of the rickettsial (rih-KET-see-ul) infections, diseases caused by bacteria from the Rickettsiaceae family. These bacteria typically spread to people through blood-sucking parasites* such as ticks and fleas. In Rocky Mountain spotted fever, the bacterium *Rickettsia rickettsii* lives and reproduces in the Ixodidae (ik-SAH-dih-day) family of hard-bodied ticks, such as the American dog tick and the Rocky Mountain wood tick, before it infects people. Once it does infect a person, it enters cells lining the blood vessels and can cause serious disease.

Several of the disease's first symptoms can be confused with those of other infections. As the condition grows worse, it often causes a

KEYWORDS
for searching the Internet and other reference sources

Ixodidae ticks

Rickettsia rickettsii

Rickettsial infections

Zoonoses

* **tick** is a small blood-sucking creature that may transmit disease-causing germs from animals to humans through its bite.

* **parasites** (PAIR-uh-sites) are organisms such as protozoa (one-celled animals), worms, or insects that must live on or inside a human or other organism to survive.

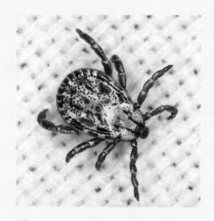

▲

The Rocky Mountain wood tick, *Dermacentor andersoni*, is one of the species of hard-bodied ticks responsible for spreading the bacterium that causes Rocky Mountain spotted fever. Once infected, a tick can carry the bacterium for life. ©*S.J. Krasemann/Peter Arnold, Inc.*

* **abdominal** (ab-DAH-mih-nul) refers to the area of the body below the ribs and above the hips that contains the stomach, intestines, and other organs.

* **hallucinations** (ha-loo-sin-AY-shuns) occur when a person sees or hears things that are not really there. Hallucinations can result from nervous system abnormalities, mental disorders, or the use of certain drugs.

* **antibodies** (AN-tih-bah-deez) are protein molecules produced by the body's immune system to help fight specific infections caused by microorganisms, such as bacteria and viruses.

widespread rash, which led people to call RMSF "black measles" when it was described in the late nineteenth century. If the infection is not treated, it can damage several organ systems and sometimes lead to death.

How Common Is It?

Despite its name, the infection is not limited to the Rocky Mountains. It is found throughout the United States, and most cases actually occur in the southeastern part of the country. The disease also has been found in southern Canada, Mexico, some countries in Central America, and parts of South America. According to the U.S. Centers for Disease Control and Prevention, between 250 and 1,200 cases are reported in the United States each year, with most in children under the age of 15. About 5 percent of Rocky Mountain spotted fever cases are fatal, usually because a person does not receive treatment quickly.

Is It Contagious?

RMSF is not contagious from person to person. It can spread only from a tick to a person, usually through the tick's bite when it feeds. Rarely, people can become infected when they come into contact with tick droppings or dead ticks that have been crushed. The bacterium lives in the tick and survives from one generation of the parasite to the next. Female ticks can pass it to their eggs, and male ticks can pass it to females when they mate.

What Are the Infection's Signs and Symptoms?

Symptoms of infection include severe headache, fever, confusion, chills, nausea (NAW-zee-uh), vomiting, loss of appetite, and muscle pain. Many infections have these symptoms, so they may not be immediately identified as RMSF. As the disease worsens, it may cause joint pain, abdominal* pain, extreme thirst, hallucinations*, diarrhea (dye-uh-REE-uh), and a rash. The rash usually appears 3 to 6 days after the start of symptoms. It typically starts as small, pink spots that crop up on the wrists, lower part of the arms, and ankles. The rash does not itch, and over time the spots become raised. In many patients, a red, spotted rash develops that looks like dots of blood under the skin, often on the palms of the hands and the soles of the feet. Even though this rash is one of the most distinctive symptoms, it is not seen in every patient. As many as 10 percent to 20 percent of patients do not have the typical rash.

How Do Doctors Diagnose Rocky Mountain Spotted Fever?

Doctors usually identify the infection based on symptoms seen during an examination, reports of the disease in the area, and knowledge of a recent tick bite. Fever, rash, and history of a tick bite are considered the classic features of RMSF. The doctor also may take a blood sample to look for antibodies* to the bacteria.

What Is the Treatment?

People with RMSF often need to be in the hospital, where they can receive supportive care. The disease is treated with antibiotics, which are given as soon as a doctor suspects that a patient might have RMSF. Waiting until laboratory tests confirm the diagnosis could put the patient at greater risk, because the infection can progress so quickly. Patients continue taking the medicine for at least 3 days after the fever goes away.

What Medical Complications Can Occur?

Treatment typically takes 5 to 10 days, but it can last much longer. Without treatment or with delayed treatment, severe cases of illness can lead to death. In addition, the disease can cause problems with the central nervous system*, the kidneys, the digestive system*, and the respiratory tract*. This can lead to partial paralysis*, hearing loss, meningitis*, heart failure, brain damage, kidney failure, and shock*.

How Can Rocky Mountain Spotted Fever Be Prevented?

It is important to take precautions to limit the risk of tick bites: for example, by avoiding walks through brush and dense vegetation in areas with lots of ticks. When a person spends time outside, it is a good idea to wear long pants, long sleeves, and socks, with the pants tucked into the socks. Light-colored clothing makes ticks easier to see, and insect repellent can protect exposed skin. After being outside in tick-infested areas, it is wise to remove clothing and check the body, including the hair, thoroughly for the parasites. Doctors recommend that any ticks that are found be removed right away; the longer the tick stays attached, the greater the chance that the RMSF bacterium can enter the body.

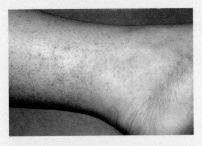

The rash associated with Rocky Mountain spotted fever usually starts as small pink spots, which, over time, become raised. ©*Ken E. Greer*

* **central nervous** (SEN-trul NER-vus) **system** is the part of the nervous system that includes the brain and spinal cord.

* **digestive system** is the system that processes food. It includes the mouth, esophagus, stomach, intestines, colon, and rectum and other organs involved in digestion, including the liver and pancreas.

* **respiratory tract** includes the nose, mouth, throat, and lungs. It is the pathway through which air and gases are transported down into the lungs and back out of the body.

* **paralysis** (pah-RAH-luh-sis) is the loss or impairment of the ability to move some part of the body.

* **meningitis** (meh-nin-JY-tis) is an inflammation of the meninges, the membranes that surround the brain, and the spinal cord. Meningitis is most often caused by infection with a virus or a bacterium.

* **shock** is a serious condition in which blood pressure is very low and not enough blood flows to the body's organs and tissues. Untreated, shock may result in death.

DR. RICKETTS

Even if you have heard about Rocky Mountain spotted fever, you may not know the name Howard T. Ricketts. Dr. Ricketts discovered the bacterium behind the disease and figured out that it spreads to people through tick bites. In recognition of that work, *Rickettsia rickettsii*, the RMSF bacterium, received its double Ricketts name. Dr. Ricketts also did research on typhus (TY-fis), another rickettsial infection. He died of typhus in 1910.

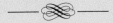

Resources

Organization

U.S. Centers for Disease Control and Prevention (CDC), 1600 Clifton Road, Atlanta, GA 30333. The CDC provides a fact sheet and other information on rickettsial infections.
Telephone 800-311-3435
http://www.cdc.gov

Website

KidsHealth.org. KidsHealth is a website created by the medical experts of the Nemours Foundation and is devoted to issues of children's health. It contains articles on a variety of health topics, including Rocky Mountain spotted fever.
http://www.KidsHealth.org

► See also
Ehrlichiosis
Rickettsial Infections
Tick-borne Infections
Zoonoses

KEYWORDS
for searching the Internet
and other reference sources

Exanthem subitum

Human herpesvirus type 6

Human herpesvirus type 7

* **acute** describes an infection or other illness that comes on suddenly and usually does not last very long.

* **mononucleosis** (mah-no-nu-klee-O-sis) is an infectious illness caused by a virus that often leads to fever, sore throat, swollen glands, and tiredness.

* **cytomegalovirus** (sye-tuh-meh-guh-lo-VY-rus), or CMV, infection is very common and usually causes no symptoms. It poses little risk for healthy people, but it can lead to serious illness in people with weak immune systems.

* **herpes simplex** (HER-peez SIM-plex) is a virus that can cause infections of the skin, mouth, genitals, and other parts of the body.

Roseola Infantum

Roseola infantum (ro-see-O-luh in-FAN-tum) is a viral infection seen in young children that produces a rash and high fever.

What Is Roseola Infantum?

Also known as exanthem subitum (eg-ZAN-thum SU-bih-tum), roseola infantum is an acute* viral infection that mainly affects children between the ages of 6 months and 3 years and is characterized by high fever followed by a rash. The disease stems from infection with human herpesvirus (her-peez-VY-rus) type 6 (HHV 6) or human herpesvirus type 7 (HHV 7). Both of these are part of the same family of viruses as varicella zoster (var-uh-SEH-luh ZOS-ter), which causes chicken pox; Epstein-Barr (EP-steen BAR) virus, which causes mononucleosis*; cytomegalovirus*; and herpes simplex* virus.

How Common Is It?

HHV 6 and HHV 7 affect almost all children who are between 6 months and 3 years of age, but not all of these infections produce the illness recognized as roseola infantum. Roseola rarely is seen in children more than 4 years old, and the illness appears most often during the spring and fall.

Is Roseola Infantum Contagious?

Roseola spreads from person to person, most likely through tiny drops of fluid expelled from the mouth and nose of an infected child when he or she laughs, coughs, sneezes, or talks.

What Are the Signs and Symptoms?

Symptoms of roseola infantum usually appear between 5 and 15 days after exposure to the virus. Children may first have a mild respiratory tract* illness, followed by a high fever that can reach 105 degrees Fahrenheit and last from 2 to 5 days. When the fever subsides, a rash appears, starting on the trunk of the body and spreading to the limbs, face, and neck. The rash of raised red and pink splotches, which fade to white when pressed, lasts from 1 to 3 days. Additional symptoms of the infection can include tiredness, swollen eyelids, a runny nose, swollen lymph nodes* in the neck, and irritability. In up to 10 percent of children, the high fever associated with roseola infantum causes febrile seizures*.

How Is Roseola Infantum Diagnosed?

To diagnose roseola, doctors look for physical symptoms and signs such as rash and swollen lymph nodes, particularly those in the back of the scalp. A medical history may show that the child has been exposed to others with the disease at home or in a child care setting. Because the rash appears after the fever, roseola often is diagnosed after the child has begun to recover from the illness.

How Is the Infection Treated?

Most cases of roseola infantum respond well to treatment at home. Acetaminophen* can help lower a fever, and drinking lots of clear fluids can prevent dehydration*. Children usually feel ill only while they still have a fever and probably will be less active during that time. By the time the rash appears, a child's behavior may be almost back to normal.

Are There Complications?

Most cases of infection resolve in 4 to 6 days without additional problems. Seizures are the most common complication, but this does not mean that the child will have an increased risk of a long-term seizure problem. In rare cases, the disease may lead to the development of meningitis (meh-nin-JY-tis, which is inflammation of the membranes covering the brain and spinal cord) or encephalitis (en-seh-fuh-LYE-tis, which is inflammation of the brain).

Can Roseola Infantum Be Prevented?

There is no simple way for children to avoid exposure to HHV6 and HHV7 completely. Young children have lots of close contact with each other. Adults rarely contract this illness, possibly indicating that having roseola as a child provides lifelong immunity* to the viruses. Some children do experience a second bout of the disease, but this occurs infrequently. Like other viruses in this family, HHV6 and HHV7 can reactivate after the first infection and cause illness, but this happens primarily in people who have a weakened immune system.

* **respiratory tract** includes the nose, mouth, throat, and lungs. It is the pathway through which air and gases are transported down into the lungs and back out of the body.

* **lymph** (LIMF) **nodes** are small, bean-shaped masses of tissue that contain immune system cells that fight harmful microorganisms. Lymph nodes may swell during infections.

* **seizures** (SEE-zhurs) are sudden bursts of disorganized electrical activity that interrupt the normal functioning of the brain, often leading to uncontrolled movements in the body and sometimes a temporary change in consciousness. A febrile seizure is a type of seizure, seen in infants and young children, that is triggered by fever.

* **acetaminophen** (uh-see-teh-MIH-noh-fen) is a medication commonly used to reduce fever and relieve pain.

* **dehydration** (dee-hi-DRAY-shun) is a condition in which the body is depleted of water, usually caused by excessive and unreplaced loss of body fluids, such as through sweating, vomiting, or diarrhea.

* **immunity** (ih-MYOON-uh-tee) is the condition of being protected against an infectious disease. Immunity often develops after a germ is introduced to the body. One type of immunity occurs when the body makes special protein molecules called antibodies to fight the disease-causing germ. The next time that germ enters the body, the antibodies quickly attack it, usually preventing the germ from causing disease.

KEYWORDS
for searching the Internet and other reference sources

Congenital rubella syndrome

German measles

MMR

Vaccination

* **miscarriage** is the ending of a pregnancy through the death of the embryo or fetus before birth.

* **premature delivery** is when a baby is born before it has reached full term.

* **cataracts** (KAH-tuh-rakts) are areas of cloudiness of the lens of the eye that can interfere with vision.

* **microcephaly** (my-kro-SEH-fah-lee) is the condition of having an abnormally small head, which typically results from having an underdeveloped or malformed brain.

* **epidemic** (eh-pih-DEH-mik) is an outbreak of disease, especially infectious disease, in which the number of cases suddenly becomes far greater than usual. Usually epidemics are outbreaks of diseases in specific regions, whereas worldwide epidemics are called pandemics.

300

Resource

Website

KidsHealth.org. KidsHealth is a website created by the medical experts of the Nemours Foundation and is devoted to issues of children's health. It contains articles on a variety of health topics, including roseola infantum.
http://www.KidsHealth.org

Rubella (German Measles)

Rubella (roo-BEH-luh) is a viral illness that causes a rash. Many people know the disease by its other common name, German measles.

What Is Rubella?

Rubella is caused by the virus of the same name. The word "rubella" comes from the Latin word for "little red," which originally described the infection's telltale rash. It also is known by the names German measles and three-day measles, because of its short duration.

Rubella infection usually is not serious. Most people have mild symptoms and a faint rash. However, if a woman develops rubella during the early stages of her pregnancy, it can cause miscarriage*, premature delivery*, and multiple birth defects, known as congenital (kon-JEH-nih-tul) rubella syndrome (CRS). Babies born with CRS may have cataracts* and other eye problems, microcephaly*, mental retardation, deafness, heart defects, enlarged liver or spleen, and other problems.

How Common Is Rubella?

In the United States, the disease was widespread before the current rubella vaccine was introduced. A rubella epidemic* in 1964 and 1965 spawned an estimated 12.5 million cases and 20,000 cases of CRS, according to the U.S. Centers for Disease Control and Prevention (CDC). In 1969, the year the vaccine became available, 57,686 cases of rubella were reported to the CDC. Since then, the number of U.S. cases each year has dropped steadily. The CDC reports that most cases of rubella since the mid-1990s have been seen in young Latino adults who did not receive the vaccine as children. In 2001, there were only 19 cases of rubella reported in the United States, versus 1,400 a decade earlier. The CDC credits global immunization efforts, particularly in Latin America, for the decline.

Is Rubella Contagious?

The illness is contagious and spreads through contact with tiny drops of fluid from the mouth and nose of someone who is infected. The drops

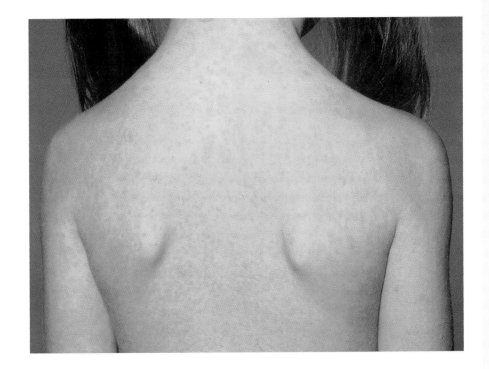

This child has the characteristic rash of rubella. The rubella vaccine has greatly decreased the number of cases in the United States since it was put into use in 1969. Although rubella is generally not serious in otherwise healthy people, in pregnant women it is associated with birth defects and miscarriage. *Custom Medical Stock Photo, Inc.*

leave the mouth and nose when the person sneezes, coughs, or talks. Then other people may inhale the drops, or the drops may land on something that other people touch. Once people get the drops on their hands, they can infect themselves by touching their mouth or nose. The virus enters through the mucous membranes* there and takes hold in the body. Pregnant women also can pass the infection to the fetus* in the womb.

What Happens When Someone Has Rubella?

Signs and symptoms   Symptoms of the illness are often mild, particularly in children. In fact, between one third and one half of all cases may not even be identified as rubella because the symptoms go unnoticed or cannot be distinguished from those of a common, mild respiratory illness such as a cold.

Children with rubella usually develop a distinctive rash. It starts on the face as pink or light red spots and then spreads downward on the body. The rash is fainter than a measles rash, usually does not itch, and lasts from 1 to 3 days. Older children and adults may have symptoms of a viral illness before the rash appears, including swollen lymph nodes* (particularly in the area behind the ears and in the back of the neck), mild fever, runny nose, and conjunctivitis*. Adults also may experience joint and muscle pain and stiffness along with their other symptoms.

Making the diagnosis   If a patient is suspected of having rubella, the doctor can confirm the diagnosis by taking samples of fluid from the mouth or nose with a swab. Samples of blood and, rarely, cerebrospinal fluid*

* **mucous membranes** are the moist linings of the mouth, nose, eyes, and throat.

* **fetus** (FEE-tus) is the term for an unborn human after it is an embryo, from 9 weeks after fertilization until childbirth.

* **lymph** (LIMF) **nodes** are small, bean-shaped masses of tissue that contain immune system cells that fight harmful microorganisms. Lymph nodes may swell during infections.

* **conjunctivitis** (kon-jung-tih-VY-tis), often called "pinkeye," is an inflammation of the thin membrane that lines the inside of the eyelids and covers the surface of the eyeball. Conjunctivitis can be caused by viruses, bacteria, allergies, chemical irritation, and other conditions or diseases that cause inflammation.

* **cerebrospinal** (seh-ree-bro-SPY-nuhl) **fluid** is the fluid that surrounds the brain and spinal cord.

▶ *See also*
Congenital Infections
Conjunctivitis
Encephalitis
Vaccination (Immunization)

may be collected as well. All of these will be examined for signs of the virus. The blood sample also may be tested for antibodies* to the virus.

Treatment There is no treatment for the disease, and it is generally so mild that specific treatment is unnecessary. Over-the-counter medication such as acetaminophen (uh-see-teh-MIH-noh-fen) can lower a fever and ease pain in the muscles and joints. Infants born with CRS will be treated for any defects they may have developed.

Recovery Most patients recover completely in 1 to 2 weeks, and in many patients the disease runs its course in as little as 3 days.

Complications tend to occur more often in adults than in children. Temporary arthritis*, which can last up to a month, is common in adults who have rubella. Other, rare complications include inflammation of the brain (encephalitis, en-seh-fuh-LYE-tis), inflammation of nerves (neuritis, nuh-RYE-tis), and abnormal bleeding. If the infection occurs in a pregnant woman, it can lead to miscarriage, premature delivery, or congenital rubella syndrome.

How Can Rubella Be Prevented?

Vaccination is the best way to prevent rubella infection. The vaccine for rubella is given as part of a combined vaccination for measles*, mumps*, and rubella called MMR. Children receive the MMR vaccine in two doses, usually at age 15 months and 5 years, before entering kindergarten. Doctors recommend that women who are old enough to have children be tested for immunity* to rubella, and if the woman is not immune to the virus, she should be vaccinated.

Resources

Organization

U.S. Centers for Disease Control and Prevention (CDC), 1600 Clifton Road, Atlanta, GA 30333. The CDC is the U.S. government authority for information about infectious and other diseases. It provides information about rubella at its website.
Telephone 800-311-3435
http://www.cdc.gov

Website

KidsHealth.org. KidsHealth is a website created by the medical experts of the Nemours Foundation and is devoted to issues of children's health. It contains articles on a variety of health topics, including rubella.
http://www.KidsHealth.org

Rubeola *See* Measles (Rubeola)

S

Schistosomiasis

Schistosomiasis (shis-tuh-so-MY-uh-sis) is an illness caused by parasitic* worms. The worms must spend part of their life cycle growing in freshwater snails before they enter and cause infestations* in humans.

What Is Schistosomiasis?

Schistosomiasis is a parasitic disease that is not directly contagious from person to person. Five types of *Schistosoma* worm, also called blood flukes, can infest people and cause schistosomiasis: *S. mansoni, S. japonicum, S. mekongi, S. intercalatum,* and *S. haematobium.* These parasites have a complex life cycle; they have to go through several separate stages on their way to adulthood, and both snails and humans play important roles in that cycle. Another name for the disease is bilharziasis (bil-har-ZYE-uh-sis) or "snail fever."

The worm starts life as an egg in a freshwater source such as a pond, lake, or stream. It hatches into a larva*, and if the right type of aquatic snails live in that water, the larva will find and enter a snail. There it passes through several stages of development. During the last phase in the snail, the parasite turns into a larva that can swim. It then leaves the snail and returns to the water, where it may come into contact with a person; the larva can survive in the water for up to 2 days without a human host. When people bathe, wade, swim, or wash clothes in the water, the parasite can burrow into bare skin and enter the bloodstream. Once it is in the blood, it matures into an adult worm.

Depending on the species, the female adult worms lay their eggs within blood vessels near the person's bladder or liver. The eggs gradually move to the urinary tract, liver, and intestines*. Over time, some eggs pass through the urinary tract and intestines and are excreted when the person urinates or has a bowel movement. If feces (excreted waste) from an infested person contaminate a freshwater source such as a pond, the eggs can enter the water and begin the parasite life cycle all over again.

How Common Is Schistosomiasis?

Schistosomiasis is not seen in the United States. However, the disease has a major impact on millions of people around the world in developing countries. According to the World Health Organization, more than

KEYWORDS
for searching the Internet and other reference sources

Bilharziasis

Blood flukes

Flatworms

Parasites

Schistosomes

Snail fever

Zoonoses

* **parasitic** (pair-uh-SIH-tik) refers to organisms such as protozoa (one-celled animals), worms, or insects that can invade and live on or inside human beings and may cause illness. An animal or plant harboring a parasite is called its host.

* **Infestations** refer to illnesses caused by multi-celled parasitic organisms, such as tapeworms, roundworms, or protozoa.

* **larva** (LAR-vuh) is the immature form of an insect or worm that hatches from an egg.

* **intestines** are the muscular tubes that food passes through during digestion after it exits the stomach.

200 million people worldwide are infested with the worms, with 20 million of those having serious symptoms.

The disease is most common in tropical parts of the world, where it is a leading cause of illness. The parasites that cause schistosomiasis can be found in southern China, parts of the Middle East, and some countries in the Caribbean, South America, Africa, and southeast Asia. People from the United States who travel to those areas sometimes develop schistosomiasis if they swim or wade in tainted water, but they rarely get the severe, chronic* form of the disease.

What Are the Signs and Symptoms of Schistosomiasis?

A rash and itchy skin, particularly at the spot where the parasite burrowed into the body, may develop within a few days. The worms then mature and spread through the bloodstream, and 1 to 2 months later patients may have muscle aches, fever, chills, and cough. It is not uncommon, however, for people to not show any symptoms during this early stage of infestation. Over time, as the worms spread into the liver and intestines, patients can experience diarrhea (dye-uh-REE-uh), liver enlargement, vomiting, and abdominal* pain.

How Do Doctors Diagnose and Treat Schistosomiasis?

If the doctor suspects schistosomiasis, he or she will collect a urine or stool (bowel movement) sample to look for the worm's eggs. Several samples may need to be examined before the worms can be identified. The doctor also may take a sample of blood for testing, although the blood test may not show evidence of the infestation unless it is done 6 to 8 weeks after the patient's contact with the parasite. Occasionally, a tissue biopsy* will be done to check for signs of the parasite in organs such as the liver.

Doctors can prescribe medicine to treat the infestation. Patients usually need to take pills for only 1 to 2 days. Without treatment, and with continued use of the same tainted water source, the illness can last for years.

Can Schistosomiasis Cause Complications?

People who become re-infested with schistosomiasis again and again over many years can develop damage to the bladder, lungs, intestines, and liver; the disease is one of the leading causes of cirrhosis* in the world. In some cases, scarring of the liver is so severe that blood flowing through the organ becomes partly blocked, causing a condition known as portal hypertension. Severe portal hypertension can make veins in the esophagus* and stomach swell and bleed, sometimes to the point that the bleeding is fatal.

* **chronic** (KRAH-nik) means continuing for a long period of time.

* **abdominal** (ab-DAH-mih-nul) refers to the area of the body below the ribs and above the hips that contains the stomach, intestines, and other organs.

* **biopsy** (BI-op-see) is a test in which a small sample of skin or other body tissue is removed and examined for signs of disease.

* **cirrhosis** (sir-O-sis) is a condition that affects the liver, involving long-term inflammation and scarring, which can lead to problems with liver function.

* **esophagus** (eh-SAH-fuh-gus) is the soft tube that, with swallowing, carries food from the throat to the stomach.

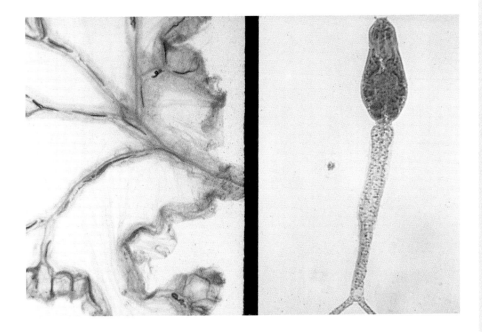

Flatworm flukes: on the left, *Schistosoma japonicum*; on the right, *Schistosoma mansoni*. These parasites can enter the human body through the skin and then develop into an adult worm in the bloodstream. *Custom Medical Stock Photo, Inc.*

◀

Other complications of the disease arise when the worm's eggs travel through the bloodstream to the spinal cord or brain, where they can cause seizures*, inflammation of the spinal cord, or paralysis*.

How Can Schistosomiasis Be Prevented?

Experts advise that travelers visiting countries where schistosomiasis occurs avoid wading, swimming, or bathing in any body of fresh water such as ponds, rivers, or lakes. Filtering or boiling drinking water for at least 1 minute will kill parasites, including the *Schistosoma* worms. The U.S. Centers for Disease Control and Prevention also recommends heating bathing water to 150 degrees Fahrenheit for at least 5 minutes to make sure it is free of potential parasites.

To reduce the spread of schistosomiasis, health officials focus on educating people who live in areas where the worms are found. They teach the public how the parasites spread and encourage people not to urinate or have bowel movements in rivers and ponds.

* **seizures** (SEE-zhurs) are sudden bursts of disorganized electrical activity that interrupt the normal functioning of the brain, often leading to uncontrolled movements in the body and sometimes a temporary change in consciousness.

* **paralysis** (pah-RAH-luh-sis) is the loss or impairment of the ability to move some part of the body.

Resources

Organizations

U.S. Centers for Disease Control and Prevention (CDC), 1600 Clifton Road, Atlanta, GA 30333. The CDC is the U.S. government authority for information about infectious and other diseases. The organization provides information about schistosomiasis at its website. Telephone 800-311-3435
http://www.cdc.gov

World Health Organization (WHO), Avenue Appia 20, 1211 Geneva 27, Switzerland. WHO provides information about schistosomiasis at its website.
Telephone 011-41-22-791-2111
http://www.who.int

Sepsis

Sepsis is a serious systemic infection caused by bacteria in the blood-stream.

What Is Sepsis?

Sepsis is caused most commonly by bacteria in the bloodstream, a condition known as bacteremia (bak-tuh-REE-me-uh). These bacteria produce toxins* that provoke a response by the body's immune system. The effect of the toxins combined with the response of the immune system brings about the disease. Bacteremia may resolve on its own or it can lead to sepsis if the bacteria are not removed by the immune system. Although bacteremia and sepsis frequently coexist, each can be present without the other. The bacteria may come from a local infection, like pneumonia* or a urinary tract* infection, or they may come from the nose, skin, or intestines*, where bacteria live without causing problems unless they enter the bloodstream. The most common sources of infection that lead to sepsis are the lungs, skin, intestine, urinary tract, and gall bladder*.

Sepsis is most dangerous to people with weak immune systems, such as infants, the elderly, people with HIV/AIDS or cancer, or those who have undergone organ transplantation. In infants younger than 3 months, any fever may be a sign of sepsis or another serious infection. Doctors advise immediate evaluation of these infants and prompt treatment with antibiotics if sepsis is suspected. Group B streptococcus (strep-tuh-KAH-kus) bacteria passed from mother to baby during birth are a major cause of sepsis in infants. *Streptococcus pneumoniae* (strep-tuh-KAH-kus nu-MO-nye) and *Neisseria meningitidis* (nye-SEER-e-uh meh-nin-JIH-tih-dis) bacteria are associated with sepsis in older children and in adults. Sepsis in adults most often is seen after surgery or another medical procedure in the hospital, but it may occur outside the hospital, particularly associated with urinary tract infection.

How Common Is Sepsis?

Sepsis is not very common. According to the U.S. National Library of Medicine, sepsis develops in about 2 of every 10,000 people in the general population. In infants, sepsis occurs in fewer than 1 to 2 per 1,000

▶ *See also*
Intestinal Parasites
Zoonoses

KEYWORDS
for searching the Internet and other reference sources

Bacteremia

Group B streptococcus

Septic shock

Streptococcus pneumoniae

*****toxins** are poisons that harm the body.

*****pneumonia** (nu-MO-nyah) is inflammation of the lung.

*****urinary tract** (YOOR-ih-nair-e TRAKT) is the system of organs and channels that makes urine and removes it from the body. It consists of the urethra, bladder, ureters, and kidneys.

*****intestines** are the muscular tubes that food passes through during digestion after it exits the stomach.

*****gall bladder** is a small pear-shaped organ on the right side of the abdomen that stores bile, a liquid that helps the body digest fat.

live births. Sepsis is a complication in about 2 of every 100 hospitalizations, where related intravenous (IV) lines, surgical wounds or drains, and bedsores* can be entry points for bacteria.

Is Sepsis Contagious?

Sepsis itself is not contagious, but the infectious agents that can cause sepsis can be transmitted from person to person. For example, in newborns, group B streptococcus organisms can spread from mother to baby during delivery.

What Are the Signs and Symptoms of the Disease?

Early symptoms of sepsis may include fever, shaking chills, rapid breathing and heartbeat, confusion, delirium*, and rash. As the infection spreads, a person's blood pressure drops, leading to a condition known as shock*. Body organs that have important functions, including the liver, lungs, and kidneys, may begin to shut down. The blood-clotting* system also may be affected. Sepsis in young children may be more difficult to diagnose at first, because it has fewer obvious symptoms. Children may have a fever or changing temperature, a change in heart rate, or difficulty breathing. They also might be irritable or sluggish, and they may lose interest in eating.

How Do Doctors Make the Diagnosis?

A diagnosis of sepsis is made based on a person's symptoms. Blood tests are performed to identify the bacteria and to look for a low platelet* count (an indicator of the blood-clotting problems seen with sepsis) and an abnormally low or high white blood cell count (both can occur with sepsis). Other tests can help show damage to vital organs, such as the kidneys.

Can Sepsis Be Treated?

As soon as a diagnosis of sepsis is suspected, treatment with intravenous antibiotics begins. Patients with sepsis are hospitalized in an intensive care unit, where they may be given oxygen, intravenous fluids, and medication to stabilize blood pressure, treat other symptoms, and kill the bacteria responsible for the condition. Dialysis* may be necessary if the patient's kidneys fail. If respiratory failure* occurs, patients usually are placed on a respirator, a machine that aids their breathing until they can breathe again on their own. If the patient survives, recovery from sepsis can take weeks.

What Are the Complications of the Disease?

Septic shock* may occur in patients with sepsis. Disseminated intravascular coagulation is a complication associated with sepsis in which the

* **bedsores**, also called pressure sores, are skin sores caused by prolonged pressure on the skin and typically are seen in people who are confined by illness or paralysis to beds or wheelchairs.

* **delirium** (dih-LEER-e-um) is a condition in which a person is confused, is unable to think clearly, and has a reduced level of consciousness.

* **shock** is a serious condition in which blood pressure is very low and not enough blood flows to the body's organs and tissues. Untreated, shock may result in death.

* **clotting** is the body's way of thickening blood to stop bleeding.

* **platelets** (PLATE-lets) are tiny disk-shaped particles within the blood that play an important role in clotting.

* **dialysis** (dye-AL-uh-sis) is a process that removes waste, toxins (poisons), and extra fluid from the blood; usually it is done when a person's kidneys are unable to perform these functions normally.

* **respiratory failure** is a condition in which breathing and oxygen delivery to the body is dangerously altered. This may result from infection, nerve or muscle damage, poisoning, or other causes.

* **septic shock** is shock due to overwhelming infection and is characterized by decreased blood pressure, internal bleeding, heart failure, and, in some cases, death.

307

body's blood-clotting system is out of control; this can lead to serious internal bleeding. This complication usually improves when the cause of sepsis is treated. Sepsis can be fatal, depending on the infectious agent and on the age and overall health of the patient. Quick diagnosis and treatment can improve outcomes and save lives.

How Is Sepsis Prevented?

Sepsis may not be preventable in many cases, but an early response to symptoms may stop a bacterial infection from progressing to sepsis. This is particularly important with regard to people with weak immune systems. Among hospitalized patients, efforts are made to limit the use of intravenous and urinary catheters*, which are both common entry points for sepsis-causing bacteria. Following a recommended vaccination* schedule for children can lessen their risk of contracting certain infections that might lead to sepsis. Immunization against *Streptococcus pneumoniae* is recommended for infants and for adults and children at high risk due to age or medical problems. This vaccine is highly effective in preventing pneumonia and sepsis caused by this organism.

Pregnant women typically are tested to determine whether they are carrying group B streptococcus bacteria in their vagina*. Treating these women with antibiotics during pregnancy may reduce the risk of passing the bacterium from mother to child. People with medical conditions, such as sickle-cell disease*, that put them at greater risk for developing serious bacterial infections are prescribed antibiotics to decrease the chance that sepsis can develop.

Resources

Organization

U.S. National Library of Medicine, 8600 Rockville Pike, Bethesda, MD 20894. The National Library of Medicine has a website packed with information on diseases (including sepsis) and public health, consumer resources, dictionaries and encyclopedias of medical terms, and directories of doctors and helpful organizations.
Telephone 888-346-3656
http://www.nlm.nih.gov

Website

KidsHealth.org. KidsHealth is a website created by the medical experts of the Nemours Foundation and is devoted to issues of children's health. It contains articles on a variety of health topics, including sepsis.
http://www.KidsHealth.org

* **catheters** (KAH-thuh-ters) are small plastic tubes placed through a body opening into an organ (such as the bladder) or through the skin directly into a blood vessel. They are used to give fluids to or drain fluids from a person.

* **vaccination** (vak-sih-NAY-shun), also called immunization, is giving, usually by an injection, a preparation of killed or weakened germs, or a part of a germ or product it produces, to prevent or lessen the severity of the disease caused by that germ.

* **vagina** (vah-JY-nah) is the canal, or passageway, in a woman that leads from the uterus to the outside of the body.

* **sickle-cell disease** is a hereditary condition in which the red blood cells, which are usually round, take on an abnormal crescent shape and have a decreased ability to carry oxygen throughout the body.

▶ *See also*

Pneumonia

Skin and Soft Tissue Infections

Streptococcal Infections

Urinary Tract Infections

Vaccination (Immunization)

Sexually Transmitted Diseases

Sexually transmitted diseases (STDs) are infections that pass from one person to another through sexual contact, which includes oral, genital, or anal intercourse.

What Are STDs?

STDs can be caused by bacteria, viruses, or parasites. Although the symptoms of a particular STD depend on the specific infection, many STDs cause vaginitis (vah-jih-NYE-tis), an inflammation of the vagina often accompanied by an abnormal discharge (fluid released from the body), and urethritis (yoo-ree-THRY-tis), an inflammation of the urethra (the tube through which urine passes from the bladder to the outside of the body), which can make urination painful. Several STDs can produce blisters or sores on the penis, vagina, rectum, or buttocks. In women, some STDs may spread to the cervix*, a condition called cervicitis (sir-vih-SYE-tis), or to the uterus* and fallopian tubes*, a condition known as pelvic inflammatory disease (PID). In men STDs may spread to the testicle (causing epididymitis*) or prostate* (causing prostatitis, inflammation of the prostate). It is not uncommon for several STDs to occur in the same person, and the presence of an STD can increase the risk of contracting infection with human immunodeficiency (ih-myoo-no-dih-FIH-shen-see) virus (HIV), the virus that causes acquired immunodeficiency syndrome (AIDS), from an infected partner.

How Common Are They?

STDs are common in the United States; between 13 million and 15 million new cases are diagnosed every year. Despite the fact that much information is available about preventing these infections and limiting their spread, the number of people infected is growing, and about two-thirds of cases are reported in people under the age of 25 years.

Are STDs Contagious?

STDs are contagious and are transmitted through sexual contact that involves vaginal, anal, or oral sex. The diseases can spread between people of the opposite sex or people of the same sex. The germs that cause many STDs move from person to person through semen (the sperm-containing whitish fluid produced by the male reproductive tract), vaginal (VAH-jih-nul) fluids, or blood. Other STDs, like herpes and genital warts, can spread by intimate skin-to-skin contact, often with sores the disease causes. Certain STDs can pass from a mother to her baby during pregnancy or childbirth. STDs do not pass from one person to another by simply hugging, shaking hands, or sharing utensils.

KEYWORDS
for searching the Internet and other reference sources

Acquired immunodeficiency syndrome (AIDS)

Cervicitis

Chlamydia

Epididymitis

Genital warts

Gonorrhea

Herpes simplex virus

Human immunodeficiency virus (HIV)

Pelvic inflammatory disease

Prostatitis

Syphilis

Trichomoniasis

Urethritis

Vaginitis

* **cervix** (SIR-viks) is the lower, narrow end of the uterus that opens into the vagina.

* **uterus** (YOO-teh-rus) is the muscular, pear-shaped internal organ in a woman where a baby develops until birth.

* **fallopian** (fah-LO-pee-uhn) **tubes** are the two slender tubes that connect the ovaries and the uterus in females. They carry the ova, or eggs, from the ovaries to the uterus.

* **epididymitis** (eh-pih-dih-duh-MY-tis) is a painful inflammation of the epididymis, a structure attached to the testicles.

* **prostate** (PRAH-state) is a male reproductive gland located near where the bladder joins the urethra. The prostate produces the fluid part of semen.

What Are Some Common STDs?

Gonorrhea Gonorrhea (gah-nuh-REE-uh) is caused by the bacterium *Neisseria gonorrhoeae* (nye-SEER-e-uh gah-no-REE-eye). It may not produce any symptoms in women who are infected. When symptoms are present, they include vaginal discharge and pain when urinating. Lower belly pain usually occurs when the infection has spread past the cervix and caused PID. Most men with gonorrhea have a discharge from the penis and pain when they urinate. Gonorrhea is treated with antibiotics that kill the bacteria.

Syphilis Syphilis (SIH-fih-lis) is caused by the bacterium *Treponema pallidum* (treh-puh-NEE-muh PAL-ih-dum). It is different from many other STDs, because there are distinct stages to the illness. In the first stage, a small, hard sore called a chancre (SHANG-ker) appears where the bacteria entered the body. In the next stage, a red or brown rash develops, sometimes on the palms of the hands and soles of the feet; in some cases, patients also may have a fever, swollen lymph nodes*, muscle aches, and headaches. If the disease goes untreated, it can progress to the third and most serious stage, when it may damage the bones, organs, and nervous system, which can result in blindness, paralysis*, dementia*, heart problems, and sometimes even death. Like gonorrhea, syphilis can be treated effectively with antibiotics. More than 31,000 cases of syphilis were reported in the United States in 2000.

Herpes simplex virus Herpes simplex (HER-peez SIM-plex) virus causes herpes. There are two types of herpes, type1 and type 2. Type 2 usually spreads through sexual contact and causes genital herpes. In a person with genital herpes, small, painful blisters develop on the vagina, cervix, penis, buttocks, or thighs. Once infection occurs, the herpes virus remains in the body and can recur throughout a person's life. Antiviral medications may shorten outbreaks of symptoms and make them less severe, but they do not kill the virus. In the United States an estimated 45 million people over the age of 12 have genital herpes infection.

Chlamydia Chlamydia (kla-MIH-dee-uh) is caused by the bacterium *Chlamydia trachomatis* (kla-MIH-dee-uh truh-KO-mah-tis), and in many infected people it produces no symptoms. The most common symptoms in both men and women are discharge and pain when urinating. Because infection with chlamydia may not be noticed, it can spread and produce other symptoms, including epididymitis in men and PID in women. More than 700,000 cases were reported in the United States in 2000, but the actual number of new cases could be 3 million to 4 million per year. A person with chlamydia can be treated effectively with antibiotics.

HIV Infection with HIV damages immune system cells in the body that normally fight infections, leaving the body unable to defend itself

*lymph (LIMF) nodes are small, bean-shaped masses of tissue that contain immune system cells that fight harmful microorganisms. Lymph nodes may swell during infections.

*paralysis (pah-RAH-luh-sis) is the loss or impairment of the ability to move some part of the body.

*dementia (dih-MEN-sha) is a loss of mental abilities, including memory, understanding, and judgment.

against a variety of illnesses. A person can be infected with HIV and not have AIDS, although most people with HIV do end up developing AIDS. The first symptoms of HIV infection include fever, muscle aches, sore throat, and, in some cases, a rash that looks somewhat like that of measles*. Other symptoms usually take much longer to appear, perhaps years, and may include rapid weight loss, recurring fever, a dry cough, night sweats, pneumonia*, white spots on the tongue or throat, long-lasting diarrhea, and skin rashes and yeast infections. A person with AIDS also may have memory loss, depression, and extreme tiredness.

In the United States, there were more than 40,000 new cases of AIDS reported in 2000, and more than 850,000 people were living with HIV in 2000. There have been more than 460,000 reported deaths related to AIDS in the United States since the disease was first identified in the early 1980s. There is no cure for AIDS, but a combination of medications can help a person live longer and have a better quality of life.

Human papillomavirus Genital and anal warts are caused by human papillomavirus (pah-pih-LO-mah-vy-rus), or HPV, a very common virus. The warts are soft and skin-colored, and they can grow alone or in bunches on the genitals; on the skin around the genitals, rectum, or buttocks; or in the vagina or cervix. Like herpes, genital warts can reappear again and again, because once this type of virus enters the body, it remains there for life. Doctors can remove genital warts by freezing, burning, or cutting them off or by coating them with medication that destroys the warts. In women, infection with HPV can affect the cells of the cervix, which may lead to cervical cancer.

Trichomoniasis Trichomoniasis (trih-ko-mo-NYE-uh-sis) is a very common STD that is caused by a parasite. Most women with trichomoniasis have a frothy, yellow, foul-smelling vaginal discharge, along with itching and irritation in the vagina and discomfort during sex and urination. Men with this STD typically do not have symptoms; those who do have symptoms may feel irritation in the penis or a burning sensation after they urinate or ejaculate*. More than 2 million cases are diagnosed each year in the United States. Trichomoniasis can be treated with antibiotics.

Can STDs Be Prevented?

The only sure way to prevent STDs is not to have sexual contact with anyone. In most cases, it is impossible or very difficult to tell whether another person has an STD. People may not always tell the truth about their sexual past, or they may have an STD and not know it. For people who do have sex, the safest choices are to limit the number of sexual partners and to use latex condoms. Latex condoms lower the risk of contracting many STDs, including HIV infection. Certain STDs such as genital warts and herpes may present additional problems, because the

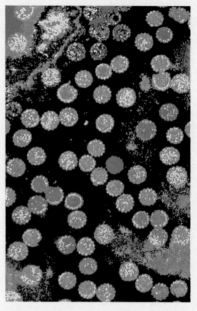

Human papillomavirus, or HPV, of which there are over 50 types. HPV causes genital warts and is strongly associated with cervical and penile cancers. *Custom Medical Stock Photo, Inc.*

*measles (ME-zuls) is a viral respiratory infection that is best known for the rash of large, flat, red blotches that appear on the arms, face, neck, and body.

*pneumonia (nu-MO-nyah) is inflammation of the lung.

*ejaculate (e-JAH-kyoo-late) means to discharge semen from the penis.

warts or herpes blisters can be on the skin around the genitals and condoms do not protect against them if the sores are not covered by the condom. Avoiding skin-to-skin contact is the best option for preventing these kinds of STDs.

Resources

Organization

U.S. Centers for Disease Control and Prevention (CDC), 1600 Clifton Road, Atlanta, GA 30333. The CDC provides fact sheets and other information on STDs at its website.
Telephone 800-311-3435
http://www.cdc.gov

Website

KidsHealth.org. KidsHealth is a website created by the medical experts of the Nemours Foundation and is devoted to issues of children's health. It contains articles on a variety of health topics, including sexually transmitted diseases.
http://www.KidsHealth.org

Sinusitis

Sinusitis (sy-nyoo-SY-tis) is an inflammation of the sinuses (SY-nuh-ses), the hollow chambers or cavities located in the bones of the face that surround the nose.

What Causes Sinusitis?

There are four pairs of paranasal sinuses (the sinuses surrounding the nose):

- The frontal sinuses are in the forehead and over the eyebrows.
- The ethmoid (ETH-moyd) sinuses are between the eyes at the bridge of the nose.
- The sphenoid (SFEE-noyd) sinuses are behind the ethmoid sinuses.
- The maxillary (MAX-ih-lary) sinuses are in the cheekbones.

The sinuses and the narrow tube-like structures that link them to the nasal passages are lined with the same mucous membranes* that line the nose. Colds, allergies, and exposure to some chemicals can cause swelling and inflammation in the lining of the sinus passages and block sinus drainage. Bacteria (such as *Streptococcus pneumoniae*, strep-tuh-KAH-kus

KEYWORDS
for searching the Internet and other reference sources

Allergies

Asthma

Paranasal sinuses

Respiratory infections

Sinuses

Streptococcus pneumoniae

*mucous membranes are the moist linings of the mouth, nose, eyes, and throat.

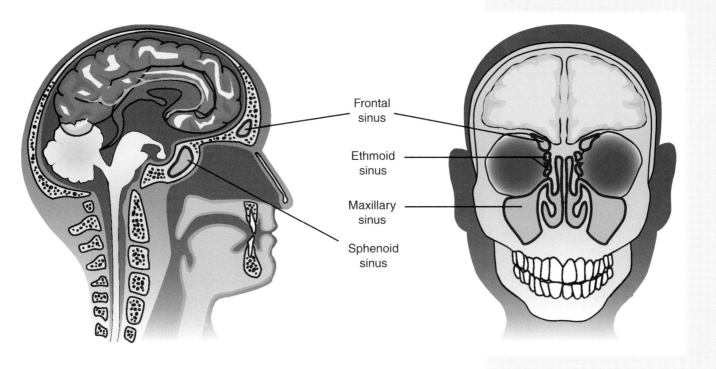

Frontal
sinus

Ethmoid
sinus

Maxillary
sinus

Sphenoid
sinus

There are four pairs of sinuses in the human skull.

nu-MO-nye), viruses, and fungi that live in the body may become trapped, multiply, and invade the inflamed sinuses.

People with allergies, asthma, and cystic fibrosis* are more likely to have sinus infections. So are people with a weakened immune system, such as those who have AIDS or cancer; people with narrow sinus passages or with growths or blockages in the nasal area, such as tumors or polyps*; and people with previously broken or deformed nasal bones. The risk of sinusitis also is higher when people swim or dive, because of the pressure this activity puts on the sinus cavities.

Are There Different Types of Sinusitis?

Physicians classify sinusitis in three ways:

◼ Acute* sinusitis often develops after a person has had a cold, with symptoms lasting less than 3 weeks.

◼ Chronic* sinusitis can last 3 to 8 weeks or longer; it often occurs in people who have allergies or asthma.

◼ Recurrent sinusitis consists of several acute episodes of sinusitis in 1 year.

How Common Is Sinusitis?

The National Institute of Allergy and Infectious Diseases estimates that every year 37 million people in the United States have sinusitis.

* **cystic fibrosis** (SIS-tik fy-BRO-sis) is a disease that causes the body to produce thick mucus that clogs passages in many of the body's organs, including the lungs.

* **polyps** (PAH-lips) are bumps or growths usually on the lining or surface of a body part (such as the nose or intestine). Their size can range from tiny to large enough to cause pain or obstruction. They may be harmless, but they also may be cancerous.

* **acute** describes an infection or other illness that comes on suddenly and usually does not last very long.

* **chronic** (KRAH-nik) means continuing for a long period of time.

313

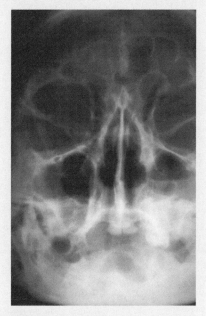

This X ray shows, on the right side of the X ray, an example of the inflammation associated with sinusitis. If the patient's sinusitis is severe, the doctor may recommend surgery to help drainage of the sinus cavities. *Custom Medical Stock Photo, Inc.*

---

* **respiratory tract** includes the nose, mouth, throat, and lungs. It is the pathway through which air and gases are transported down into the lungs and back out of the body.

* **mucus** (MYOO-kus) is a thick, slippery substance that lines the insides of many body parts.

* **computerized tomography** (kom-PYOO-ter-ized toe-MAH-gruh-fee) or CT, also called computerized axial tomography (CAT), is a technique in which a machine takes many X rays of the body to create a three-dimensional picture.

* **acetaminophen** (uh-see-teh-MIH-noh-fen) is a medication commonly used to reduce fever and relieve pain.

Is Sinusitis Contagious?

No one can catch a sinus infection from another person, but the viruses and bacteria that cause colds and other respiratory tract* infections that can trigger sinusitis may spread from person to person in drops of fluid from the nose or mouth. When people cough, sneeze, laugh, or talk, they can transmit germs to their hands, to the surfaces around them, and into the air. Other people can breathe in the germs or touch contaminated surfaces with their hands and spread the germs to their noses and mouths.

What Are the Symptoms of Sinusitis?

Symptoms of a cold (runny nose and low fever) often give way to pain and pressure in the sinuses, which are usually the first signs of sinusitis. Other symptoms include pain or puffiness around the eyes; a bad-smelling, yellow-green discharge from the nose; bad breath; a headache in the morning; aching in the upper jaw and the back teeth; weakness or extreme tiredness; and coughing, especially at night. People with sinusitis occasionally develop earaches, neck pain, or a sore throat caused by mucus* draining into the throat.

How Is Sinusitis Diagnosed?

Sinusitis is suspected if cold symptoms last for more than 10 days or if sinusitis symptoms are present. A doctor may order X rays or a computerized tomography* (CT) scan to determine whether the sinuses are inflamed.

How Is Sinusitis Treated?

Bacterial sinusitis usually clears up after treatment with antibiotics. There is no specific treatment for sinusitis caused by a virus. People can try to relieve the symptoms of sinusitis in several ways. They can take acetaminophen* to help ease the pain and use nonprescription decongestants (dee-kon-JES-tents), taken by mouth or in sprays, to lessen stuffiness. Using a decongestant nasal spray for more than a few days, however, may itself cause swelling of the sinuses and slow recovery. Saline or salt sprays also may reduce swelling in the sinuses. Placing a warm compress over the infected sinuses, using a steam vaporizer*, or sitting in a warm, steamy bathroom can help as well. Doctors may prescribe special nasal sprays or oral (by mouth) medications for people with chronic sinusitis who have allergies that contribute to the infection. In some cases, people with severe chronic sinusitis may undergo surgery to enlarge their sinus passages, to remove a polyp, or to fix a deviated septum* that might be blocking sinus drainage.

How Long Will It Last?

Acute sinusitis usually clears up within 3 weeks, or within 1 to 2 weeks with treatment. Chronic sinusitis lasts 3 to 8 weeks or longer and may require longer courses of antibiotics and other treatments to resolve the condition.

Are There Complications?

Complications of sinusitis are rare, although they do occur. Sinusitis can cause osteomyelitis* when the infection from the sinus spreads into the bones of the face or skull, or it can lead to an infection of brain tissue or meningitis (inflammation of the meninges*). A sinus infection also can spread to invade the tissues surrounding the eyes.

Can Sinusitis Be Prevented?

Because there is no practical way to prevent all colds or to eliminate all allergies, sinusitis is not entirely preventable. People can limit their exposure to the viruses and bacteria that cause the infections by washing their hands thoroughly and frequently and by not sharing eating or drinking utensils. Not smoking and avoiding exposure to tobacco smoke also can help limit the risk of sinusitis. It is wise for people with allergies to avoid the things that trigger their allergy symptoms and to control their allergies with the treatment recommended by their doctors. Drinking plenty of fluids and keeping the air in the house moist by using a vaporizer can help thin mucus and prevent its buildup in the sinuses. Limiting alcohol consumption also may help, because alcohol can cause nasal membranes to swell.

Resources

Organization

National Institute of Allergy and Infectious Diseases (NIAID), Building 31, Room 7A-50, 31 Center Drive MSC 2520, Bethesda, MD 20892. The NIAID, part of the National Institutes of Health, publishes pamphlets and a fact sheet about sinusitis at its website, along with links to other websites offering more information. http://www.niaid.nih.gov

Skin and Soft Tissue Infections

Skin and soft tissue infections are infections involving the layers of the skin and the soft tissues beneath it.

What Causes Skin and Soft Tissue Infections?

Viruses, bacteria, and fungi generally cause skin and soft tissue infections by entering the body at a spot where a cut, scrape, bite, or other wound has broken the skin; some infections are even the result of bacteria that normally live on the body. These infections can affect the layers of the skin or deeper tissues, such as muscle and connective tissue (the interlacing framework of tissue that forms ligaments, tendons, and

*****vaporizer** is a device that converts water (or a liquid medication) into a vapor, a suspension of tiny droplets that hang in the air and can be inhaled.

*****deviated septum** is a condition in which the wall of tissue between the nasal passages, the septum, divides the passageways unevenly, sometimes causing breathing difficulties and blockage of sinus drainage.

*****osteomyelitis** (ah-stee-o-my-uh-LYE-tis) is a bone infection that is usually caused by bacteria. It can involve any bone in the body, but it most commonly affects the long bones in the arms and legs.

*****meninges** (meh-NIN-jeez) are the membranes that enclose and protect the brain and the spinal cord.

▶ *See also*
Common Cold
Influenza
Meningitis
Osteomyelitis
Sore Throat
Streptococcal Infections

* **pus** is a thick, creamy fluid, usually yellow or greenish in color, that forms at the site of an infection. Pus contains infection-fighting white cells and other substances.

other supporting structures of the body), and they may bring about symptoms in other parts of the body.

Many infections like varicella (chicken pox) and measles (rubeola) affect the skin, but these infections involve the whole body and do not primarily arise within the skin or soft tissues.

What Are Some Types of Skin and Soft Tissue Infections?

Dermatophyte infections   Dermatophytes (dur-MAH-toh-fites) are fungi that live on the dead outer layer of skin. Sometimes they can produce symptoms of infection. Tinea (TIH-nee-uh) infections, commonly called ringworm (although they have nothing to do with worms), usually are caused by the *Trichophyton* group of these organisms. They include tinea pedis (PEE-dis), or athlete's foot; tinea cruris (KRU-ris), or jock itch; tinea capitis (KAH-pih-tis), or ringworm of the scalp; tinea unguium (UN-gwee-um), or ringworm of the nails; and tinea corporis (KOR-poor-us), or ringworm of the body. Damaged skin is more vulnerable to infection, as is skin in warm, moist areas of the body. When the fungus takes hold, it typically causes a ring-like rash of red, flaking skin. The border of the rash may be raised, as if a worm were under the skin. The rash's shape and this raised edge led people to call the infection ringworm. When the nails are infected, they usually become yellow, thickened, and brittle.

Tinea versicolor, or pityriasis (pih-tih-RYE-uh-sis) versicolor, is caused by the fungus *Malassezia furfur.* Symptoms include scaly patches of skin, ranging in color from light to dark. The patches occur on the chest, neck, back, underarms, and upper arms. Hot, humid weather encourages the growth of tinea versicolor. These fungal skin infections typically are treated with antifungal creams or ointments. In severe cases or when the infections do not improve with this therapy, several antifungal medications are available that may be given by mouth.

Impetigo   Impetigo (im-pih-TEE-go) refers to a skin infection in which there are red blister-like bumps that contain a yellowish fluid or pus*. After the blisters break open, they crust over. Impetigo is most common on the face, especially around the nose and mouth. Usually, either streptococcus (strep-tuh-KAH-kus) or staphylococcus (stah-fih-lo-KAH-kus) bacteria are the cause of the infection. Impetigo can spread easily, especially among children, who may scratch the lesions and then touch other areas of their skin or another person. People also can contract impetigo from handling clothing or blankets that have been in contact with infected skin.

Doctors prescribe antibiotics to treat impetigo. The infection generally clears up without leaving permanent skin damage.

Skin abscesses   Skin abscesses (AB-seh-sez) may occur in areas of the skin where the body has been fighting a bacterial infection. To isolate the infection, the body forms a wall of tissue around the collection of pus, and this area is the abscess. Abscesses are usually round, raised, and red, and they may feel warm and tender. A furuncle (FYOOR-ung-kul), or boil, is an abscess that forms at the base of a hair follicle*. A carbuncle (KAR-bung-kul) forms when the infection spreads to include several follicles and the surrounding skin and deeper tissues. Like furuncles, carbuncles are red, raised, and sore to the touch.

Most skin abscesses eventually burst to allow the pus to drain out, but treatment with antibiotics may be needed to clear up the infection in some cases. Skin abscesses that do not improve on their own need to be lanced (punctured and drained) by a doctor.

Cellulitis

Cellulitis (sel-yoo-LYE-tis) is an inflammation of the skin and/or the tissues beneath it. The culprits behind the infection are almost always group A streptococcus or *Staphylococcus aureus* (stah-fih-lo-KAH-kus ARE-ree-us) bacteria. Cellulitis may occur in people with diabetes* or those who have immune system problems even if they do not have a skin injury. The infection can occur anywhere on the body, but it is found most frequently on the face and lower legs. It appears as tender, red, swollen areas of skin. The skin in the infected area may feel stretched and warm. A few days after the first symptoms, patients may experience fever, chills, and muscle aches. Red streaks also may appear on the skin, signaling the spread of the infection.

Antibiotics are used to treat cellulitis. Even after the infection is gone, the skin may look different for several weeks. Complications are rare, but they can include sepsis*, gangrene*, and lymphangitis*. Cellulitis may involve infection of deeper tissue called the fascia (FAY-she-uh). Infection in this layer can be very serious or even life threatening and often requires surgery to remove the infected tissue.

Necrotizing fasciitis

Necrotizing fasciitis (NEH-kro-tie-zing fash-e-EYE-tis), also called flesh-eating disease, is a rare but potentially fatal disease caused by group A streptococcus bacteria infection. It affects the deeper layers of skin and tissues beneath the skin. Necrotizing fasciitis starts with sudden painful swelling and discoloration (red, purple, or bronze) of the skin. Often, the appearance of the affected skin does not reflect how far the infection has spread into the deeper layers of tissue. The disease can spread rapidly, with the infected area growing larger and darker. The ability to feel in the infected area disappears as the skin tissue dies. As the infection quickly progresses, the patient can become very ill. Early treatment with antibiotics and surgery to remove the damaged tissue is extremely important. Recovery may take several months.

Molluscum contagiosum

Molluscum contagiosum (moh-LUS-kum kon-tay-jee-O-sum), caused by a virus, produces small, solid, dome-shaped bumps on the surface of the skin. They are flesh-colored and

* **hair follicle** (FAH-lih-kul) is the skin structure from which hair develops and grows.

* **diabetes** (dye-uh-BEE-teez) is a condition in which the body's pancreas does not produce enough insulin or the body cannot use the insulin it makes effectively, resulting in increased levels of sugar in the blood. This can lead to increased urination, dehydration, weight loss, weakness, and a number of other symptoms and complications related to chemical imbalances within the body.

* **sepsis** is a potentially serious spreading of infection, usually bacterial, through the bloodstream and body.

* **gangrene** (GANG-green) is the decay or death of living tissue caused by a lack of oxygen supply to the tissue and/or bacterial infection of the tissue.

* **lymphangitis** (lim-fan-JIE-tis) is inflammation of the lymphatic system, the system that carries lymph through the body. Lymph is a clear fluid that contains white blood cells.

*genitals (JEH-nih-tuls) are the external sexual organs.

pearly with a dimple in the center. The growths are similar to warts. Viruses cause both conditions—poxvirus in the case of molluscum contagiosum and human papillomavirus in the case of warts. Growths can be single, but they most often appear in groups on the trunk, arms, legs, and genitals* and occasionally on the face.

The disease usually clears up by itself over several months, although new growths may arise on the skin if the virus spreads through contact with infected areas. Doctors may recommend home treatment with over-the-counter medications or removal of the growths by freezing, surgery, laser therapy, or acid treatments.

Herpes Simplex Virus There are two types of the herpes simplex virus (HSV): HSV-1 and HSV-2. Both can show up as skin infections. HSV-1 can cause small, clear blisters (also known as cold sores, fever blisters, or oral herpes) on the face, and HSV-2 can cause blisters in the genital area. These blisters can break, bleed, and crust over, leaving red spots of healing skin.

There is no cure for either HSV-1 or HSV-2. Currently, antiviral medications can help control outbreaks of herpes virus and are used to treat genital herpes or sometimes recurrent cold sores from HSV-1.

Warts Warts are caused by human papillomavirus (pah-pih-LO-mah-vy-rus), or HPV. They can be skin-colored, pink, tan, or white, and they may appear anywhere on the body. Common warts usually are seen on the hands (especially around the nails), feet, and face, because the virus spreads most easily to those areas. Common warts are rough and raised, but plantar warts, found on the soles of the feet, are flat. Unlike other warts, plantar warts can be painful.

Many warts disappear by themselves after months or even years. Treatments are available for those that do not, including over-the-counter medications or professional treatment by freezing, surgery, laser therapy, or acid treatments.

Are Skin and Soft Tissue Infections Contagious?

Necrotizing fasciitis, cellulitis, and abscesses are not contagious from person to person, but the bacteria that can cause these infections can spread between people. Dermatophytes, warts, and molluscum contagiosum spread fairly easily through skin-to-skin contact.

How Are Skin and Soft Tissue Infections Diagnosed?

A doctor examines the size, shape, and color of the affected area and checks it for tenderness and warmth. The doctor may order blood tests for cellulitis to assess the extent of the infection; tests of skin scrapings for suspected fungal infections or molluscum contagiosum; or tests on a tissue sample for necrotizing fasciitis. Doctors can use a special type of filtered ultraviolet light to check for tinea capitis because the fungi that cause it glow a characteristic color when the light is shined on the infected area.

Can Skin and Soft Tissue Infections Be Prevented?

The best way to prevent skin and soft tissue infections is to avoid getting cuts, scrapes, bites, or any kind of open wound. Frequent hand washing can curb the spread of bacteria. Doctors also advise keeping any opening in the skin clean and dry. It is wise to consult a doctor if the area around the wound becomes reddened, hot, or painful or if the infected person develops a fever. Dermatophyte infection is best avoided by keeping the skin dry, such as in areas where sweating occurs.

Resources

Organization

American Academy of Dermatology, P.O. Box 4014, Schaumburg, IL 60168. The American Academy of Dermatology offers fact sheets and general information about various skin problems on its website. Information for young people can be found through the Kids' Connection at the website.
Telephone 847-330-0230
http://www.aad.org

Website

KidsHealth.org. KidsHealth is a website created by the medical experts of the Nemours Foundation and is devoted to issues of children's health. It contains articles on a variety of health topics, including cellulitis, impetigo, tinea, warts, and other bacterial, fungal, and viral infections. http://www.KidsHealth.org

Skin Parasites

Skin parasites (PAIR-uh-sites) are tiny organisms that invade the skin, often causing irritation and itching.

What Are Skin Parasites?

Parasites live off other living things (including people), often living, feeding, and reproducing on them. Some parasites thrive on human blood and cannot live long without it. When these parasites latch onto someone's skin, they may lay their eggs there. Before long, that person could become the host (an organism that provides another organism, such as

▶ *See also*

Abscesses

Fungal Infections

Gangrene

Herpes Simplex Virus Infections

Impetigo

Ringworm

Sepsis

Skin Parasites

Staphylococcal Infections

Streptococcal Infections

Warts

KEYWORDS
for searching the Internet and other reference sources

Chiggers

Lice

Mites

Nits

Pediculosis

Pediculus humanus capitis

Phthirus pubis

Pubic lice

Sarcoptes scabiei

Scabies

319

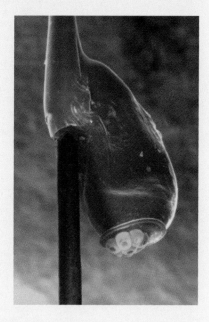

This image shows a magnification of one of the eggs laid by head lice. These eggs, called "nits," are visible to the naked eye. The term "nit-pick," which means to be concerned with insignificant details, derives from the process of taking the tiny eggs out of the hair by hand, a method used for centuries before more effective treatment was widely available. *Custom Medical Stock Photo, Inc.*

*hair follicles (FAH-lih-kulz) are the skin structures from hair develops and grows.

*hives are swollen, itchy patches on the skin.

a parasite or virus, with a place to live and grow) for hundreds or more of the parasites.

Skin parasites are found worldwide and infest large numbers of people. For example, as many as 6 to 12 million people worldwide contract head lice every year, according to the U.S. Centers for Disease Control and Prevention. Head lice most often affect children in school and daycare settings.

What Are Some Common Skin Parasites?

There are many parasites that infest human skin, but lice, scabies (SKAY-beez), and chiggers are among the most common.

Head lice Also known as *Pediculus humanus capitis* (peh-DIH-kyoo-lus HYOO-mah-nus KAH-pih-tis), head lice are six-legged parasites with tiny claws that cling to hairs. They are found on the scalp, neck, and behind the ears. Lice lay visible, whitish eggs called nits. In about 7 days, the nits hatch into young called nymphs (NIMFS). Nymphs grow up fast, and in just 1 week they mature into adult lice that must feed on blood to stay alive. Head lice may not cause any symptoms immediately, but as with other insect bites the body reacts to the invaders, leading to itching and sores from scratching.

Pubic lice Pubic lice, or *Phthirus pubis* (THEER-us PYOO-bus), invade the pubic hair and sometimes other body hair such as beards, eyebrows, eyelashes, and armpit hair. They often are called "crabs" because of their crab-like appearance. Pubic lice cause intense itching, especially at night, when they feed by burying their heads into hair follicles*. The nits or adult lice can be seen on pubic hairs or surrounding skin.

Scabies Microscopic *Sarcoptes scabiei* (sar-KOP-teez SKAY-be-eye) mites cause an infestation called scabies. The mites work their way under the top layer of skin and lay their eggs. Most people are not even aware of the intruders until intense itching begins 2 to 6 weeks later. Red, pimple-like bumps appear on the skin, and there may be wavy lines on the skin tracing the mites' paths, especially in the webbing between the fingers and in the skin folds at the back of the knees and the inside of the elbows.

Chiggers Chiggers are mites that tend to live in weeds, tall grass, or wooded areas. The chigger larvae (LAR-vee, immature mites) feed on a variety of animals, including humans. The larvae crawl onto the skin of passersby and can use their tiny claws to grab onto human hair. They then attach to the skin, usually at the ankles or waist or in skin folds, with hooked mouthparts and feed on skin cells. Unlike lice and scabies, chiggers only feed on their host for a couple of days, then let go and fall off. Chigger bites can cause a red bump that continues to grow in size, a skin rash, hives*, and severe itchiness. Sometimes the larvae are visible in the center of the bump.

How Are Skin Parasites Spread?

Despite what many believe, people do not get skin parasites because of poor hygiene. Instead, skin parasites tend to spread in situations where they can walk or fall from one person to another (or in the case of chiggers, from vegetation to human skin). The parasites often require relatively prolonged and close contact to move between people, and they spread most easily in crowded conditions, from sharing personal items, and from skin-to-skin contact.

Head lice in particular fall easily onto their next victims in close quarters. They also can infest hairbrushes, barrettes, hats, and sometimes clothes or bed linens. If other people use these items, they can become infested as well. Pubic lice spread mostly through sexual contact, but people also can get them from bed linens and clothes.

Scabies spreads quickly in crowded living conditions or in places with lots of skin-to-skin contact (such as daycare centers and nursing homes). Like lice, scabies can be passed through sexual contact and by sharing clothes, towels, and bed linens.

Diagnosis and Treatment

Doctors often diagnose skin parasite infestations just by spotting the parasites, their eggs, larvae, or characteristic red bumps on the skin. With scabies, a skin scraping might be taken to check for mites, eggs, and mite feces (FEE-seez, or bowel movements). However, this test is not always accurate because the mites may have moved from the spot that was scraped.

Over-the-counter and prescription lotions and shampoos (known as pediculicides, peh-DIH-kyoo-lih-sides) can be used to kill head lice. In some cases, treatment may need to be repeated or replaced with stronger medications because lice are becoming resistant to some treatments. Other people living in the same house with the infested person may be treated at the same time.

Pubic lice also are treated with a pediculicide, similar to the treatment of head lice. If the infestation includes the eyelashes, petroleum jelly is applied several times a day to the eyelids for a week or more.

Patients with scabies are given medicated lotions to apply over the entire body, and the lotion must stay on for 8 to 12 hours. Chigger bites do not require any special treatment to heal, but antihistamines* may ease itching.

Infestation with lice and scabies can persist until they are treated properly. Once treatment begins, patients usually are no longer contagious after a day or two, but sores and itching may not disappear for a couple of weeks. Chigger bites heal quickly.

Can Skin Parasites Cause Medical Complications?

Complications of skin parasites are rare. Frequent or rough scratching of bites or sores can lead to bacterial infections, such as impetigo*. If

* **antihistamines** (an-tie-HIS-tuh-meens) are drugs used to combat allergic reactions and relieve itching.

* **impetigo** (im-pih-TEE-go) is a bacterial skin infection that usually occurs around the nose and mouth and causes itching and fluid-filled blisters that often burst and form yellowish crusts.

321

lice spread to eyebrows or eyelashes, the eyelids may become infected. Norwegian or crusted scabies is a form of scabies that can be severe in people with weak immune systems, such as those with a chronic* illness and elderly people.

How Can People Prevent Infestation with Skin Parasites?

To avoid skin parasites, experts recommend that people:

■ shower daily, wash hands frequently, and wear clean clothes

■ avoid anyone who has lice or scabies until that person is treated

■ never share brushes, hats, bed linens, or clothes

■ practice abstinence (not having sex); birth control does not prevent pubic lice or scabies

■ avoid chigger-infested areas and wear socks, long pants, and long sleeves in wooded or grassy areas

To prevent the spread of parasites in a home when a family member has been diagnosed with an infestation, it is wise to:

■ wash bed linens, towels, and clothes in hot water, then dry them on high heat

■ vacuum the entire house, then throw the vacuum cleaner bag away

■ disinfect combs and hair items

■ seal items that cannot be cleaned in airtight plastic bags for 2 weeks; at the end of that time, any parasites on those items will have died

In addition, children who have skin parasites should stay home from school or daycare until a day or two after they begin their treatment.

Resources

Organization

U.S. Centers for Disease Control and Prevention (CDC), 1600 Clifton Road, Atlanta, GA 30333. The CDC is the U.S. government authority for information about infectious and other diseases. It posts fact sheets about various parasitic infestations and diseases at its website. Telephone 800-311-3435
http://www.cdc.gov

Website

KidsHealth.org. KidsHealth is a website created by the medical experts of the Nemours Foundation and is devoted to issues of children's health. It contains articles on a variety of health topics, including lice, scabies, and chiggers.
http://www.KidsHealth.org

▶ *See also*
Skin and Soft Tissue Infections

Smallpox

Smallpox is a contagious and often fatal infection caused by the variola (ver-e-O-luh) virus.

What Is Smallpox?

What do Queen Mary II of England, King Louis XV of France, and Czar Peter II of Russia have in common? Other than being royalty, they all died from smallpox, one of the deadliest diseases in history. This devastating illness first surfaced thousands of years ago, and many believe smallpox killed more people than all other diseases combined before it was wiped out in the late 1970s. The variola (from the Latin word *varus*, meaning "spotted") virus causes two types of smallpox: variola major and variola minor. Variola major (the type discussed in this chapter) is extremely serious and can be fatal in up to 30 percent of cases. The milder variola minor is fatal in less than 1 percent of patients.

How Common Is the Disease?

Thanks to the vaccine* developed by Edward Jenner in 1796 and the World Health Organization's (WHO) intensified immunization program begun in 1967, smallpox is no longer found in the world; the last naturally occurring case was reported in Somalia in Africa in 1977. Before this successful eradication program, the illness affected millions of people of all ages every year. Those who survived the severe period of infection often were left scarred or blinded.

Is It Contagious?

Smallpox is so contagious that just one infected person can launch an epidemic*. As soon as the first symptoms of the disease appear, an infected person can spread the virus by coughing, sneezing, or even talking. This expels tiny virus-packed drops of moisture into the air. When a healthy person breathes in these drops, the virus finds a new home. Less often, touching patients' sores or even just their bed linens or clothes can spread the infection. Smallpox is typically most contagious during the first week of illness. Outbreaks of the disease in a community have tended to occur at 2- to 3-week intervals.

Signs and Symptoms

Once the virus enters the body, it quickly reproduces and takes over healthy cells. An infected person usually is not even aware of the viral intruders for at least a week. Then the first wave of smallpox symptoms appears, often resembling those of a cold or the flu: fever, extreme tiredness, headache, backache, and occasionally, nausea (NAW-zee-uh) and vomiting. These symptoms can last up to a week. About 2 to 3 days

KEYWORDS
for searching the Internet and other reference sources

Biological weapon

Edward Jenner

Vaccinia vaccine

Variola major

Variola minor

Vesicles

* **vaccine** (vak-SEEN) is a preparation of killed or weakened germs, or a part of a germ or product it produces, given to prevent or lessen the severity of the disease that can result if a person is exposed to the germ itself. Use of vaccines for this purpose is called immunization.

* **epidemic** (eh-pih-DEH-mik) is an outbreak of disease, especially infectious disease, in which the number of cases suddenly becomes far greater than usual. Usually epidemics are outbreaks of diseases in specific regions, whereas worldwide epidemics are called pandemics.

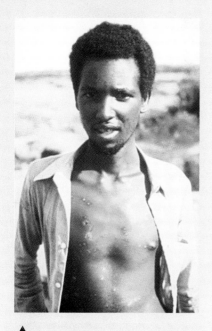

Ali Maow Maalin, of Somalia. He is the last person known to have contracted smallpox, in 1977. *Science VU/CDC/Visuals Unlimited*

* **lesions** (LEE-zhuns) is a general term referring to sores or damaged or irregular areas of tissue.

* **pus** is a thick, creamy fluid, usually yellow or greenish in color, that forms at the site of an infection. Pus contains infection-fighting white cells and other substances.

* **biological warfare** is a method of waging war by using harmful microorganisms to purposely spread disease to many people.

* **immunology** (ih-myoo-NOL-uh-jee) is the science of the system of the body composed of specialized cells and the substances they produce that help protect the body against disease-causing germs.

after the onset of symptoms, a rash of red blisters or lesions* appears suddenly on the face, arms, and palms. Within a few days, the lesions fill with fluid and pus* and spread to other parts of the body, including the inside of the nose and mouth. The sores can expand and break open, causing pain. Eventually, scabs form and later fall off. During its early stages, smallpox can be confused with chicken pox, which is caused by a different virus (varicella zoster, var-uh-SEH-luh ZOS-ter). Chicken pox produces a much milder rash that usually develops on the body and is less prominent on the face, arms, and hands.

How Do Doctors Make the Diagnosis?

Because smallpox was wiped out in the last quarter of the twentieth century, very few doctors practicing today have ever seen a case. With the heightened awareness of the possibility that smallpox could be used as a weapon in biological warfare*, doctors are being trained to recognize the disease. To make a diagnosis of smallpox, tests would be done on blood and fluid from a patient's lesions to identify the virus. To prevent a widespread outbreak, the patient most likely would be isolated, and those in close contact with the person would be vaccinated. If just one case of smallpox were diagnosed today, it could cause a public health emergency.

What Is the Treatment for Smallpox?

There is no known cure for smallpox. Receiving the smallpox vaccine within 4 days of being exposed to someone who has the disease may prevent infection or lessen symptoms. Scientists are looking for new medicines as possible treatments for the disease. Public health agencies rec-

BIRTH OF A VACCINE

Edward Jenner often is called the father of modern immunology* because of his major contribution to ending smallpox. As an English country doctor, Jenner was fascinated that milkmaids exposed to cowpox (a disease that affects cows and is caused by a virus similar to variola) did not contract smallpox. He developed a vaccine containing live cowpox virus and injected it into an 8-year-old boy. The boy did not contract smallpox, and vaccinations for the disease quickly became standard. Following Jenner's discovery, fatalities from smallpox dropped significantly. Jenner believed that his vaccine provided lifelong immunity to the disease. It is now thought, however, that the vaccine may not protect people for more than 10 years.

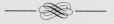

ommend that patients who have symptoms of smallpox be isolated immediately—either in a special unit of a hospital or at home—so that the infection will not spread to others. Health care workers are advised to take careful precautions when treating these patients. In the absence of a cure, treatment focuses on easing symptoms and preventing further infections. Patients may receive intravenous fluids (fluids injected directly into a vein), pain relievers, and antibiotics (to combat bacterial infections that can develop in the open sores) while the disease runs its course.

What to Expect

Smallpox infection can last from 3 to 4 weeks or until the last scabs fall off. The lesions often leave behind deep, pitted scars. When smallpox is fatal, patients usually die during the second week of illness. Smallpox can lead to serious complications, including these:

- hemorrhagic (heh-muh-RAH-jik) smallpox (which is associated with bleeding in the skin and body membranes)
- malignant smallpox (in which the sores are flat and close together)
- blindness
- bacterial infections
- pneumonia*
- encephalitis*

How Can Smallpox Be Prevented?

Widespread vaccination in the United States for smallpox ended in 1972. In 1980 WHO declared the disease eradicated. It is unknown how long vaccine-generated immunity* lasts. Experts believe that it prevents infection for at least 10 years, but scientists think that few people in the world today are still immune to smallpox.

Today there are two official facilities that store samples of the virus: the U.S. Centers for Disease Control and Prevention (CDC) in Atlanta, Georgia, and the Russian State Research Center of Virology and Biotechnology in Koltsovo. In the unlikely event that bioterrorists were to get access to any of these stored samples, it is possible that they might use the virus to launch a biological attack. If this were to happen, vaccines would be in high demand. To prepare for such a potential emergency, mass production of the vaccine is under way in the United States.

Owing to possible side effects of the smallpox vaccine, the CDC suggests that it be given only to those at greatest risk of being exposed to the virus, including military personnel and "first responders," for example, medical care providers, law enforcement personnel, and laboratory workers. About one in a million people who are vaccinated die from the effects of the vaccine, and a small percentage experience scarring or serious infections.

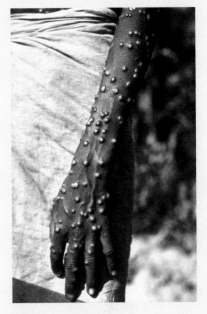

▲

Though most often spread by drops of moisture expelled through an infected person's cough, smallpox may also be acquired through direct contact with the person's sores. *Phototake*

* **pneumonia** (nu-MO-nyah) is inflammation of the lung.

* **encephalitis** (en-seh-fuh-LYE-tis) is an inflammation of the brain, usually caused by a viral infection.

* **immunity** (ih-MYOON-uh-tee) is the condition of being protected against an infectious disease. Immunity often develops after a germ is introduced to the body. One type of immunity occurs when the body makes special protein molecules called antibodies to fight the disease-causing germ. The next time that germ enters the body, the antibodies quickly attack it, usually preventing the germ from causing disease.

Resources

Organizations

Center for Civilian Biodefense Strategies, Johns Hopkins University, 111 Market Place, Suite 830, Baltimore, MD 21202. The Center for Civilian Biodefense Strategies has fact sheets on smallpox and its place in bioterrorism.
Telephone 410-223-1667
http://www.hopkins-biodefense.org

U.S. Centers for Disease Control and Prevention (CDC), 1600 Clifton Road, Atlanta, GA 30333. The CDC provides fact sheets and vaccine information on smallpox.
Telephone 800-311-3435
http://www.cdc.gov

World Health Organization (WHO), Avenue Appia 20, 1211 Geneva 27, Switzerland. The WHO website has links to fact sheets and information on the prevention and control of smallpox.
Telephone 011-41-22-791-2111
http://www.who.int

▶ See also

Bioterrorism

Encephalitis

Pneumonia

Public Health

Varicella (Chicken Pox) and Herpes Zoster (Shingles)

KEYWORDS
for searching the Internet and other reference sources

Adenovirus

Common cold

Group A streptococci

Influenza

Mononucleosis

Pharyngitis

Strep throat

Streptococcal infections

Viral infections

* **influenza** (in-floo-EN-zuh), also known as the flu, is a contagious viral infection that attacks the respiratory tract.

* **adenovirus** (ah-deh-no-VY-rus) is a type of virus that can produce a variety of symptoms, including upper respiratory disease, when it infects humans.

Sore Throat

The pain and discomfort of a sore throat, also called pharyngitis (fair-un-JY-tis), are usually the result of inflammation due to infection or irritation.

What Is a Sore Throat?

A sore throat can be a symptom of many infectious diseases. Viral infections such as the common cold, influenza*, adenovirus* infection, and infectious mononucleosis* cause most sore throats. Bacterial infections are less common, but the sore throats they produce usually are more severe. Group A beta hemolytic streptococci (he-muh-LIH-tik strep-tuh-KAH-kye) are the most common bacterial culprits, and they cause strep throat. Rarely, fungal infections can cause a sore throat, usually in people with weakened immune systems. Non-infectious causes of sore throat include allergies, postnasal drip (the dripping of mucus from the back of the nose into the throat), and too much yelling or straining the voice. Smoking and other irritants also can cause a sore throat.

Are Sore Throats Common?

Sore throats are very common, especially in children. It is not unusual for children between the ages of 5 and 10 to develop several sore throat infections over the course of a year. Most of these illnesses are common viral respiratory infections. About 15 percent of all sore throats are caused by group A streptococci.

All of the infections that cause sore throats are contagious. They can spread through contact with drops of fluid from an infected person that can be coughed or sneezed into the air. The drops can be inhaled or transferred by the hand to the mouth or nose. The infections that cause sore throats also can spread through direct contact with an infected person, such as through kissing.

What Are the Signs and Symptoms of a Sore Throat?

Sore throats are painful, sometimes swollen, and red. Many viral infections that cause sore throats are associated with other symptoms, including hoarseness, runny nose, cough, and diarrhea (dye-uh-REE-uh).

Streptococcal infections frequently produce a bright red throat, trouble swallowing, and swollen, often tender lymph nodes* in the neck. The tonsils* often are enlarged, there may be white specks and pus* on them, or they may be covered with a gray or white coating. Other symptoms of strep throat include high fever, headache, and abdominal* pain.

Sore throat is a common symptom of infectious mononucleosis, a viral infection caused by the Epstein-Barr (EP-steen BAR) virus. The tonsils become very swollen and, as in strep throat, may have white patches or an extensive coating. Swallowing is difficult and, in a few cases, the tonsils enlarge enough to cause difficulty breathing. Other signs and symptoms of mononucleosis include swollen lymph nodes in the neck, fever, extreme tiredness, muscle aches, and an enlarged spleen.

How Do Doctors Diagnose the Cause of a Sore Throat?

If the doctor suspects that a patient might have a strep throat infection, the doctor will use a cotton swab to take a sample from the throat and tonsils for a culture*. Often, the doctor will do a rapid strep test in the office, but this quick test is not as reliable as a culture.

Infectious mononucleosis is diagnosed by examining blood samples for antibodies* to the virus. Nasal and throat swabs can be tested to detect other causes of a sore throat, if necessary. If a patient's sore throat and other symptoms match those of a common viral cold or respiratory infection, the doctor may base the diagnosis on the physical symptoms alone.

How Is a Sore Throat Treated?

Treatment of a sore throat depends on the diagnosis. If it stems from a common cold caused by a virus, treatment is aimed at relieving symptoms until the illness disappears. Drinking plenty of fluids can help

* **mononucleosis** (mah-no-nu-klee-O-sis) is an infectious illness caused by a virus with symptoms that typically include fever, sore throat, swollen glands, and tiredness.

* **lymph** (LIMF) **nodes** are small, bean-shaped masses of tissue that contain immune system cells that fight harmful microorganisms. Lymph nodes may swell during infections.

* **tonsils** are paired clusters of lymph tissue in the throat that help protect the body from bacteria and viruses that enter through a person's nose or mouth.

* **pus** is a thick, creamy fluid, usually yellow or greenish in color, that forms at the site of an infection. Pus contains infection-fighting white cells and other substances.

* **abdominal** (ab-DAH-mih-nul) refers to the area of the body below the ribs and above the hips that contains the stomach, intestines, and other organs.

* **culture** (KUL-chur) is a test in which a sample of fluid or tissue from the body is placed in a dish containing material that supports the growth of certain organisms. Typically, within days the organisms will grow and can be identified.

* **antibodies** (AN-tih-bah-deez) are protein molecules produced by the body's immune system to help fight specific infections caused by microorganisms, such as bacteria and viruses.

dehydration (dee-hi-DRAY-shun) is a condition in which the body is depleted of water, usually caused by excessive and unreplaced loss of body fluids, such as through sweating, vomiting, or diarrhea.

mucus (MYOO-kus) is a thick, slippery substance that lines the insides of many body parts.

rheumatic (roo-MAH-tik) **fever** is a condition associated with fever, joint pain, and inflammation affecting many parts of the body, including the heart. It occurs following infections with certain types of strep bacteria.

kidney is one of the pair of organs that filter blood and remove waste products and excess water from the body in the form of urine

abscesses (AB-seh-sez) are localized or walled off accumulations of pus caused by infection that can occur in the skin and anywhere within the body.

prevent dehydration* and clear out mucus* in the back of the throat. Water, ginger ale, warm tea with honey, and soups are good choices, but not acidic juices (such as lemonade or orange juice), because they can irritate the throat. Gargling with warm salt water can help soothe a sore throat, and over-the-counter pain relievers and throat drops can help ease symptoms as well. Antibiotics are not effective for treating viral infections such as colds. Most viral sore throats go away on their own without complications, and they generally clear up within a few days to a week.

When strep throat has been diagnosed, a 10-day course of antibiotics usually is prescribed; all of the antibiotics should be taken as directed to prevent complications. Strep throat can lead to rheumatic fever*, kidney* problems, or throat abscesses*, and prompt treatment with antibiotics can prevent some of these complications. Symptoms of strep throat usually improve within 1 to 2 days of starting antibiotics.

The best treatment for infectious mononucleosis is rest. In addition, over-the-counter medications such as acetaminophen (uh-see-teh-MIH-noh-fen) can help relieve pain and fever. Infectious mononucleosis can take from 1 to 2 months to subside, and other symptoms from the illness, such as tiredness, can remain for months after.

Can Sore Throats Be Prevented?

Many respiratory infections are spread through contact with respiratory fluids from infected people. The best prevention strategy is basic hygiene, which includes covering the mouth when sneezing or coughing and washing hands regularly. If someone has an infection or has been in close contact with someone who does, it is wise not to share utensils, food, and drinking glasses with that person.

Resources

Organizations

National Institute of Allergy and Infectious Diseases (NIAID), Building 31, Room 7A-50, 31 Center Drive MSC 2520, Bethesda, MD 20892. The NIAID, part of the National Institutes of Health, posts information about sore throats at its website. http://www.niaid.nih.gov

U.S. National Library of Medicine, 8600 Rockville Pike, Bethesda, MD 20894. The National Library of Medicine has a website packed with information on diseases and conditions such as sore throat. It also offers consumer resources, dictionaries and encyclopedias of medical terms, and directories of doctors and helpful organizations. Telephone 888-346-3656 http://www.nlm.nih.gov

Website

KidsHealth.org. KidsHealth is a website created by the medical experts of the Nemours Foundation and is devoted to issues of children's health. It contains articles on a variety of health topics, including sore throat.
http://www.KidsHealth.org

Staphylococcal Infections

Staphylococcal (stah-fih-lo-KAH-kul) infections are infections caused by Staphylococcus aureus *(stah-fih-lo-KAH-kus ARE-ree-us) and related species of bacteria.*

What Are Staphylococcal Infections?

They cannot be seen with the naked eye, but bacteria cover the skin's surface. *Staphylococcus aureus* bacteria, also called staph bacteria, often live on people's skin, particularly around openings such as the nose, mouth, genitals*, and rectum* and sometimes inside the nose and mouth, without causing disease. But when a person's skin is broken or cut, the bacteria can enter the wound and cause an infection. Staph infections range from minor skin infections to joint, bone, or lung infections to widespread or systemic infections. Some strains* of staph produce a toxin (or poison) that causes illness.

Newborns, elderly people, and people with immune systems weakened by diseases such as cancer and AIDS* are at greater risk of serious staph infections. Some serious infections can be acquired in a hospital when a patient is being treated for another condition.

How Common Are They?

Some species of staph bacteria are present on people's skin all the time. The more dangerous *Staphylococcus aureus* may come and go regularly from people's noses and skin. Skin infections caused by staph, such as boils, are quite common. Many staph infections are minor and do not require treatment; serious staph infections are less common.

Are They Contagious?

Sometimes staph infections of the skin are contagious. If a person touches another person who has a staph infection of the skin and then touches his or her own mouth or nose or an area of broken skin, the staph infection can spread. A person also can spread the bacteria from one part of the body to another through touch. Staph can be transmitted via contaminated surfaces and food and through the air as well.

 See also

Common Cold

Influenza

Laryngitis

Mononucleosis, Infectious

Sinusitis

Streptococcal Infections

KEYWORDS
for searching the Internet and other reference sources

Antibiotic resistance

Cellulitis

Food poisoning

Impetigo

Methicillin-resistant staphylococcus aureus (MRSA)

Scalded skin syndrome

Staphylococcus aureus

Toxic shock syndrome

Vancomycin intermediate staphylococcus aureus (VISA)

* **genitals** (JEH-nih-tuls) are the external sexual organs.

* **rectum** is the final portion of the large intestine, connecting the colon to the anus.

* **strains** are various subtypes of organisms, such as viruses or bacteria.

* **AIDS**, or acquired immunodeficiency (ih-myoo-no-dih-FIH-shen-see) syndrome, is an infection that severely weakens the immune system; it is caused by the human immunodeficiency virus (HIV).

The Evolution of Antibiotic-Resistant Staph

Antibiotics are used widely to treat infections such as those caused by staph. Over time, staph bacteria may become stronger so that the antibiotics may not be as effective against the germ, which is known as antibiotic resistance. When Alexander Fleming discovered penicillin in 1928, staph bacteria were highly sensitive to it. Now, few staph bacteria are killed by penicillin. These bacteria often are resistant to many antibiotics. The more important strains of antibiotic-resistant staph are known as methicillin-resistant staphylococcus aureus (MRSA). MRSA is resistant to commonplace antibiotics, but it is still susceptible to the last-resort, more powerful medications. A more serious strain of staph infection, vancomycin intermediate staphylococcus aureus (VISA), can resist vancomycin, one of the most powerful (and last-resort) antibiotics available. Although all strains of the bacteria found so far have been treatable with some type of antibiotic, VISA potentially could defy all medication currently available to treat such infections. MRSA and VISA infections usually develop only in a hospital or health care facility, where prolonged treatment of patients with several antibiotics is common.

* **pus** is a thick, creamy fluid, usually yellow or greenish in color, that forms at the site of an infection. Pus contains infection-fighting white cells and other substances.

* **hair follicle** (FAH-lih-kul) is the skin structure from which hair develops and grows.

What Are Some Types of Staph Infections?

Impetigo (im-pih-TEE-go) is a skin infection that usually occurs around the nose and mouth. In impetigo, fluid-filled blisters develop and often burst and form yellowish crusts. Impetigo is a contagious infection that can spread if a person scratches the blisters and then scratches or touches another area of the body.

Carbuncles (KAR-bung-kulz) and furuncles (FYOOR-ung-kulz), also known as boils, are staph infections that produce a red, swollen bump filled with pus* in the skin surrounding a hair follicle*. With boils pus forms in a single hair follicle, whereas carbuncles form from grouped furuncles and have several small chambers, like a series of connected boils.

Cellulitis (sel-yoo-LYE-tis) is an infection of the deeper layers of the skin and the connective tissues below the skin's surface. People with cellulitis usually have an area of red, swollen, tender, warm skin. They also may have fever, swollen lymph nodes*, and a general feeling of illness. Cellulitis is most common on the face and lower legs.

Scalded skin syndrome (also known as Ritter disease) is a staph infection that typically occurs in infants and children less than 5 years old and causes large portions of skin to be shed from the body. In this condition the staph bacteria produce a toxin that damages skin. Fluid collects beneath the skin and loosens it so that large portions slip off when rubbed. When the skin slips off, it leaves raw areas that eventually crust over. When the area under the skin is exposed, the child is at risk of excessive fluid loss and additional bacterial infections. Other symptoms include fever and skin redness and tenderness. Babies with this condition may become extremely ill.

Toxic shock syndrome (TSS) is a severe infection that, like scalded skin syndrome, is caused by a toxin produced by staph bacteria. It was first recognized in the late 1970s and early 1980s, mostly among women who were using certain types of very absorbent tampons, but it can occur in people of both sexes and in both children and adults. Because this type of absorbent tampon is no longer available, TSS now usually develops after surgery or in wounds that, in most cases, do not look infected but contain the toxin-producing staph. Skin abscesses* or other staphylococcal infections also may lead to TSS. Symptoms of TSS include sudden fever, low blood pressure, very red rash, vomiting, diarrhea (dye-uh-REE-uh), and muscle pain.

Staph bacteria can produce other types of toxins that cause food poisoning if a person eats contaminated food (usually meats, poultry, eggs, and dairy products) that has not been heated or refrigerated at the proper temperature. Symptoms include belly pain, nausea (NAW-zee-uh), and vomiting. If the food poisoning is severe, a person may experience headaches, muscle aches, and blood pressure changes.

Some staph infections affect internal organs. Staph is a common cause of the bone infection osteomyelitis (ah-stee-o-my-uh-LYE-tis). Staph infections also may cause pneumonia (nu-MO-nyah), an inflammation of the lungs; blood infection (sepsis); and, more rarely, meningitis (meh-nin-JY-tis), an inflammation of the membranes that surround the brain and the spinal cord (the meninges, meh-NIN-jeez). The bacteria may spread from an infection elsewhere in the body, or they can come from a medical device, such as a catheter*, that has been colonized* by staph bacteria. *Staphylococcus aureus* also may infect the heart valves, where it causes inflammation and gives rise to a condition called endocarditis (en-do-kar-DYE-tis).

How Is a Staph Infection Diagnosed?

A doctor may diagnose and treat a staph infection based on its appearance, but a definite diagnosis is made by identifying the organism under a microscope or by culture*. Samples are taken from the site of the infection, which may be the skin, the blood, or an abscess. Staph food poisoning generally is diagnosed based on symptoms, dietary history, and sometimes illness in other people who have eaten the same food or eaten at the same place.

What Is the Treatment for Staph Infections?

Minor skin infections caused by staph bacteria often can be treated with an over-the-counter antibiotic ointment, or they can heal on their own. If a person has an abscess that stems from a staph infection, surgery to drain the pus may be necessary in addition to antibiotics, to allow the infection to heal.

More serious staph infections, such as endocarditis, osteomyelitis, TSS, and scalded skin syndrome, usually require hospitalization and supportive care, such as antibiotics, intravenous fluids to prevent dehydration, and other medications. Endocarditis caused by staph may require surgery in which the infected, damaged heart valve is removed and an artificial valve is inserted.

Because antibiotics are used widely to treat both minor and serious infections caused by staph and other bacteria, some strains of bacteria have become resistant to common antibiotics. New medications and forms of treatment will be important in the future, and scientists are working to develop a *Staphylococcus aureus* vaccine that might help people with weakened immune systems resist staph infection.

How Long Does Infection Last?

Minor skin infections caused by staph bacteria usually clear up within a week, whereas more serious widespread illnesses may take several weeks to more than a month to get better.

What Are the Complications of Staph Infection?

Minor staph skin infections rarely result in complications, but some can produce more widespread infection, such as sepsis, a serious systemic infection caused by bacteria invading the bloodstream. TSS can lead to

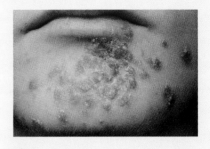

▲

The staph infection called impetigo most often involves the face. Impetigo is more common among young children. In young adults, it may be a complication of other skin problems. *Custom Medical Stock Photo, Inc.*

* **lymph** (LIMF) **nodes** are small, bean-shaped masses of tissue that contain immune system cells that fight harmful microorganisms. Lymph nodes may swell during infections.

* **abscesses** (AB-seh-sez) are localized or walled off accumulations of pus caused by infection that can occur anywhere within the body.

* **catheter** (KAH-thuh-ter) is a small plastic tube placed through a body opening into an organ (such as the bladder) or through the skin directly into a blood vessel. It is used to give fluids to or drain fluids from a person.

* **colonized** means that a group of organisms, particularly bacteria, are living on or inside the body without causing symptoms of infection.

* **culture** (KUL-chur) is a test in which a sample of fluid or tissue from the body is placed in a dish containing material that supports the growth of certain organisms. Typically, within days the organisms will grow and can be identified.

*shock is a serious condition in which blood pressure is very low and not enough blood flows to the body's organs and tissues. Untreated, shock may result in death.

shock*, organ failure, and death. Scalded skin syndrome can give rise to other infections, dehydration, and sepsis. Osteomyelitis can cause permanent bone damage and may require surgical treatment.

Can Staph Infections Be Prevented?

There are several ways to help prevent the spread of staph infections:

- washing hands before eating and after using the toilet, or touching the nose
- washing any cuts, scrapes, or open sores
- keeping wounds covered with a clean bandage

Food poisoning can be prevented by washing hands before food preparation, storing food properly before cooking, cooking food to the appropriate temperatures, using clean utensils and dishes, and refrigerating or freezing food as soon as possible after cooking. To lessen the risk of TSS, women are advised to use less-absorbent tampons, to change them frequently, and not to use only tampons during a menstrual period, or to avoid tampons altogether.

Resource

Organization

U.S. Centers for Disease Control and Prevention (CDC), 1600 Clifton Road, Atlanta, GA 30333. The CDC provides information about infections such as staph, how often they occur, and how to prevent them.
Telephone 800-311-3435
http://www.cdc.gov

► *See also*

Abscesses

Endocarditis, Infectious

Intestinal Infections

Meningitis

Osteomyelitis

Sepsis

Skin and Soft Tissue Infections

KEYWORDS
for searching the Internet and other reference sources

Alpha-hemolytic streptococci

Beta-hemolytic streptococci

Cellulitis

Group A streptococcal (GAS) infections

Group B streptococcal (GBS) infections

Impetigo

Necrotizing fasciitis

Scarlet fever

Sepsis

Strep throat

Toxic shock syndrome

Streptococcal Infections

Streptococcal (strep-tuh-KAH-kul) infections are caused by various strains* of Streptococcus (strep-tuh-KAH-kus) bacteria.

What Are Streptococcal Infections?

Streptococci (strep-tuh-KAH-kye) are common bacteria that live in the human body, including the nose, skin, and genital tract. These bacteria can destroy red blood cells, damage them, or cause no damage at all. The amount of damage they do is used to classify streptococcus strains. The ones that destroy red blood cells are known as beta-hemolytic (he-muh-LIH-tik), and these strains are categorized as groups A through G.

Groups A and B streptococci are most often associated with disease. Group A strep (GAS) infections range from superficial skin infections and strep throat to serious and life-threatening illnesses such as toxic shock syndrome and necrotizing fasciitis (NEH-kro-tie-zing fash-e-EYE-tis). Group B strep (GBS) is the leading cause of life-threatening infections in newborns. In pregnant women, GBS can lead to bladder infections, infections of the womb, and death of the fetus*.

Alpha-hemolytic streptococci are strains that damage red blood cells but do not destroy them. Two important strains are *S. viridans* (VEER-ih-dans), which is found in the mouth and is involved in tooth decay and endocarditis*, and *S. pneumoniae* (nu-MO-nye), which can cause pneumonia*, middle ear infection, and meningitis*.

Group A Streptococcus (GAS) Infections

How common are they? According to the National Institute of Allergy and Infectious Diseases (NIAID), more than 10 million cases of mild GAS infections, such as skin and throat infections, are diagnosed each year. Between 9,000 and 10,000 cases of more serious infections, including toxic shock syndrome and necrotizing fasciitis, occur annually. People with immune systems weakened by diseases such as diabetes or cancer, are at a greater risk for developing serious GAS infections.

Are they contagious? GAS bacteria are contagious and spread through contact with fluid from the mouth or nose of an infected person or contact with infected skin lesions*.

Some GAS infections

- Strep throat, or streptococcal pharyngitis (fair-un-JY-tis), is a painful inflammation of the throat. Symptoms include a sore throat with white patches on the tonsils*, swollen lymph nodes* in the neck, fever, and headache.

- Scarlet fever often occurs along with strep throat or other strep infections. It is caused by strains of group A strep that produce a toxin (or poison) that results in a very red rash and a bright red tongue, along with a high fever.

- Impetigo (im-pih-TEE-go) is a superficial skin infection common in young children. Symptoms include fluid-filled blisters (one or more) surrounded by red skin. The blisters eventually break and form a honey-colored crust.

- Cellulitis (sel-yoo-LYE-tis) is an inflammation of the skin and/or its underlying soft tissues. Symptoms include skin that is red, tender, and painful to the touch; fever; and chills.

- Bacteremia (bak-tuh-REE-me-uh) is the presence of bacteria in the bloodstream, which can spread infection to other organs. Bacteremia that causes symptoms, which is known as sepsis, is

* **strains** are various subtypes of organisms, such as viruses or bacteria.

* **fetus** (FEE-tus) is the term for an unborn human after it is an embryo, from 9 weeks after fertilization until childbirth.

* **endocarditis** (en-do-kar-DYE-tis) is an inflammation of the valves and internal lining of the heart, known as the endocardium (en-doh-KAR-dee-um), usually caused by an infection.

* **pneumonia** (nu-MO-nyah) is inflammation of the lung.

* **meningitis** (meh-nin-JY-tis) is an inflammation of the meninges, the membranes that surround the brain and the spinal cord. Meningitis is most often caused by infection with a virus or a bacterium.

* **lesions** (LEE-zhuns) is a general term referring to sores or damaged or irregular areas of tissue.

* **tonsils** are paired clusters of lymphatic tissue in the throat that help protect the body from bacteria and viruses that enter through a person's nose or mouth.

* **lymph** (LIMF) **nodes** are small, bean-shaped masses of tissue that contain immune system cells that fight harmful microorganisms. Lymph nodes may swell during infections.

* **shock** is a serious condition in which blood pressure is very low and not enough blood flows to the body's organs and tissues. Untreated, shock may result in death.

* **arthritis** (ar-THRY-tis) refers to any of several disorders character-ized by inflammation of the joints.

* **culture** (KUL-chur) is a test in which a sample of fluid or tissue from the body is placed in a dish containing material that supports the growth of certain organisms. Typically, within days the organisms will grow and can be identified.

* **intravenous** (in-tra-VEE-nus), or IV, means within or through a vein. For example, medications, fluid, or other substances can be given through a needle or soft tube inserted through the skin's surface directly into a vein.

associated with fever, rapid heart rate, and low blood pressure that may lead to shock*.

■ Toxin-producing strains of GAS can cause a rare but serious illness called streptococcal toxic shock syndrome. The infection may occur anywhere in the body, and the toxin (poison) is released into the bloodstream, causing low blood pressure and shock.

■ Necrotizing fasciitis (or flesh-eating disease) is a rare, rapidly progressing infection of the deeper layers of skin, muscle and other tissues. Symptoms usually start at the site of an injury, where the skin becomes painful, swollen, discolored (such as red, purple, or bronze), and hot to the touch. The skin gradually becomes darker and blisters can form while the tissues beneath the skin are being damaged. Fever, shock, and multiple organ damage may accompany this serious infection.

■ Rheumatic (roo-MAH-tik) fever, a syndrome involving arthritis* and inflammation of the heart, is actually a complication of untreated strep throat. Rashes and neurological problems also may occur, and people with rheumatic fever may have permanent damage to one or more heart valves.

Making the diagnosis With skin infections, a doctor may take a sample from the affected area to culture*. For other types of suspected infections, blood samples are drawn and swabs of fluid from the patient's nose and throat are cultured for bacteria. A rapid strep test on a sample taken with a throat swab can also be done in a doctor's office.

Treatment Superficial skin infections often are treated with topical (on the skin) antibiotic ointments. Other GAS infections are treated with oral (by mouth) or intravenous* (IV) antibiotics. Serious GAS infections require hospitalization, where patients receive IV fluids and antibiotics. In some cases, such as with necrotizing fasciitis, surgical removal of dam-aged tissue is necessary. Treatment of rheumatic fever depends on the severity of the disease but includes using antibiotics to treat strep infec-tions, anti-inflammatory medicines such as high-dose aspirin, and med-ications to treat heart complications.

What to expect Symptoms of strep throat usually improve within 1 to 2 days after starting antibiotics. Skin infections often clear up within a week, but more serious infections can take weeks or even months to heal. Complications from serious bacterial infections include sepsis, shock, organ damage and failure, and death.

Prevention Maintaining good health and hygiene can help reduce the risk of bacterial infection. Not sharing food or eating utensils, washing hands frequently, and cleaning and bandaging cuts and scrapes can help prevent the spread of bacteria.

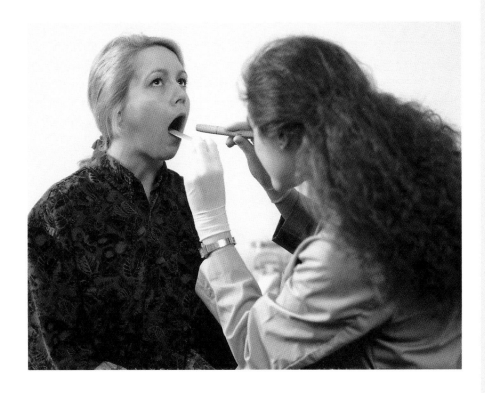

A doctor examines a patient's sore throat. Most sore throats are caused by infections, however, they can also be caused by allergies and environmental irritants such as smoke. *Custom Medical Stock Photo, Inc.*

Group B Streptococcus (GBS) Infections

How common are they? According to the Centers for Disease Control and Prevention, GBS is the most frequent cause of life-threatening infections in newborns. Early screening of pregnant women for GBS and treatment have reduced infection rates by approximately 70 percent. Currently, 17,000 cases of GBS infection occur annually in the United States.

Are they contagious? GBS infections are contagious and can pass from mother to child before or during birth. At least 25 percent of women are carriers of GBS at some point in their life but do not become ill from it. The bacteria can be found in the bowel, vagina*, bladder, and throat.

Some GBS infections

■ Newborns can develop sepsis, pneumonia, and meningitis due to infection with GBS. Symptoms of GBS infection in newborns include fever, irritability, extreme sleepiness, breathing difficulties, and poor feeding.

■ GBS bacteria in pregnant women can cause urinary tract infections* as well as chorioamnionitis (kor-e-o-am-nee-on-EYE-tis, infection of the womb and membranes surrounding the fetus) and stillbirth (a fetus that is dead at birth). Symptoms of urinary tract infection include fever, pain, and a burning sensation during urination. Women with chorioamnionitis often

* **vagina** (vah-JY-nah) is the canal, or passageway, in a woman that leads from the uterus to the outside of the body.

* **urinary** (YOOR-ih-nair-e) **tract infection**, or UTI, is an infection that occurs in any part of the urinary tract. The urinary tract is made up of the urethra, bladder, ureters, and kidneys.

Shaking Hands with Semmelweis

Ignaz Philipp Semmelweis (1818—1865) was a Hungarian physician who suspected that doctors could spread disease by not washing their hands thoroughly after working with cadavers before delivering babies. At the time, up to 30 percent of women who gave birth in hospitals died of puerperal (pyoo-ER-puh-rul) fever, a group A strep bacterial infection that occurred after childbirth. Semmelweis noticed that women who delivered their babies with midwives were less likely to become ill. He had his student doctors wash their hands with an antiseptic, which is a solution that prevents the growth of bacteria. Because the idea that germs could cause disease had not yet been introduced, Semmelweis' ideas about hand washing were not well received until many years later.

---

* **cerebrospinal** (seh-ree-bro-SPY-nuhl) **fluid** is the fluid that surrounds the brain and spinal cord.

* **rectum** is the final portion of the large intestine, connecting the colon to the anus.

* **vaccines** (vak-SEENS) are preparations of killed or weakened germs, or a part of a germ or product it produces, given to prevent or lessen the severity of the disease that can result if a person is exposed to the germ itself. Use of vaccines for this purpose is called immunization.

* **sinuses** (SY-nuh-ses) are hollow, air-filled cavities in the facial bones.

do not show symptoms of infection until after childbirth. Symptoms include fever, belly pain, and rapid pulse.

- The most common GBS infections in other people are urinary tract infections, sepsis, tissue infections, and pneumonia. GBS infections, including pneumonia and sepsis, are more likely to be found in people with weakened immune systems or chronic diseases, such as diabetes.

Making the diagnosis   GBS infections are diagnosed by performing cultures of blood, urine, or cerebrospinal fluid* to identify the bacteria.

Treatment   GBS infections are treated with antibiotics, often intravenously, and they usually require a hospital stay, particularly for newborns. Pregnant women with urinary tract infections usually are treated with antibiotics as well.

What to expect   Recovery can take several weeks. Complications in infants, particularly those with meningitis, include hearing and vision loss and brain damage. Approximately 5 percent of cases of GBS disease in newborns are fatal.

Prevention   Most newborn cases can be prevented by testing women in the thirty-fifth to thirty-seventh week of pregnancy for the bacteria. A culture of fluid from the vagina and rectum* can determine whether a woman has GBS. If she does, giving IV antibiotics during labor reduces the risk of passing GBS to the baby. Vaccines* to prevent GBS infections during pregnancy are being developed.

Alpha-Hemolytic Streptococcus Infections

How common are they?   Infections with alpha-hemolytic strep bacteria are common; many strains live naturally in humans.

Some alpha-hemolytic strep infections

S. PNEUMONIAE (NU-MON-YI) INFECTIONS

- Bacterial pneumonia is an inflammation of the lungs that often occurs after or along with an upper respiratory infection. Symptoms may develop quickly and can include fever, chills, cough, rapid breathing, chest pain, belly pain, and vomiting. Before antibiotics were developed, bacterial pneumonia was the most common cause of death in adults.
- Otitis (o-TIE-tis) media is an inflammation of the middle ear. The infection usually is associated with ear pain and sometimes with fever.
- Sinusitis (sy-nyoo-SY-tis) is an inflammation of the sinuses*, usually due to infection. Symptoms include a stuffy nose,

colored discharge (green, yellow, or tinged with blood) from the nose, tenderness around the eyes, and headache or a feeling of pressure in the head.

- Meningitis is an inflammation of the membranes covering the brain and the spinal cord. Symptoms include fever, weakness, vomiting, irritability, and stiff neck.

S. VIRIDANS (VEER-IH-DANZ) INFECTION

- Endocarditis is an infection of the inner surface of the heart or heart valves that can be caused by *S. viridans* and other bacteria. Bacteria can enter the bloodstream (during a dental procedure, for example) and attach to already damaged heart tissue or an abnormal heart valve, causing more damage. Symptoms include extreme tiredness, weakness, fever, chills, night sweats, and weight loss. The infection can progress, resulting in problems with heart function in some cases.

Making the diagnosis   Depending on the type of infection, a diagnosis is made by testing blood, sputum*, or cerebrospinal fluid samples for signs of the bacteria.

Treatment   Oral or IV antibiotics are used, depending on the severity of the infection. A hospital stay may be needed, particularly in cases of pneumonia or meningitis. Long courses of antibiotics, lasting several weeks or more, may be required to treat endocarditis.

Prevention   Vaccines against *S. pneumoniae* are now given routinely to infants and the elderly, as well as to children and adults with weakened immune systems or certain medical conditions. People with abnormal or damaged heart valves are given courses of antibiotics when they have some types of surgical procedures, including dental work, to help prevent endocarditis from developing from the shedding of bacteria into the bloodstream that occurs with these procedures.

Resources

Organizations

U.S. Centers for Disease Control and Prevention (CDC), 1600 Clifton Road, Atlanta, GA 30333. The CDC posts information about streptococcal infections at its website.
Telephone 800-311-3435
http://www.cdc.gov

U.S. National Library of Medicine, 8600 Rockville Pike, Bethesda, MD 20894. The National Library of Medicine has a website packed with information on diseases (including streptococcal infections),

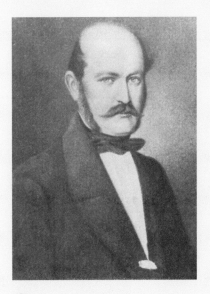

▲

After Hungarian physician Ignaz Semmelweis (1818–1865) had the physicians at a Vienna, Austria, hospital wash their hands regularly with an antiseptic, the hospital's mortality rate fell dramatically. *Library of Congress*

* **sputum** (SPYOO-tum) is a substance that contains mucus and other matter coughed out from the lungs, bronchi, and trachea.

KEYWORDS
for searching the Internet and other reference sources

Chancre

Congenital infections

Sexually transmitted disease (STD)

Treponema pallidum

---

* **paralysis** (pah-RAH-luh-sis) is the loss or impairment of the ability to move some part of the body.

* **chancre** (SHANG-ker) is a usually painless sore or ulcer that forms where a disease-causing germ enters the body, such as with syphilis.

* **fetus** (FEE-tus) is the term for an unborn human after it is an embryo, from 9 weeks after fertilization until childbirth.

* **congenital** (kon-JEH-nih-tul) means present at birth.

consumer resources, dictionaries and encyclopedias of medical terms, and directories of doctors and helpful organizations.
Telephone 888-346-3656
http://www.nlm.nih.gov

Website

KidsHealth.org. KidsHealth is a website created by the medical experts of the Nemours Foundation and is devoted to issues of children's health. It contains articles on a variety of health topics, including streptococcal infections.
http://www.KidsHealth.org

Syphilis

Syphilis (SIH-fih-lis) is a sexually transmitted disease that, if untreated, can lead to serious lifelong problems throughout the body, including blindness and paralysis*.

What Is Syphilis?

Syphilis is a disease that is caused by the bacterium *Treponema pallidum* (treh-puh-NEE-muh PAL-ih-dum). The disease develops in three distinct phases. The first, or primary, stage is marked by a chancre*. In the secondary stage, a rash develops. By the third, or tertiary, stage the disease can cause widespread damage to the body, affecting the brain, nerves, bones, joints, eyes, and heart and other organs. Syphilis does not advance to this point in all infected people, and it does so only if it has not been treated adequately during either of the two earlier stages.

Without treatment, syphilis can be fatal. It also can have serious consequences for babies who become infected in the womb, before birth. If a pregnant woman has syphilis, she can pass it to her fetus*, a condition known as congenital* syphilis. Because the immune system of a baby is not developed fully until the infant is well into the first year of life, infection with syphilis bacteria can lead to severe complications. If pregnant women who are infected are not treated, more than a third of their infants may die before or shortly after birth.

How Common Is Syphilis?

Before the introduction of the antibiotic penicillin in the 1940s, syphilis was rampant in the United States. Although the disease is still relatively common, the number of cases today is far below the high rate of infection early in the twentieth century. According to the U.S. Centers for Disease Control and Prevention (CDC), 31,575 cases (or about 12 per 100,000 people) were reported in 2000 (although the number of actual infections is likely higher, because many cases go unnoticed at first). Of those, 529 were cases of congenital syphilis. Compare that with 485,560 cases overall (or 368 per 100,000 people) in 1941, the first year that the government began tracking syphilis rates.

Is Syphilis Contagious?

Syphilis is a sexually transmitted disease that spreads from person to person through vaginal*, oral*, or anal* intercourse. A pregnant female also can pass the disease to her fetus. People are most contagious during the second stage of the infection.

What Are the Signs and Symptoms of Infection?

Syphilis has been called "the great imitator," because its symptoms can resemble those of many other diseases. Not all people have obvious symptoms, but in those who do, signs of disease appear 10 to 90 days after being infected. The first symptom is a small, usually painless sore known as

* **vaginal** (VAH-jih-nul) refers to the vagina, the canal in a woman that leads from the uterus to the outside of the body.

* **oral** means by mouth or referring to the mouth.

* **anal** refers to the anus, the opening at the end of the digestive system through which waste leaves the body.

HOW SYPHILIS CHANGED THE FACE OF MEDICAL RESEARCH

Just a few decades ago syphilis was the subject of the most infamous public health study ever carried out in the United States. From 1932 to 1972 the U.S. Public Health Service conducted a study in Macon County, Alabama, to learn more about the long-term consequences of the disease. Six hundred poor African-American men, 399 infected with syphilis, participated in the study in exchange for free medical exams, free meals, and burial insurance.

The Tuskegee Syphilis Study became notorious because local doctors who participated in the study were instructed not to treat the men's infections, even after an easy cure with penicillin became widely available in 1947. Although the men had agreed to be part of the project, they were never told they would not be treated fully for their condition. They were simply told that they were part of a study of "bad blood," a local term used for several illnesses.

Public outrage erupted in 1972 when it became known that men with syphilis in the study had been allowed to remain untreated so that doctors could investigate the progression of the disease, and the project was stopped. But that came too late for the men; many were disabled permanently or had died. In the wake of the study, the government moved quickly to adopt policies that protect people who take part in research programs. In 1974, a new law created a national commission to set basic ethical standards for research. New rules also required that participants in government-funded studies be made fully aware of how a study will proceed and voluntarily agree to take part in it. Any study that involves humans also is reviewed before it begins to ensure that it meets ethical standards.

Of course, these changes could not reverse the physical and emotional harm done to the men in the Tuskegee Syphilis Study and to their families. In recognition of that harm, in 1997, President Bill Clinton offered an apology to the survivors, families, and descendants of those men on behalf of the U.S. government.

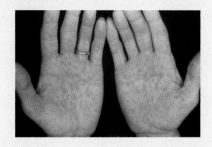

▲

An example of secondary syphilis. If syphilis is not treated in its first phase, it can progress to its second stage a month or two later in which a rash may appear on the palms of the hands and the soles of the feet. *Custom Medical Stock Photo, Inc.*

* **vagina** (vah-JY-nah) is the canal, or passageway, in a woman that leads from the uterus to the outside of the body.

* **rectum** is the final portion of the large intestine, connecting the colon to the anus.

* **lymph** (LIMF) **nodes** are small, bean-shaped masses of tissue that contain immune system cells that fight harmful microorganisms. Lymph nodes may swell during infections.

* **ulcers** are open sores on the skin or the lining of a hollow body organ, such as the stomach or intestine. They may or may not be painful.

* **mucous membranes** are the moist linings of the mouth, nose, eyes, and throat.

* **genitals** (JEH-nih-tuls) are the external sexual organs.

* **lesions** (LEE-zhuns) is a general term referring to sores or damaged or irregular areas of tissue.

a chancre that appears where the syphilis bacterium entered the body, such as on the penis or the lips of the vagina*. Without treatment, chancres will heal on their own within 6 weeks. A person who is infected may never even notice a chancre, especially if it is inside the vagina or the rectum*.

When the chancre fades, the disease moves to its second stage 1 to 2 months later. In this phase, a rash of rough reddish or brownish spots appears on the body, including the soles of the feet and the palms of the hands. The rash may be so faint that it is barely noticeable. Second-stage symptoms of syphilis also may include fever, headache, extreme tiredness, sore throat, muscle aches, swollen lymph nodes*, weight loss, hair loss, and ulcers* on mucous membranes* in the mouth and on the genitals*. Wartlike lesions* may appear on the vagina or anus. This stage of the infection also disappears on its own, fooling many people into thinking that they have had a common viral illness.

After the second-stage symptoms clear up, the disease enters a latent, or hidden, period in which there are no signs of illness. The latent period can last for many years, and in some infected people the bacteria do no further damage. In about one-third of people who reach the latent period, the disease progresses to its final stage. This phase has no symptoms at first, but as the bacteria invade and damage nerves, bones, and the heart and other organs, the patient may experience dizziness, headaches, seizures*, dementia*, loss of coordination, numbness, increasing blindness, and paralysis. The disease also can eat away at tissue in the mouth and nose, disfiguring the face. This last stage of the disease can begin 2 to 40 years after a person is first infected.

Babies who are born with syphilis may have symptoms right away or may show signs of the disease within a few weeks or months. Those symptoms include failure to thrive*, irritability, fever, rash, a nose without a bridge (known as saddle nose), bloody fluid from the nose, and a rash on the palms, soles, or face. As these children grow older, they may become blind and deaf and have notched teeth (called Hutchinson teeth). Bone lesions may arise, and lesions and scarring may appear around the mouth, genitals, and anus.

How Is the Diagnosis of Syphilis Made?

If a patient has a chancre or other lesion, the doctor collects a sample of fluid from the sore to examine under a special microscope. Syphilis bacteria in the fluid are visible under magnification. The doctor also may take a blood sample to look for antibodies* to the bacterium. If neurosyphilis (nur-o-SIH-fih-lis, syphilis that has progressed to the point that it affects the brain, spinal cord, and nerves) is suspected, the spinal fluid also may be tested for antibodies. Pregnant women are screened for syphilis during routine prenatal care.

How Is Syphilis Treated?

Even though visible signs of the infection will clear up on their own, patients with syphilis are treated to prevent the disease from progressing to the late, potentially much more harmful stage, or to prevent a pregnant woman's infant from being damaged by the infection. Early-stage syphilis is treated easily with antibiotics. People who are infected with syphilis are advised to notify all their recent sexual partners so that they, too, can be tested for the disease. Patients with advanced cases of the disease often need to be hospitalized. They also receive antibiotics, although medications cannot reverse damage already done to the body.

How Long Does Infection Last?

A single dose of antibiotics can clear up syphilis infections that are less than a year old. Longer-term cases require longer courses of treatment. Congenital syphilis also needs a longer course of treatment. Without treatment, the disease can last for years or even decades.

Does the Disease Have Complications?

Untreated cases of syphilis can lead to destructive tissue lesions known as gummas on the skin, bones, and organs; seizures; damage to the spine that can result in paralysis; heart problems; damage to blood vessels that can lead to stroke*; and death. According to the CDC, a person with syphilis has a two to five times greater risk of acquiring human immunodeficiency (ih-myoo-no-dih-FIH-shen-see) virus (HIV), the virus that causes acquired immunodeficiency syndrome (AIDS), an infection that weakens the immune system. The reason for this increased risk is that open sores make it easier for HIV to enter the body during sexual contact. Also, people infected with HIV are more likely to experience neurological* complications of syphilis. In infants, syphilis can lead to hearing loss, blindness, neurological problems, and death.

Can Syphilis Be Prevented?

Using latex condoms or not having sex, especially with someone who is known to be infected, can prevent the spread of syphilis and other sexually transmitted diseases. To be effective, the condom has to cover all syphilis sores. Contact with sores in the mouth or on areas such as the rectum that may not be covered by a condom can spread the disease. Doctors advise pregnant women to be tested and, if needed, treated for syphilis to minimize the risk of passing it to the developing fetus.

Resources

Organizations

American Social Health Association, P.O. Box 13827, Research Triangle Park, NC 27709. The American Social Health Association has information and fact sheets concerning sexually transmitted diseases, including syphilis, at its website.
Telephone 919-361-8400
http://www.ashastd.org

* **seizures** (SEE-zhurs) are sudden bursts of disorganized electrical activity that interrupt the normal functioning of the brain, often leading to uncontrolled movements in the body and sometimes a temporary change in consciousness.

* **dementia** (dih-MEN-sha) is a loss of mental abilities, including memory, understanding, and judgment.

* **failure to thrive** is a condition in which an infant fails to gain weight and grow at the expected rate.

* **antibodies** (AN-tih-bah-deez) are protein molecules produced by the body's immune system to help fight specific infections caused by microorganisms, such as bacteria and viruses.

* **stroke** is a brain-damaging event usually caused by interference with blood flow to the brain. A stroke may occur when a blood vessel supplying the brain becomes clogged or bursts, depriving brain tissue of oxygen. As a result, nerve cells in the affected area of the brain, and the specific body parts they control, do not properly function.

* **neurological** refers to the nervous system, which includes the brain, spinal cord, and the nerves that control the senses, movement, and organ functions throughout the body.

U.S. Centers for Disease Control and Prevention (CDC), 1600 Clifton Road, Atlanta, GA 30333. The CDC provides fact sheets and other information on syphilis at its website.
Telephone 800-311-3435
http://www.cdc.gov

Website

KidsHealth.org. KidsHealth is a website created by the medical experts of the Nemours Foundation and is devoted to issues of children's health. It contains articles on a variety of health topics, including syphilis.
http://www.KidsHealth.org

▶ *See also*

AIDS and HIV Infection

Congenital Infections

Sexually Transmitted Diseases

T

Tetanus (Lockjaw)

Tetanus (TET-nus) is a serious bacterial infection that affects the body's central nervous system*. Tetanus, also known as lockjaw, can lead to muscle rigidity, convulsions*, and death.

What Is Tetanus?

Tetanus is a disease caused by infection with *Clostridium tetani* (klos-TRIH-dee-um teh-TAH-nye) bacteria, which are found all over the world in soil, dust, and some animal feces (FEE-seez, or bowel movements) and even on human skin. The bacteria can enter the body through any type of wound, such as a scratch or deep cut. Infection begins after bacterial spores* have moved deep within the body and become active. *Clostridium tetani* bacteria are anaerobic (ah-nuh-RO-bik), meaning that they grow best in places with very little oxygen—so the deeper they travel into the body, the better their chances to survive.

Once tetanus spores become active, the bacteria begin producing a toxin (a poisonous substance) called tetanospasmin (teh-tuh-no-SPAZ-min), which attaches to the nerves around the area of the wound. The tetanus toxin also can spread and attach to the ends of nerves of the spinal cord and at neuromuscular junctions (where nerves meet muscles). The toxin blocks the release of a neurotransmitter (nur-o-trans-MIH-ter), a chemical that carries a signal from nerves to other nerves or muscles. This affects the messages that the muscles receive, resulting in severe muscle spasms* that can be powerful enough to tear muscles apart.

There are three types of tetanus infection. Local tetanus is limited to the area of the wound; cephalic (seh-FAH-lik) tetanus is an uncommon form that affects the nerves of the face after a head injury or, rarely, a long-lasting ear infection; and generalized tetanus affects much of the body and accounts for the majority of tetanus cases. Neonatal tetanus is a generalized form of the infection that occurs in newborns. It is caused by bacteria contaminating the stump of the umbilical cord*, particularly if the cord has been cut with an instrument that has not been sterilized*.

How Common Is It?

Tetanus occurs around the world but is found frequently in densely populated areas that have hot, damp climates. The disease is rare in the United States, primarily because of vaccination. Nearly all reported cases

KEYWORDS
for searching the Internet and other reference sources

Clostridium tetani

Lockjaw

Tetanospasmin

Trismus

* **central nervous system** (SEN-trul NER-vus SIS-tem) is the part of the nervous system that includes the brain and spinal cord.

* **convulsions** (kon-VUL-shuns), also called seizures, are involuntary muscle contractions caused by electrical discharges within the brain and are usually accompanied by changes in consciousness.

* **spores** are a temporarily inactive form of a germ enclosed in a protective shell.

* **spasms** (SPAH-zumz) are involuntary muscular tightenings or contractions.

* **umbilical** (um-BIH-lih-kul) **cord** is the flexible cord that connects a baby to the placenta, the organ that unites the unborn child to the mother's uterus, the organ in which the baby develops.

* **sterilize** (STAIR-uh-lyze) is to eliminate all live bacteria or microorganisms from something, usually through the use of heat, pressure, chemicals, or other antimicrobial agents.

*intravenous (in-tra-VEE-nus), or IV, means within or through a vein. For example, medications, fluid, or other substances can be given through a needle or soft tube inserted through the skin's surface directly into a vein.

*abdominal (ab-DAH-mih-nul) refers to the area of the body below the ribs and above the hips that contains the stomach, intestines, and other organs.

*culture (KUL-chur) is a test in which a sample of fluid or tissue from the body is placed in a dish containing material that supports the growth of certain organisms. Typically, within days the organisms will grow and can be identified.

*immune globulin (ih-MYOON GLAH-byoo-lin), also called gamma globulin, is the protein material that contains anti-bodies.

*respiratory system, or respiratory tract, includes the nose, mouth, throat, and lungs. It is the pathway through which air and gases are transported down into the lungs and back out of the body.

*respirator is a machine that helps people breathe when they are unable to breathe adequately on their own.

of tetanus occur in people who have never been vaccinated or who have not had a booster shot in the previous 10 years. Neonatal tetanus infection is rare in developed countries because of improved surgical techniques, but there are hundreds of thousands of deaths from tetanus annually worldwide, mostly in developing countries. Intravenous* drug abusers, such as people who inject heroin, are at a higher risk of contracting the disease.

Is Tetanus Contagious?

Tetanus is not spread from person to person. Bacterial spores must enter a wound for the infection to spread.

What Are the Signs and Symptoms of Infection?

Symptoms of tetanus appear from 3 to 21 days or longer after infection, but usually they develop within 7 days. In about 50 percent of generalized cases of tetanus, the first sign is trismus, or stiffness in the jaw muscles (also known as lockjaw), followed by a stiff neck, shoulder, or back; trouble swallowing; and fever. Spasms can soon spread to the abdominal* muscles, upper arms, and thighs. Other symptoms include sweating, high blood pressure, and periods of rapid heartbeat. The closer the infection is to the central nervous system, the sooner the symptoms appear. The earlier the symptoms begin to appear, the greater the risk of death.

How Do Doctors Make the Diagnosis?

The diagnosis is made based on the presence of symptoms and the patient's history (for example, getting a wound by stepping on a soil-contaminated nail). Laboratory tests are not useful in determining whether a patient has tetanus. A culture* of the wound can be done, but these cultures generally do not show the bacteria.

What Is the Treatment for Tetanus?

Typically, tetanus infection is treated in a hospital. Treatment begins with giving the patient tetanus immune globulin* to control or reverse the effects of toxin that has not yet attached itself to nerve endings. Penicillin or other antibiotics also may be given to kill the bacteria. Cleaning the wound and removing dead tissue, in some cases by surgery, is important in ridding the body of invading bacteria. Muscle spasms can be treated with muscle relaxants. Respiratory system* support, provided by a respirator*, may be necessary to help maintain breathing if the respiratory muscles have been affected.

How Long Does Tetanus Last?

Symptoms may last 3 to 4 weeks, although complete recovery can take several months. Tetanus can be mild, but in most cases the illness is severe and death may occur even after treatment has begun. Tetanus usually requires a long stay in the intensive care unit of the hospital.

What Are the Complications?

Complications of the illness include spasms of the vocal cords and the muscles that control breathing, which can lead to difficulty breathing; fractures in the long bones or the spine from severe muscle spasms and convulsions; high blood pressure; abnormal heart rhythm; secondary infections, such as sepsis* and pneumonia (inflammation of the lung); a blood clot* in the lungs; and death. In the United States, 11 percent of reported tetanus cases are fatal. Unvaccinated children and the elderly are at greater risk of dying if they become infected with tetanus bacteria.

Can Tetanus Be Prevented?

Immunization is the best means of preventing tetanus. The vaccination usually is given in combination with other vaccines: the DTaP (diphtheria*/ tetanus/acellular pertussis*) form for children and the Td (tetanus/diphtheria) form for adults. A series of shots is required to develop immunity to tetanus toxin, followed by booster shots every 10 years. In some cases of unclean wounds, a booster will be given after the injury to help prevent tetanus.

Resources

Organization

U.S. Centers for Disease Control and Prevention (CDC), 1600 Clifton Road, Atlanta, GA 30333. The CDC provides fact sheets and other information on tetanus at its website.
Telephone 800-311-3435
http://www.cdc.gov

Website

KidsHealth.org. KidsHealth is a website created by the medical experts of the Nemours Foundation and is devoted to issues of children's health. It contains articles on a variety of health topics, including tetanus.
http://www.KidsHealth.org

Tick-borne Infections

A tick-borne infection is an infection that is transmitted through the bite of a tick.

What Are Tick-borne Infections?

Ticks can spread bacteria or parasites through their bites. A tick becomes infected when it bites an animal, and then the tick can pass the

---

* **sepsis** is a potentially serious spreading of infection, usually bacterial, through the bloodstream and body.

* **blood clot** is a thickening of the blood into a jelly-like substance that helps stop bleeding. Clotting of the blood within a blood vessel can lead to blockage of blood flow.

* **diphtheria** (dif-THEER-e-uh) is an infection of the lining of the upper respiratory tract (the nose and throat). It is a serious disease that can cause breathing difficulty and other complications, including death.

* **pertussis** (per-TUH-sis) is a bacterial infection of the respiratory tract that causes severe coughing.

▶ *See also*
Skin and Soft Tissue Infections
Vaccination (Immunization)

KEYWORDS
for searching the Internet and other reference sources

Babesiosis

Borreliosis

Ehrlichiosis

Lyme disease

Rickettsial diseases

Rocky Mountain spotted fever

Tips for Removing a Tick

Using tweezers, grasp the tick as close to the head as possible.

Pull firmly and steadily until the tick lets go (do not squeeze or twist).

Put the tick in a jar of alcohol in case it is needed for diagnosis.

Swab the bite area with alcohol.

Petroleum jelly and lit matches do not help in tick removal and should not be used.

*host is an organism that provides another organism (such as a parasite or virus) with a place to live and grow.

infection to humans when it bites them. Tick-borne infections cannot pass from human to human; they need time in the host* animal to develop.

Ticks can spread a number of different diseases, including Rocky Mountain spotted fever, ehrlichiosis (air-lik-e-O-sis), Lyme (LIME) disease, and babesiosis (bah-bih-sye-OH-sis).

Rocky Mountain spotted fever   Despite its name, most cases of Rocky Mountain spotted fever (RMSF) are not found in the Rocky Mountains but in the southeastern states. It also appears throughout the contintental United States and in Canada, Mexico, and Central and South America. RMSF is one of the most dangerous tick-borne infections because it can be difficult to diagnose and has severe complications. Caused by the *Rickettsia rickettsii* (rih-KET-see-uh rih-KET-see-eye) bacterium, the disease spreads to humans through bites from the wood tick, dog tick, and Lone Star tick.

Symptoms of RMSF include high fever, headache, aching in the muscles, nausea (NAW-zee-uh), vomiting, and diarrhea (dye-uh-REE-uh). A rash may appear first at the wrists, ankles, palms, and soles and then on the forearms, neck, face, and trunk. RMSF is fatal in about 5 percent of cases. This may be due to delays in diagnosing and treating the disease.

Ehrlichiosis   Several types of bacteria in the genus *Ehrlichia* (air-LIH-kee-uh) cause ehrlichiosis. In the United States, the Lone Star tick, the blacklegged tick, and the western blacklegged tick spread the illness. People have long known that ehrlichiosis causes disease in animals, but the first case in humans in the United States was not identified until the 1980s. Ehrlichiosis is found in most parts of the country.

Symptoms of ehrlichiosis resemble those of the flu: fever, chills, extreme tiredness, headache, muscle and joint pain, nausea, and vomiting. There is usually no rash in adults, but many children develop a rash. Some people have no symptoms or only mild symptoms. Complications, although rare, can occur in the elderly and people with weakened immune systems.

Lyme disease   Lyme disease gets its name from the town in Connecticut where doctors discovered the disease in 1977. It is the most common tick-borne illness in the United States. The majority of cases appear in the northeastern, north central, and northwestern states.

The bacterium *Borrelia burgdorferi* (buh-REEL-e-uh burg-DOR-fe-ree), transmitted through deer ticks, causes Lyme disease. In most cases, the first sign of infection is the erythema migrans (air-uh-THEE-muh MY-granz) rash. It usually appears at the site of the tick bite, although it can develop anywhere on the body. The rash can be round, oval, or shaped like a bull's-eye with a red center surrounded by a clear area and then by a ring of red. Other early signs of the disease, such as extreme tiredness, headache, muscle aches, and fever, are similar to those of many infections, making diagnosis difficult. Not everyone who has Lyme disease develops the rash, and some people never show any symptoms.

The early disseminated* stage of the disease typically comes weeks to months later in people who have not received treatment. Symptoms at this stage include multiple rashes, meningitis*, radiculitis*, Bell's palsy*, and in some cases abnormalities of the heart rhythm. Lyme disease is not usually fatal, but if the illness remains untreated it can cause symptoms even years later. They can include arthritis, confusion, lack of coordination, difficulty in sleeping, and mood changes.

Babesiosis Babesiosis is a rare disease that appears mainly in the northeastern United States. It spreads through the bite of a deer tick that has been infected with a *Babesia* (buh-BE-she-uh) parasite, which attacks red blood cells. Because the deer tick also can spread Lyme disease, some people become infected with both diseases at the same time.

In healthy people, babesiosis infection may cause no symptoms. In others, early symptoms are extreme tiredness, lack of appetite, and a general feeling of being sick. Later symptoms include high fever, sweating, muscle aches, headache, and dark urine. The symptoms of babesiosis are similar to those of malaria*. Infected people also may have anemia* because of the parasite's attack on their red blood cells. The disease is not often fatal, but it can cause complications in the elderly, pregnant women, people with weakened immune systems, and people who have had their spleen removed.

How Common Are Tick-borne Infections?

About 16,000 cases of Lyme disease occur in the United States each year. RMSF is the second most common type of tick-borne illness, with the U.S. Centers for Disease Control and Prevention receiving as many as 1,200 reports of RMSF cases each year.

In contrast to these diseases, both ehrlichiosis and babesiosis are rare, with about 1,200 reports of ehrlichiosis over an 11-year period and several hundred cases of babesiosis since it was first reported in 1966.

How Are Tick-borne Infections Diagnosed and Treated?

Diagnosing a tick-borne illness can be difficult because the symptoms of many of the illnesses resemble those of the flu or other infections. One of the best clues is a recent tick bite, but many people do not remember being bitten.

Doctors often diagnose these diseases based on the patient's history of symptoms and activities, where the patient lives or became sick, and a physical examination that includes looking for rashes. A doctor may order a blood test to check for antibodies* to the organism causing the infection, but these tests usually are not helpful in the early stages of the illness. Skin biopsy* from a rash area may confirm a diagnosis.

* **disseminated** describes a disease that has spread widely in the body.

* **meningitis** (meh-nin-JY-tis) is an inflammation of the meninges, the membranes that surround the brain and the spinal cord. Meningitis is most often caused by infection with a virus or a bacterium.

* **radiculitis** (ruh-dih-kyoo-LYE-tis) is numbness, tingling, or burning sensation along the course of a nerve due to irritation or inflammation of the nerve.

* **Bell's palsy** (PAWL-zee) is a condition in which there is weakness or loss of function of muscles on one side of the face.

* **malaria** (mah-LAIR-e-uh) is a disease spread to humans by the bite of an infected mosquito.

* **anemia** (uh-NEE-me-uh) is a blood condition in which there is a decreased amount of oxygen-carrying hemoglobin in the blood and, usually, fewer than normal numbers of red blood cells.

* **antibodies** (AN-tih-bah-deez) are protein molecules produced by the body's immune system to help fight specific infections caused by microorganisms, such as bacteria and viruses.

* **biopsy** (BI-op-see) is a test in which a small sample of skin or other body tissue is removed and examined for signs of disease.

Antibiotics are effective against the bacterial infections. Anti-parasitic medicines work well for babesiosis. In most cases, patients recover at home. Sometimes, however, especially in cases of RMSF, patients may need hospitalization for more intensive antibiotic therapy and supportive care.

What Should People Expect if They Have a Tick-borne Infection?

In almost all cases of tick-borne illnesses, quick treatment brings a complete cure, although it may take several months before all symptoms disappear. Untreated cases of Lyme disease can cause problems years after the tick bite.

Complications, while rare, can occur. For example:

- RMSF can cause paralysis*, hearing loss, and nerve damage.
- Ehrlichiosis can cause kidney* failure, respiratory problems, seizures*, and coma*.
- Long-term complications from Lyme disease include chronic* arthritis and nervous system problems.
- Babesiosis can cause respiratory problems, seizures, kidney failure, and other organ failure.

Can People Prevent Tick-borne Infections?

Avoiding areas where ticks are found is the best way to prevent the diseases they carry. If people venture into areas where ticks are likely to live, experts suggest that they wear long pants and long-sleeved shirts in light colors (to make it easier to find ticks) when going outside and that they tuck their pant legs into their socks. Applying insect repellents also can be helpful. Checking for ticks after being outside is also wise. Studies show that ticks may not infect people until they have been attached for 2 days, so quickly removing ticks can help prevent illness. When ticks are found, they should be removed, and people should watch for signs of infection, such as rash or fever.

Resources

Organizations

American Lyme Disease Foundation, Inc., Mill Pond Offices, 293 Route 100, Somers, NY 10589. The American Lyme Disease Foundation provides information on Lyme disease and other tick-borne illnesses on its website.
Telephone 914-277-6970
http://www.aldf.com

Lyme Disease Foundation, Inc., One Financial Plaza, Hartford, CT 06103. The Lyme Disease Foundation offers information on tick-borne illnesses and avoiding tick bites on its website.

*paralysis (pah-RAH-luh-sis) is the loss or impairment of the ability to move some part of the body.

*kidney is one of the pair of organs that filter blood and remove waste products and excess water from the body in the form of urine.

*seizures (SEE-zhurs) are sudden bursts of disorganized electrical activity that interrupt the normal functioning of the brain, often leading to uncontrolled movements in the body and sometimes a temporary change in consciousness.

*coma (KO-ma) is an unconscious state in which a person cannot be awakened and cannot move, see, speak, or hear.

*chronic (KRAH-nik) means continuing for a long period of time.

Telephone 860-525-2000
http://www.lyme.org

Website

KidsHealth.org. KidsHealth is a website created by the medical experts of the Nemours Foundation and is devoted to issues of children's health. It contains articles on a variety of health topics, including tick-borne infections.
http://www.KidsHealth.org

▶ *See also*
Ehrlichiosis
Lyme Disease
Malaria
Rickettsial Infections
Rocky Mountain Spotted Fever
Zoonoses

Toxoplasmosis

Toxoplasmosis (tox-o-plaz-MO-sis), often called toxo, is a parasitic infection that usually causes no symptoms in healthy people, but it can be serious in people with weak immune systems and in unborn babies.

KEYWORDS
for searching the Internet and other reference sources
Parasitic diseases
Toxoplasma gondii
Zoonoses

What Is Toxoplasmosis?

The parasite *Toxoplasma gondii*, the organism behind toxoplasmosis, is found in soil and can infect humans and many species of animals. It is often found in cats, and is passed in cat feces (FEE-seez, or bowel movements). Touching dirty litter from a cat's litter box is one common way that people contract the parasite. Eating undercooked meat or accidentally eating contaminated soil are other ways that people become infected.

Many people who have toxoplasmosis have no symptoms or symptoms that are very mild. However, women who become infected when they are pregnant can pass the organism to the fetus*. In an unborn child, the parasite can cause congenital* toxoplasmosis, a condition that can range from mild to severe and may involve developmental problems and mental retardation, seizures*, and vision problems. Toxoplasmosis also can take a heavy toll on people with weakened immune systems, such as those with AIDS* or cancer, or those who have had an organ or bone marrow* transplant. Toxoplasmosis may affect the brain in these people.

How Common Is Toxoplasmosis?

The U.S. Centers for Disease Control and Prevention estimates that as many as 60 million people in the United States have been infected with *T. gondii*, but cases of actual disease are much less common. Most people who carry the parasite have no symptoms of illness.

Is Toxoplasmosis Contagious?

Pregnant women who are infected during pregnancy can pass the organism to the unborn child, but this is the only way that it spreads from person to person. Many people contract toxoplasmosis from eating raw or undercooked meat containing the parasite's cysts*, especially pork and

* **fetus** (FEE-tus) is the term for an unborn human after it is an embryo, from 9 weeks after fertilization until childbirth.

* **congenital** (kon-JEH-nih-tul) means present at birth.

* **seizures** (SEE-zhurs) are sudden bursts of disorganized electrical activity that interrupt the normal functioning of the brain, often leading to uncontrolled movements in the body and sometimes a temporary change in consciousness.

* **AIDS**, or acquired immunodeficiency (ih-myoo-no-dih-FIH-shen-see) syndrome, is an infection that severely weakens the immune system; it is caused by the human immunodeficiency virus (HIV).

* **bone marrow** is the soft tissue inside bones where blood cells are made.

* **cysts** (SISTS) are shell-like enclosures that contain a small organism in a resting stage.

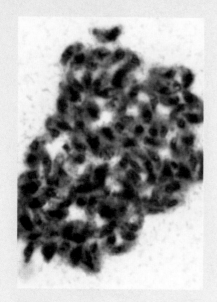

A microscopic view of the *Toxoplasma gondii* parasite. More than 60 million Americans have been infected with this single-celled parasite, though usually only people with weakened immune systems become ill. ©*Arthur M. Siegelman*

* **lymph** (LIMF) **nodes** are small, bean-shaped masses of tissue that contain immune system cells that fight harmful microorganisms. Lymph nodes may swell during infections.

* **retina** (REH-tih-nuhz) is the tissue that forms the inner surface of the back of the eyeballs; it receives the light that enters the eye and transmits it through the optic nerves to the brain to produce visual images.

* **miscarriage** is the ending of a pregnancy through the death of the embryo or fetus before birth.

* **jaundice** (JON-dis) is a yellowing of the skin, and sometimes the whites of the eyes, caused by a buildup in the body of bilirubin, a chemical produced in and released by the liver. An increase in bilirubin may indicate disease of the liver or certain blood disorders.

lamb. Others unknowingly ingest the parasite's eggs after touching cat feces, soil, or anything that has come into contact with cat feces. The eggs can stick to a person's hands and may eventually end up in the mouth, where they can be swallowed.

What Happens to People with Toxoplasmosis?

Most people with the infection have no symptoms. When symptoms do occur, they may include swollen lymph nodes*, muscle aches, headache, and sore throat. For people with weakened immune systems (especially those with AIDS), toxoplasmosis can cause severe infection of the brain or, less commonly, the lungs or heart. As a result, symptoms are worse, and they may include fever, headache, confusion, seizures, blurred vision from inflammation of the retina*, psychosis (sye-KO-sis, form of mental illness in which an individual becomes disconnected from reality), and problems with speech or movement. Severe disease can be fatal.

In some cases, infection in a pregnant woman induces a miscarriage*. Congenital infection in newborns may be marked by small body and head size, jaundice*, rash, fever, anemia*, inflamed retinas, and an enlarged spleen and liver. These children may develop blindness, mental retardation, learning disabilities, and other problems with the central nervous system (the part of the nervous system that includes the brain and spinal cord), such as seizures and difficulty controlling movements. Sometimes the developmental disabilities are present from birth and sometimes they do not appear for many months or years.

How Do Doctors Diagnose Toxoplasmosis?

If a doctor suspects toxoplasmosis, he or she will draw a blood sample and test it for evidence of the parasite. An eye doctor may use a special lamp called a slit lamp to check the eyes for abnormalities of the retinas. People with weakened immune systems who are more likely to develop a severe infection might have magnetic resonance imaging* (MRI), a computerized tomography* (CT) scan of the head, or rarely, a brain biopsy (removing a small sample of brain tissue to examine) to look for signs of damage caused by the parasite. Infants with congenital toxoplasmosis also will need a CT scan of the head and thorough examination of other areas of the body possibly affected by the parasite.

What is the Treatment for Toxoplasmosis?

People who have toxoplasmosis but are otherwise healthy do not need any treatment. However, people with weak immune systems, pregnant women, and newborns with the congenital infection are treated with medication. Patients with AIDS often continue taking the medicine even after the infection clears up to keep it from returning.

Healthy people usually have symptoms for only a few days, if at all. In newborns and patients with unhealthy immune systems, the illness can last for weeks or months and cause permanent disability.

Can Toxoplasmosis Be Prevented?

Pregnant women and people whose immune systems are weak can take steps to avoid infection with *T. gondii*. First, they can be tested for the parasite. If they test positive, they will likely be started on medication for the infection, even if they do not have any symptoms. If they test negative, they can follow some simple measures to keep from becoming infected in the future, such as:

- wearing gloves when gardening and handling soil to prevent infection from parasites in the dirt

- wearing gloves when cooking or having someone who is healthy and not pregnant handle raw meat

- cooking all meat thoroughly, until the juices run clear and it is no longer pink inside

- washing all utensils and cutting boards that have come into contact with raw meat in hot water and soap

- washing hands frequently, particularly after outdoor activities, after preparing food, and before eating

** **anemia** (uh-NEE-me-uh) is a blood condition in which there is a decreased amount of oxygen-carrying hemoglobin in the blood and, usually, fewer than normal numbers of red blood cells.*

** **magnetic resonance imaging** (MRI) uses magnetic waves, instead of X rays, to scan the body and produce detailed pictures of the body's structures.*

** **computerized tomography** (kom-PYOO-ter-ized toe-MAH-gruh-fee) or CT, also called computerized axial tomography (CAT), is a technique in which a machine takes many X rays of the body to create a three-dimensional picture.*

DISEASES ASSOCIATED WITH CATS

- Cat-scratch disease: an infectious illness that can cause swollen lymph nodes and symptoms similar to those of the flu. It is caused by bacteria carried in cat saliva that usually enter the body from a cat scratch or a bite that breaks the skin.

- Cryptosporidiosis (krip-toh-spor-id-e-O-sis): an intestinal infection caused by a parasite that can live in people and animals, including cats. People pick up the parasite through contact with infected feces and typically have diarrhea and stomach pain.

- Giardiasis (jee-ar-DYE-uh-sis): an intestinal infection caused by a parasite that can live in people and animals, including cats. People become infected when they come into contact with feces from an infected person or animal and typically have diarrhea and an upset stomach.

- Lyme (LIME) disease: a bacterial infection spread to humans by the bite of infected ticks, which can

be carried by cats. The illness starts with a distinctive rash and/or symptoms like those of the flu and can progress to a more serious disease with complications affecting other body organs.

- Rabies (RAY-beez): a viral infection of the central nervous system that usually is transmitted to humans by the bite of an infected animal.

- Ringworm: a fungal infection of the skin, scalp, or nails that usually causes red, dry, flaky skin. The fungus also can infect pets such as cats, which can spread the fungus to people.

- Toxocariasis (tox-o-kah-RYE-uh-sis): an infestation in people of a type of parasitic roundworm found in cats (another species is found in dogs). As the worms move through the body, they can affect the eyes and other body organs.

- Toxoplasmosis: a parasitic infection often found in cats, and is passed to humans through contact with cat feces.

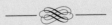

■ keeping family cats inside and feeding them only dry or canned cat food, because cats can pick up the parasite from eating raw meat

■ having someone who is healthy and not pregnant change the cat's litter box every day

■ not touching strange or stray cats or letting any cat into the home that might have lived outside or eaten raw meat

Resources

Organization

U.S. Centers for Disease Control and Prevention (CDC), 1600 Clifton Road, Atlanta, GA 30333. The CDC is the U.S. government authority for information about infectious and other diseases. It provides information about toxoplasmosis at its website. Telephone 800-311-3435
http://www.cdc.gov

Website

KidsHealth.org. KidsHealth is a website created by the medical experts of the Nemours Foundation and is devoted to issues of children's health. It contains articles on a variety of health topics, including toxoplasmosis.
http://www.KidsHealth.org

Travel-related Infections

When people travel to other countries, they are at increased risk for travel-related infections.

What Are Travel-related Infections?

When travelers go abroad, they may be exposed to many bacterial, viral, parasitic, and fungal infections that they would not come into contact with in the United States. With different climates, sanitation, and hygiene practices (such as bathing and urinating in the same water source), some diseases that are rarely or never seen in the United States are common in other parts of the world. The risk of infectious disease is greatest in tropical and subtropical countries because warm, moist climates offer an ideal environment for the survival and growth of certain organisms. Visiting developing regions of the world, particularly Africa (especially sub-Saharan Africa), southeast Asia, and Central and South Amer-

KEYWORDS
for searching the Internet and other reference sources

Cholera

Dengue fever

Ebola virus

Filariasis

Hepatitis

Leishmaniasis

Malaria

Mosquito-borne diseases

Plague

Rabies

Rickettsial infections

Schistosomiasis

Traveler's diarrhea

Trypanosomiasis

Yellow fever

ica, also puts travelers at higher risk for travel-related infections. One of the most common ailments is "traveler's diarrhea" (dye-uh-REE-uh), which can be caused by a variety of bacterial, parasitic, and viral infections. According to the U.S. Centers for Disease Control and Prevention (CDC), between 20 and 50 percent of travelers experience diarrhea.

How Are Travel-related Infections Spread?

Some travel-related infections are spread through the bites of insects, such as mosquitoes (which carry malaria, mah-LAIR-e-uh, and yellow fever) or flies (for example, the tsetse, SET-see, fly can carry trypanosomiasis, trih-pan-o-so-MY-uh-sis). Other diseases, including schistosomiasis (shis-tuh-so-MY-uh-sis), can be contracted from swimming, wading, or bathing in contaminated water. Eating or drinking contaminated food or water is another common way of contracting disease, especially traveler's diarrhea.

What Are Some Common Travel-related Infections?

Malaria   Malaria is a disease that is transmitted through a mosquito bite and affects 300 to 500 million people worldwide each year, according to the World Health Organization (WHO). When an infected mosquito bites a human, the *Plasmodium* (plaz-MO-dee-um) parasite causes fever and symptoms similar to those of the flu, such as extreme tiredness, muscle aches, nausea (NAW-zee-uh), and chills. If left untreated, malaria can cause seizures*, kidney* failure, and death. Medications can treat malaria and prevent disease in travelers.

Cholera   Cholera (KAH-luh-ruh) is a gastrointestinal* disease that causes watery diarrhea, vomiting, and other symptoms. Without treatment, it can lead to dehydration* and even death. People develop cholera by eating food or drinking water that has been contaminated with the cholera bacterium, *Vibrio cholerae* (VIH-bree-o KAH-luh-ray). Eating contaminated shellfish or coming into contact with the feces* of an infected person also could infect someone. A person with cholera is treated to replace fluids lost through vomiting or diarrhea; some antibiotics may reduce the severity and length of the illness.

Dengue fever   Dengue (DENG-gay) fever is caused by a virus from the *Flavivirus* (FLAY-vih-vy-rus) group transmitted to humans via the bite of an infected mosquito. According to the CDC, up to 100 million people worldwide develop symptoms of dengue fever each year, such as fever, severe headaches, joint pain, and rashes. Dengue hemorrhagic (heh-muh-RAH-jik) fever is a severe form of dengue that is associated with bruising easily, bleeding from the nose or gums, and bleeding internally, in addition to the other symptoms of dengue fever. No medication can treat either form of the illness. Doctors recommend that people who have

* **seizures** (SEE-zhurs) are sudden bursts of disorganized electrical activity that interrupt the normal functioning of the brain, often leading to uncontrolled movements in the body and sometimes a temporary change in consciousness.

* **kidney** is one of the pair of organs that filter blood and remove waste products and excess water from the body in the form of urine.

* **gastrointestinal** (gas-tro-in-TES-tih-nuhl) means having to do with the organs of the digestive system, the system that processes food. It includes the mouth, esophagus, stomach, intestines, colon, and rectum and other organs involved in digestion, including the liver and pancreas.

* **dehydration** (dee-hi-DRAY-shun) is a condition in which the body is depleted of water, usually caused by excessive and unreplaced loss of body fluids, such as through sweating, vomiting, or diarrhea.

* **feces** (FEE-seez) is the excreted waste from the gastrointestinal tract.

353

dengue fever drink plenty of fluids to avoid dehydration and take acetaminophen (uh-see-teh-MIH-noh-fen) for pain relief.

Filariasis   A bite from an infected mosquito can transmit filariasis (fih-luh-RYE-uh-sis), a parasitic disease that affects the lymphatic system*. When the infected mosquito feeds, tiny worms pass from it to the person, where they travel to and grow in the lymph vessels. Someone with this disease may not have noticeable symptoms, but filariasis can lead to permanent damage to the kidneys and lymphatic system. It also can progress to a condition called elephantiasis (eh-luh-fan-TIE-uh-sis), in which fluid builds up in parts of the body and causes swelling and disfigurement. The condition can be treated with medication.

Viral hepatitis   Viral hepatitis (heh-puh-TIE-tis) is a viral infection of the liver* that leads to inflammation of the organ. Infections caused by the hepatitis B and C viruses are contracted sexually or through contact with contaminated blood or other body fluids, but hepatitis A virus is more contagious and is the hepatitis virus that more commonly infects travelers. It can spread through person-to-person contact or through contaminated water and food, especially shellfish and raw vegetables and fruits. A person with hepatitis may have symptoms similar to those of the flu, such as fever, chills, and weakness. People with hepatitis A may need extra fluids and rest, but most recover without medication.

Leishmaniasis   Travelers who are bitten by an infected sand fly can develop leishmaniasis (leesh-muh-NYE-uh-sis), a disease caused by *Leishmania* (leesh-MAH-nee-uh) parasites that can affect the skin or the internal organs. People with the skin disease often have skin sores, which may spread to cause facial disfigurement. Those with the internal form of the disease experience fever and an enlarged spleen* or liver and may need to be hospitalized.

Plague   Fleas that bite rodents infected with the bacterium *Yersinia pestis* (yer-SIN-e-uh PES-tis) can transmit plague (PLAYG) to humans. Two to 6 days after becoming infected with plague, a person may have swollen and tender lymph nodes*, fever, cough, chills, and belly pain. The plague can lead to severe respiratory illness, shock*, and death if a person is not treated with antibiotics.

Rabies   Although rabies (RAY-beez) in humans is rare in the United States, people who travel to other countries may be at higher risk for infection. The virus that causes rabies, from the Rhabdoviridae (rab-doh-VEER-ih-day) family, is transmitted to humans through a bite from an infected animal, and without treatment rabies can cause paralysis*, seizures, coma*, and death. A person who has been bitten by an animal suspected of having rabies can receive injections of the rabies vaccine to prevent the infection from developing.

---

* **lymphatic** (lim-FAH-tik) **system** is a system that contains lymph nodes and a network of channels that carry fluid and cells of the immune system through the body.

* **liver** is a large organ located beneath the ribs on the right side of the body. The liver performs numerous digestive and chemical functions essential for health.

* **spleen** is an organ in the upper left part of the abdomen that stores and filters blood. As part of the immune system, the spleen also plays a role in fighting infection.

* **lymph** (LIMF) **nodes** are small, bean-shaped masses of tissue that contain immune system cells that fight harmful microorganisms. Lymph nodes may swell during infections.

* **shock** is a serious condition in which blood pressure is very low and not enough blood flows to the body's organs and tissues. Untreated, shock may result in death.

* **paralysis** (pah-RAH-luh-sis) is the loss or impairment of the ability to move some part of the body.

* **coma** (KO-ma) is an unconscious state in which a person cannot be awakened and cannot move, see, speak, or hear.

Schistosomiasis Schistosomiasis is a disease caused by parasitic *Schistosoma* (shis-tuh-SO-mah) worms that infect humans when they come into contact with contaminated water. The worms must spend part of their life cycle growing in freshwater snails before they enter and infest humans. Common symptoms include rash, fever, muscle aches, and chills. Years later, if left untreated, schistosomiasis can lead to permanent liver damage or damage to the urinary tract*.

Typhoid fever According to the CDC, typhoid (TIE-foyd) fever affects up to 16 million people worldwide each year, although only about 400 cases occur in the United States (and the majority of those contract it while traveling abroad). A person who has contact with water or food contaminated with *Salmonella typhi* (sal-muh-NEH-luh TIE-fee) bacteria may develop symptoms such as fever, weakness, rash, stomach pain, or headache. Typhoid fever is treatable with antibiotics.

Typhus Typhus (TY-fis) is transmitted by the bites of fleas or lice infected with Rickettsiae (rih-KET-see-eye) bacteria. Symptoms of typhus include an extremely high fever, rash, nausea, joint pain, and headache. Patients often become very sick, and without treatment the disease can be life threatening. However, it is treatable with antibiotics.

Viral hemorrhagic fevers Viral hemorrhagic (heh-muh-RAH-jik) fevers (VHF) are a group of rare but potentially life-threatening viral illnesses that cause symptoms ranging from fever, extreme tiredness, and dizziness to bleeding from the eyes and ears, kidney failure, and seizures. Humans contract VHF after exposure to people or animals that have been infected with one of a variety of viruses. Examples of VHF include Ebola virus infection and Lassa fever.

Yellow fever The yellow fever virus (from the flavivirus group) is transmitted to humans by a mosquito bite. Within a week of being infected, a person may experience fever, muscle aches, nausea, or vomiting. Most people recover within 3 to 4 days, but according to WHO about 15 percent of people with yellow fever go on to develop a more serious form of the disease that can cause bleeding, kidney failure, and death. An effective vaccine is available for yellow fever and is often recommended for travelers who will be visiting areas where the disease is found.

Trypanosomiasis African trypanosomiasis is a parasitic illness commonly known as sleeping sickness. The *Trypanosoma* (trih-pan-o-SO-mah) parasite is transmitted to humans through a bite from the tsetse fly, after which a person may develop a skin sore, high fever, extreme tiredness, swollen lymph nodes, and swelling around the eyes. The disease is called sleeping sickness because people who have an advanced form of it can have an uncontrollable urge to sleep. If untreated, trypanosomiasis can cause the brain and membranes around the brain to swell and become inflamed. The disease can be treated with hospitalization and medication.

> * **urinary** (YOOR-ih-nair-e) **tract** is the system of organs and channels that makes urine and removes it from the body. It consists of the urethra, bladder, ureters, and kidneys.

How Can Travelers Protect Themselves from Illness?

Travelers can take precautions to reduce their risk of contracting a disease while abroad. Experts offer the following tips for staying healthy:

- Do not swim, wade, or bathe in freshwater sources, the ocean near beaches that are contaminated with human feces, or pools that are not chlorinated.
- Use only bottled water or water that has been boiled for drinking and brushing teeth.
- Avoid drinks with ice in them, as the ice may be from unsafe water. Canned or bottled beverages are the safest drinks. Carefully wiping the top of the can or bottle before drinking from it may remove disease-causing agents.
- Do not eat raw foods, particularly meat and salad. Avoid raw fruits and vegetables unless you peel them yourself.
- Avoid shellfish and other fish, which can be toxic at certain times of the year even if they have been cooked.
- Do not buy foods from street vendors.
- Avoid unpasteurized milk (milk that has not been processed with heat to kill parasites and bacteria) and dairy products.
- Prevent insect bites by wearing long sleeves and long pants in light colors so the insects can be seen easily.
- Use repellent and sleep under mosquito netting.
- Stay inside at times when biting insects are most active, mostly dawn and dusk.

Vaccination Certain vaccinations* can help protect against infectious diseases that are common in different geographic areas. Depending on the destination and the length of the planned trip, travelers may receive immunizations for hepatitis, meningococcal infection, typhoid fever, or yellow fever, as well as any vaccinations in the regular immunization schedule that the person may have missed or may need to renew, such as those for diphtheria and tetanus. If someone plans to travel abroad, it is important to discuss travel plans with a doctor so that any necessary vaccinations can be given.

Resource

Organization

U.S. Centers for Disease Control and Prevention (CDC), 1600 Clifton Road, Atlanta, GA 30333. The CDC maintains the Travelers' Health Information pages at its website. The Travelers' Health section

* **vaccinations** (vak-sih-NAY-shunz), also called immunizations, are the giving of doses of vaccines, which are preparations of killed or weakened germs, or a part of a germ or product it produces, to prevent or lessen the severity of a disease.

▶ *See also*

Cholera

Dengue Fever

Ebola Virus Infection

Filariasis

Hepatitis, Infectious

Leishmaniasis

Malaria

Plague

Rabies

Rickettsial Infections

Schistosomiasis

Trypanosomiasis

Vaccination (Immunization)

Yellow Fever

offers information about many travel-related infections, where they are found, and the latest research on how to prevent them.
Telephone 800-311-3435
http://www.cdc.gov/travel

Trichinosis

Trichinosis (trih-kih-NO-sis) is a parasitic infection that comes from eating raw or undercooked meat. It is caused by species of the roundworm Trichinella *(trih-kih-NEH-luh).*

What Is Trichinosis?

Also called trichinellosis (trih-kih-neh-LO-sis), trichinosis can occur when people eat meat that is infected with the larvae* of *Trichinella* roundworms (also called nematodes, NEE-muh-todes); *Trichinella spiralis* (spy-RAL-is) is the most common species that causes trichinosis. People can become infected only by eating infected meat; the disease is not spread through human contact. The parasite also can spread when animals eat the infected flesh of other animals. Most often, meat infected with the parasite comes from pigs or wild game, such as bear, horse, wolf, and fox.

Trichinella larvae form cysts (SISTS, shell-like sacs that contain the larvae in a resting stage) in meat. When an animal eats this meat, the animal's stomach acid dissolves the cysts, and the worms are released into the body. They travel to the small intestine*, where they grow into adult worms and mate. After about a week, the mature female worm releases larvae, which travel through the bloodstream to the muscles. There they form the hard cysts that began the cycle. The cysts remain in the muscles, and people become infected when they eat these cysts in animal meat.

How Common Is Trichinosis?

According to the U.S. Centers for Disease Control and Prevention (CDC), there were 16 cases in 2000, down from an average of 38 cases per year from 1991 to 1996. The decline came about because people are now more aware of the dangers of eating raw or undercooked meat; better storage and freezing methods of meat are being used; and laws prohibiting the feeding of raw meat to pigs have been passed. Most trichinosis cases now are associated with eating wild game.

How Do People Know They Have Trichinosis?

The length of the period between eating the infected meat and the first symptoms of illness depends on the number of parasites in the meat and how much a person has eaten. It can range from 1 to 45 days, but symp-

KEYWORDS
for searching the Internet
and other reference sources

Nematodes

Roundworms

Trichinella

* **larvae** (LAR-vee) are the immature forms of an insect or worm that hatch from an egg.

* **small intestine** is the part of the intestine—the system of muscular tubes that food passes through during digestion—that directly receives the food when it passes through the stomach.

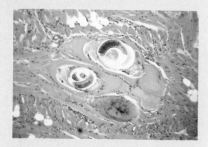

A microscopic view of the larvae of the species of worm *Trichinella* after they have become embedded in muscle, causing trichinosis. *Custom Medical Stock Photo, Inc.*

* **biopsy** (BI-op-see) is a test in which a small sample of skin or other body tissue is removed and examined for signs of disease.

* **antibodies** (AN-tih-bah-deez) are protein molecules produced by the body's immune system to help fight specific infections caused by microorganisms, such as bacteria and viruses.

* **delirium** (dih-LEER-e-um) is a condition in which a person is confused, is unable to think clearly, and has a reduced level of consciousness.

* **coma** (KO-ma) is an unconscious state in which a person cannot be awakened and cannot move, see, speak, or hear.

toms often surface in 10 to 14 days. Symptoms can be mild and even go unnoticed, but they usually start with fever, diarrhea (dye-uh-REE-uh), belly pain, nausea (NAW-zee-uh), vomiting, and extreme tiredness. Other symptoms may follow, such as headache, cough, chills, muscle and joint pain, eye swelling, and constipation. If the infection is severe, a person may have trouble with coordination as well as heart and breathing problems.

How Do Doctors Diagnose and Treat Trichinosis?

A blood test or muscle biopsy* can be done to determine whether a person has trichinosis. The blood test can detect antibodies* working to destroy the parasite, and the biopsy shows the presence of cysts in the muscles. Asking if a person has recently eaten game or traveled outside of the United States may provide information useful in making the diagnosis.

The infection can be treated with various medications to kill the worms in the intestine, but the medication does not get rid of the larvae that have produced cysts in the muscles. These larvae remain in a dormant (inactive) state in the muscle tissue. If the infection is mild, symptoms usually go away after a few months. Muscle aches and weakness may last longer. Some people require only bed rest; others need to be hospitalized and receive oxygen and intravenous (in-tra-VEE-nus) fluids (fluids injected directly into a vein). Severe complications of trichinosis include inflammation of the heart muscle, heart failure, lung problems, delirium*, and coma*. The disease can be fatal if it is not treated.

How Can Trichinosis Be Prevented?

The best way to prevent infection is to eat only thoroughly cooked meat. Curing, drying, salting, and microwaving meat may not kill *Trichinella* larvae. When cooking meat, the juices must be clear (not bloody) and the meat must reach an internal temperature of 170 degrees Fahrenheit. Freezing meat at subzero temperatures for several weeks also should kill any larvae in cysts. Raw meat can contaminate work surfaces, so it must not touch surfaces used to prepare food, and grinders and other utensils used with raw meat must be cleaned thoroughly and not used to prepare cooked meat.

Resources

Book

Gittleman, Ann Louise. *Guess What Came to Dinner? Parasites and Your Health.* New York: Avery Penguin Putnam, 2001.

Organizations

National Institute of Allergy and Infectious Diseases (NIAID), Building 31, Room 7A-50, 31 Center Drive MSC 2520, Bethesda, MD

20892. The NIAID, part of the National Institutes of Health, posts information about trichinosis and other roundworm infections at its website.
http://www.niaid.nih.gov

U.S. Centers for Disease Control and Prevention (CDC), 1600 Clifton Road, Atlanta, GA 30333. The CDC is the U.S. government authority for information about infectious and other diseases. It has a fact sheet about trichinosis at its website.
Telephone 800-311-3435
http://www.cdc.gov

▶ *See also*
Intestinal Parasites
Zoonoses

Trichomoniasis

Trichomoniasis (trih-ko-mo-NYE-uh-sis) is a common sexually transmitted disease (STD) that occurs in both women and men.

KEYWORDS
for searching the Internet and other reference sources

Sexually transmitted diseases (STDs)

Trichomonas vaginalis

What Is Trichomoniasis?

Trichomoniasis (also known as "trich") is an infection caused by the parasite *Trichomonas vaginalis* (trih-koh-MO-nas vah-jih-NAL-is). It usually affects the urethra* in men and the vagina or urethra in women.

The disease spreads from person to person through sexual contact and infects primarily women between the ages of 16 and 35. It is one of the most common STDs in young sexually active women, and the U.S. Centers for Disease Control and Prevention says that about 2 million new cases occur in women each year in the United States. As with all STDs, people who have had many sexual partners are more likely to contract trichomoniasis.

* **urethra** (yoo-REE-thra) is the tube through which urine passes from the bladder to the outside of the body.

What Are the Signs and Symptoms?

Women who contract trichomoniasis are more likely to have symptoms than men who become infected, although many people who have trichomoniasis experience no symptoms at all. If a person has symptoms, they usually appear within 6 months of becoming infected. Women often have a strong-smelling yellow-green or gray foamy vaginal discharge and itching in or around the vagina. Often, the discharge has a fishy odor. They may feel pain or burning during sex or urination and, rarely, lower abdominal* pain. Men typically have no symptoms. When they do, they may feel irritation inside the penis and burning after urination or ejaculation*. They may have a discharge from the penis as well.

* **abdominal** (ab-DAH-mih-nul) refers to the area of the body below the ribs and above the hips that contains the stomach, intestines, and other organs.

* **ejaculation** (e-jah-kyoo-LAY-shun) is the discharge of semen, a whitish fluid containing sperm, from the penis.

* **pelvic exam** is an internal examination of a woman's reproductive organs.

* **cervix** (SIR-viks) is the lower, narrow end of the uterus that opens into the vagina.

How Do Doctors Diagnose Trichomoniasis?

If a woman has symptoms of the disease, the doctor will perform a pelvic exam* to look for the tell-tale signs of inflammation on the cervix* and

359

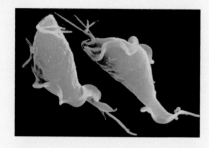

▲

A magnification of *Trichomonas vaginalis*, the parasite that causes trichomoniasis. Infection occurs in both men and women, but women have symptoms more often then men have symptoms. ©*D.M. Phillips/Visuals Unlimited*

* **Pap smear** is a common diagnostic test used to look for cancerous cells in the tissue of the cervix.

* **cultured** (KUL-churd) means subjected to a test in which a sample of fluid or tissue from the body is placed in a dish containing material that supports the growth of certain organisms. Typically, within days the organisms will grow and can be identified.

* **amniotic sac** (am-nee-AH-tik SAK) is the sac formed by the amnion, the thin but tough membrane that lines the outside of the embryo in the uterus and is filled with fluid to cushion and protect the embryo as it grows.

* **premature delivery** is when a baby is born before it has reached full term.

inner walls of the vagina. The doctor will take a sample of fluid from the vagina to look at under the microscope for evidence of the parasite. In some instances, *Trichomonas* infection may be found during a routine Pap smear* or when vaginal fluid is cultured* to diagnose infection caused by other organisms. Most cases of trichomoniasis that cause symptoms can be diagnosed in the doctor's office by examining the vaginal fluid under a microscope.

When trichomoniasis is suspected in a man, the doctor may take a sample of fluid from the man's urethra to confirm the diagnosis. If the doctor diagnoses trichomoniasis in any patient, tests for other STDs likely will be done as well, because it is common for a person to have more than one STD at the same time.

What Is the Treatment for Trichomoniasis?

Trichomoniasis is treated easily with antibiotics. Oral (by mouth) medication given over 1 week usually cures the disease. Doctors recommend that people who are infected not have sex until they have completed treatment, to limit the risk of spreading the infection. Treating all sexual partners of someone who has trichomoniasis, even if they have no symptoms, also is suggested as a way to prevent a new round of infection or the spread of the disease.

Does the Disease Have Complications?

In a pregnant woman, the infection can bring about early rupture of the amniotic sac* and premature delivery*. Trichomoniasis also may increase the risk of becoming infected with human immunodeficiency (ih-myoo-no-dih-FIH-shen-see) virus (HIV), the virus that causes acquired immunodeficiency syndrome (AIDS), which severely weakens the immune system.

Can Trichomoniasis Be Prevented?

The risk of trichomonas infection can be lowered or prevented by:

◻ practicing abstinence (not having sex)

◻ practicing safe sex by using a male latex condom

◻ reducing the number of sexual partners

Resources

Organization

U.S. Centers for Disease Control and Prevention (CDC), 1600 Clifton Road, Atlanta, GA 30333. The CDC runs the National STD and AIDS Hotline to answer questions about sexually transmitted diseases and provide referrals to doctors. It also offers information on trichomoniasis on its website. Telephone 800-311-3435

Hotline 800-227-8922

http://www.cdc.gov

Website

KidsHealth.org. KidsHealth is a website created by the medical experts of the Nemours Foundation and is devoted to issues of children's health. It contains articles on a variety of health topics, including trichomoniasis.

http://www.KidsHealth.org

Trypanosomiasis

Trypanosomiasis (trih-pan-o-so-MY-uh-sis) is a disease found in Africa and the American continents that is caused by infection with a parasite. Forms of the disease may persist for many years and have several phases, with symptoms that can vary from one stage to the next.

What Is Trypanosomiasis?

Trypanosomiasis refers to three types of infections caused by protozoa* and spread to humans through insect bites. There are two kinds of African trypanosomiasis, East African and West African. Both of these varieties also are known as sleeping sickness. The disease can affect people living on the African continent south of the Sahara Desert. American trypanosomiasis also is called Chagas (SHAH-gus) disease. It occurs only on the American continents, from Mexico to Argentina.

What Causes Trypanosomiasis?

The bite of an infected tsetse (SET-see) fly usually transmits the organisms that cause the African forms of trypanosomiasis. These flies live in the countryside in Africa, especially in bushes and thick vegetation near rivers and lakes. Tsetse flies infected with the protozoan *Trypanosoma brucei rhodesiense* (trih-pan-o-SO-mah BRU-see-eye ro-dee-see-EN-see) spread East African trypanosomiasis, the most severe form of the disease, to humans. The West African variety comes from a fly infected with *Trypanosoma brucei gambiense* (trih-pan-o-SO-mah BRU-see-eye gam-be-EN-see).

Reduviid (rih-DO-vee-id) bugs (also called assassin, cone-nose, or kissing bugs) carry the *Trypanosoma cruzi* (trih-pan-o-SO-mah KROO-zee) protozoa that cause the American variety of trypanosomiasis, or Chagas disease, named for the Brazilian doctor who discovered it. These bugs hide during the day in the cracks in mud and adobe homes. At night they crawl across sleeping people and bite them, usually on the face but sometimes on the arms, legs, or trunk. They also leave behind their feces*, which contain the protozoa. Without knowing it, people can rub

▶ *See also*
AIDS and HIV Infection
Chlamydial Infections
Gonorrhea
Sexually Transmitted Diseases

KEYWORDS
for searching the Internet and other reference sources

Chagas disease

Chagoma

Protozoa

Reduviid bug

Sleeping sickness

Trypanosoma brucei

Trypanosoma cruzi

Tsetse fly

* **protozoa** (pro-tuh-ZOH-uh) are single-celled microorganisms (tiny organisms), some of which are capable of causing disease in humans.

* **feces** (FEE-seez) is the excreted waste from the gastrointestinal tract.

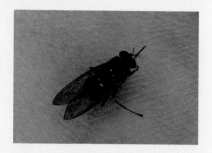

▲

The tsetse fly is responsible for spreading trypanosomiasis in Africa. ©*Rob and Ann Simpson/Visuals Unlimited, Inc.*

* **transfusion** (trans-FYOO-zhun) is a procedure in which blood or certain parts of blood, such as specific cells, is given to a person who needs it because of illness or blood loss.

* **lymph** (LIMF) **nodes** are small, bean-shaped masses of tissue that contain immune system cells that fight harmful microorganisms. Lymph nodes may swell during infections.

* **blood-brain barrier** is a biological shield in the body that helps prevent germs or other potentially harmful materials in the blood from entering the brain and spinal cord.

* **seizures** (SEE-zhurs) are sudden bursts of disorganized electrical activity that interrupt the normal functioning of the brain, often leading to uncontrolled movements in the body and sometimes a temporary change in consciousness.

* **chronic** (KRAH-nik) means continuing for a long period of time.

* **antibodies** (AN-tih-bah-deez) are protein molecules produced by the body's immune system to help fight specific infections caused by microorganisms, such as bacteria and viruses.

the infected feces into the bite, a cut or open sore, or even into their noses, mouths, or eyes.

How Common Is Trypanosomiasis?

Trypanosomiasis can infect people of every age and race, though it is uncommon in the United States. Since the late 1960s, fewer than 30 cases have been reported among U.S. citizens traveling to areas where the infection is found. In other parts of the world, however, the disease affects thousands of people. The World Health Organization estimates that as many as 500,000 people could have African trypanosomiasis, but because of poor monitoring most of these cases are not reported. Between 16 million and 18 million people in the Americas currently have Chagas disease. Approximately 50,000 may die from the disease each year.

Is Trypanosomiasis Contagious?

People cannot catch any form of trypanosomiasis in the same way that they catch a cold or the flu from other people. Only the tsetse fly spreads the African varieties, and the reduviid bug spreads Chagas disease. Rarely, a mother infected with the West African variety of trypanosomiasis or with Chagas disease can pass the illness to her unborn child. People who receive a transfusion* of blood or an organ transplant from an infected person also may contract the disease; this form of transmission tends to happen more often with Chagas disease than with the African types.

What Are the Symptoms of the Disease?

African trypanosomiasis   People who contract the African varieties of trypanosomiasis may start sleeping more, though this usually does not happen until the later stages of the disease. Sleeping sickness may start with the appearance of a sore called a chancre (SHANG-ker) at the spot where the person received the tsetse fly bite. Later symptoms include fever, extreme tiredness, severe headaches, rashes, itching, joint pain, and swelling of the hands and feet. The lymph nodes* on the back of the neck may become swollen as well. These signs typically appear 2 to 4 weeks after infection with East African trypanosomiasis.

Other symptoms can follow quickly, as the protozoa cross the blood-brain barrier* and start affecting a patient's mental functions. The later stages of sleeping sickness may bring mental confusion, changes in personality, problems with walking and talking, weight loss, and seizures*. The spleen and liver may become enlarged. Sleeping sickness gets its name from the later part of the disease, when the sick person has nighttime insomnia (in-SOM-nee-uh, an inability to sleep) but sleeps for long periods during the day. If the person does not receive treatment, the heart muscles may become inflamed or weakened, causing death from heart failure.

The early symptoms in West African trypanosomiasis are similar but may take longer to appear. Months or years may pass before an infected person becomes sick, and the disease develops more slowly, though it still can cause death if it is left untreated. The gap between infection and the start of symptoms can make this form of sleeping sickness difficult to diagnose.

Chagas disease The first sign of Chagas disease may show up a few hours after infection, when a raised red spot called a chagoma (chuh-GO-mah) appears at the site of the insect bite. Most people have no other symptoms during the early, or acute, phase of the disease, which begins a few weeks later. People who experience symptoms may have fevers, rashes, extreme tiredness, vomiting, loss of appetite, or swollen lymph nodes. The side of the face where the infected feces were rubbed into an eye or a bug bite may swell. In most people these symptoms usually disappear within 4 to 8 weeks without causing problems, but infants can die in this early stage from brain swelling. About 10 to 20 years after this first phase, approximately one-third of infected people can show symptoms of the chronic* phase of Chagas disease. They may become constipated and experience trouble swallowing. The heart may become enlarged, and patients may have altered heart rhythms or heart failure leading to death.

How Do Doctors Diagnose Trypanosomiasis?

Because all types of trypanosomiasis are rare in the United States, it is important for people who have any symptoms of the disease to let their doctor know right away if they have been traveling in areas where the disease is common. To diagnose sleeping sickness or Chagas disease, a doctor will order blood tests to look for protozoa or antibodies* to the organism. In cases where the doctor suspects sleeping sickness, a sample drawn from fluid surrounding the brain and spinal cord or tissue from swollen lymph nodes may be examined for evidence of the disease. If a patient has a suspicious-looking skin lesion*, a biopsy* will be performed to test for *Trypanosoma cruzi* protozoa.

Can Trypanosomiasis Be Treated Successfully?

There are medications available to treat all types of the disease. Doctors recommend that people with trypanosomiasis receive treatment as soon as possible. Treatment is given in a hospital. After leaving the hospital, patients typically are watched closely by a doctor for at least 2 years, to see whether they show any signs that they still have the infection.

What Happens to People with Trypanosomiasis?

East African sleeping sickness can move through the body quickly, progressing in just weeks or months to the most serious phase of illness. West African sleeping sickness takes longer to develop. People may not

Global Warming

The bite of an insect can transmit bacteria, protozoa, or even worms into a person's bloodstream, leading to a variety of illnesses. Trypanosomiasis is just one example of a tropical insect-borne disease. Here are a few others, along with the insects that spread them:

- **Malaria**   mosquitoes
  (mah-LAIR-e-uh)
- **Yellow fever**   mosquitoes
- **Elephantiasis**   mosquitoes
  (eh-luh-fan-TIE-uh-sis)
- **Leishmaniasis**   sandflies
  (leesh-muh-NYE-uh-sis)
- **Onchocerciasis,**   black flies
  (on-koh-sir-KYE-us-sis)
  or river blindness

Why are these diseases common to the tropics? It is because the hot and often rainy climate makes the tropics an ideal breeding ground for insects. Greenpeace, among other organizations dedicated to protecting the environment, has warned that global warming could create new breeding grounds for insects throughout the world. At the same time, rising temperatures could raise insect reproductive rates, increasing their numbers. As the climate in the United States and Europe becomes more "tropical," diseases such as yellow fever and malaria may become more common, bringing the tropics into our own backyards.

* **lesion** (LEE-zhun) is a general term referring to a sore or a damaged or irregular area of tissue.

* **biopsy** (BI-op-see) is a test in which a small sample of skin or other body tissue is removed and examined for signs of disease.

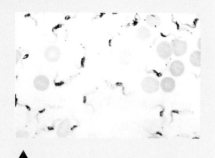

A microscopic view of blood infected with the protozoa that cause trypanosomiasis. These symptoms cause a disease known as sleeping sickness in Africa and Chagas disease in Latin America. *Custom Medical Stock Photo, Inc.*

▶ See also
Leishmaniasis
Travel-related Infections

KEYWORDS
for searching the Internet and other reference sources

Consumption

Directly observed therapy (DOT)

Lung diseases

Mantoux test

MDR tuberculosis

Mycobacterium tuberculosis

PPD test

Tuberculin skin test

reach the critical phase for months or even years. People who do not receive treatment for African trypanosomiasis can die from heart failure, and those who wait to start treatment may have permanent brain damage. Long-term complications of Chagas disease, which may not appear for 20 or more years after infection, include damage to the digestive and nervous systems, heart problems, and sudden death.

Can Trypanosomiasis Be Prevented?

There is no vaccine or medication that can prevent any form of the disease, so it is wise for people who travel in areas where the disease is common to take precautions. In Africa this includes wearing clothes of thick material, with long sleeves and long pants. Neutral colors, such as tan, are best because tsetse flies are attracted to dark and bright colors. Doctors recommend that travelers to Africa sleep under netting and avoid riding in the backs of open trucks, because dust from moving vehicles attracts the flies. It is also advisable to not walk through brush. In areas where Chagas disease is found, it is a good idea for people to avoid sleeping in mud, adobe, or thatch houses; to sleep under netting; and to use insect repellent.

Resources

Organizations

U.S. Centers for Disease Control and Prevention (CDC), 1600 Clifton Road, Atlanta, GA 30333. The CDC publishes fact sheets on all three types of trypanosomiasis at its website.
Telephone 800-311-3435
http://www.cdc.gov

World Health Organization (WHO), Avenue Appia 20, 1211 Geneva 27, Switzerland. WHO publishes information on sleeping sickness and Chagas disease at its website.
Telephone 011-41-22-791-2111
http://www.who.int

Tuberculosis

Tuberculosis (too-ber-kyoo-LO-sis) is a bacterial infection that primarily attacks the lungs but can spread to other parts of the body.

What Is Tuberculosis?

A germ known as *Mycobacterium* (my-ko-bak-TEER-e-um) *tuberculosis* causes tuberculosis (TB). Being infected with the bacterium and actually having the disease tuberculosis are very different. When most people breathe in *M. tuberculosis* bacteria, the immune system quickly seals off the invading bacteria in the lungs and protects the body from illness. These people are said to have latent, or inactive, TB (also called primary infection): their bodies carry the germs, but they have no symptoms and are not contagious. However, latent TB germs sometimes escape the immune system's barriers and cause disease.

When a person's immune system is no longer able to contain the bacteria, or if latent TB activates for other reasons, tuberculosis disease, or active TB, develops (also called secondary infection). Patients may feel sick quickly or develop symptoms gradually over weeks or months, and they may be highly contagious until treated. If TB travels through the blood to invade organs outside the lungs, it is known as disseminated TB. Many organs and bones, including the brain, pericardium (sac surrounding the heart), kidneys*, gastrointestinal* tract, and spine, can become involved and be damaged by the infection.

Is TB Common?

TB is one of the most common causes of death due to infection in the world. About 2 million people around the world die from TB each year. In the nineteenth century, TB was a major cause of death, especially among young children. Drugs to treat the disease were first developed in the 1940s, and they dramatically lowered the number of TB cases over the next few decades. Unfortunately, TB began to resurface in the 1980s, but the number of cases has been declining in recent years. Between 10 and 15 million Americans are believed to have latent TB.

There are several reasons why TB made a comeback:

- HIV/AIDS* has weakened the immune systems of many people, increasing their likelihood of contracting TB.

- Increased numbers of malnourished, poor, or homeless people live in crowded, unclean conditions and are vulnerable to infection.

- TB bacteria become more resistant to medications when patients do not take the drugs as prescribed. Multidrug-resistant (MDR) TB is difficult to treat and spreads easily.

- Immigration to the United States from countries with high rates of TB has increased.

TB can affect anyone, but it is most common among immigrants from countries with high levels of TB and people whose immune systems are weak because of chronic* illness, medications that affect the immune system, infancy, old age, poor nutrition, unclean or crowded living areas (including prisons), alcoholism, or intravenous* (IV) drug use.

In the twenty-first century, the number of TB cases is falling once again in the United States thanks to effective public health measures, in-

HIV and TB: A Lethal Combination

One of the reasons for the surge in TB cases in the 1980s was the rapid increase in the number of HIV cases. Because HIV/AIDS weakens the immune system, patients who have HIV/AIDS are at high risk for contracting TB when the germ first is breathed in. Approximately 11 million people around the globe are infected with both HIV and TB. TB is more likely to spread to other areas of the body in people with HIV, and multidrug-resistant (MDR) TB is much more dangerous in these patients. TB infection in patients who have HIV/AIDS can be cured if found and treated early.

* **kidneys** are the pair of organs that filter blood and remove waste products and excess water from the body in the form of urine.

* **gastrointestinal** (gas-tro-in-TES-tih-nuhl) means having to do with the organs of the digestive system, the system that processes food. It includes the stomach, intestines, and other organs involved in digestion, including the liver and pancreas.

* **AIDS**, or acquired immunodeficiency (ih-myoo-no-dih-FIH-shen-see) syndrome, is an infection that severely weakens the immune system; it is caused by the human immunodeficiency virus (HIV).

* **chronic** (KRAH-nik) means continuing for a long period of time.

* **intravenous** (in-tra-VEE-nus) means within or through a vein. For example, medications, fluid, or other substances can be given through a needle or soft tube inserted through the skin's surface directly into a vein.

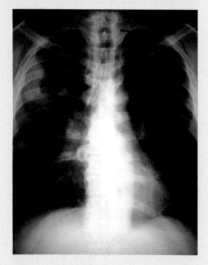

▲

An X ray of lungs infected with *Mycobacterium tuberculosis*, the bacterium that causes tuberculosis. This disease has infected humans for thousands of years. ©*B. Bates/Custom Stock Medical Photo, Inc.*

*__mucus__ (MYOO-kus) is a thick, slippery substance that lines the insides of many body parts.

cluding finding contacts of anyone known to have TB so that they may be treated as well, and directly observing that patients take medication as prescribed.

How Is TB Spread?

Active TB involving the lungs is highly contagious if untreated. Like the flu, TB is spread through the air. When a person with active TB sneezes, coughs, or talks closely to others, bacteria are passed through tiny drops of fluid from the mouth and nose that are unknowingly breathed in by others. Spending lots of time in close quarters with a person who has untreated active TB is the most common way to become infected. A brief encounter with an infected person usually does not spread TB. Touching an infected person or his or her belongings does not put a person at risk for TB. Within a few weeks of the start of effective treatment, patients are no longer contagious.

What Are the Signs and Symptoms of TB?

People with latent TB have no symptoms, but they need to be aware of signs of active TB. Active TB may begin with mild symptoms like those of the flu but quickly worsens. Possible symptoms include:

- cough that lasts a long time
- coughing up blood or lots of mucus*
- chest pain
- loss of appetite and weight loss
- weakness and exhaustion
- fever and chills
- night sweats

If TB spreads to other parts of the body, additional serious symptoms may occur, depending on the organs involved.

How Do Doctors Diagnose and Treat TB?

TB infection is detected through a skin test known as the Mantoux test or PPD (purified protein derivative) test. A tiny amount of tuberculin (too-BER-kyoo-lin) substance, a protein taken from *M. tuberculosis*, is injected into the skin of an arm. A few days later a health professional will check to see if a bump has formed at the site of the injection. If the bump is wider than a certain size (for most people, 10 to 15 millimeters or a half inch), the patient most likely has been infected by TB bacteria; this is known as a positive skin test.

Next, a doctor will determine if the patient has active TB through a physical exam and by asking about symptoms and people the patient has had close contact with recently. The doctor may hear "crackles" when listening to the lungs with a stethoscope if a person has active TB. A chest X ray will be done, and samples of sputum*, blood, and urine may be tested. It can take weeks to confirm a diagnosis, although treatment can begin based on the skin test results and the person's symptoms.

Both latent and active TB can be cured if patients closely follow their doctors' orders. Antibiotics must be taken by mouth every day for 6 months to 1 year. Hospitalization and isolation may be required in the early stages of active disease for people who are highly contagious or who have severe symptoms. Patients must continue to take medications even if they begin to feel better. If they do not, the germs that are still in the body can cause symptoms to return and drugs to stop working properly due to the development of MDR TB.

Once treatment begins, TB symptoms disappear within a few weeks. People with TB can lead normal, active lives while taking their medications over the course of several months.

What Are Some Complications of TB?

Complications of TB include:

- side effects of the drugs used to treat TB, which range from mild to severe
- lung damage and difficulty breathing
- damage to other organs from disseminated TB
- development of MDR TB
- other bacterial infections
- death

Can TB Be Prevented?

The Centers for Disease Control and Prevention recommends that people at high risk for TB (such as those with HIV infection or immigrants from areas with high rates of TB) get a skin test yearly so that treatment can begin immediately if they are found to have TB.

A TB vaccine* is given to infants and toddlers in countries with high levels of the disease. The vaccine is not commonly used in the United States because it does not always work and it may cause a positive skin test, making it more difficult to detect true TB infection.

Practical prevention tips include:

- avoiding close contact with people infected with TB until they are no longer contagious
- wearing a special type of facemask (called a respirator) that can prevent the spread of TB if close contact with someone who has TB is necessary

MDR TB

Multidrug-resistant tuberculosis (MDR TB) occurs when TB patients stop taking their prescribed medications or do not take them as directed. Patients often stop taking the drugs when they begin to feel better or to avoid side effects. However, TB bacteria can survive inside the body for several months during treatment and are ready to spring back into activity when the medication disappears.

Symptoms return with a vengeance, and infected people become highly contagious again, putting those close to them at risk. In MDR TB, germs become stronger than the antibiotics, making the drugs less effective. Patients with MDR TB need special medications, but they may not work as well. In addition, patients can spread this highly dangerous form of the disease to others.

One way to fight this problem is through directly observed therapy (DOT). In DOT, patients must take their medications regularly in the presence of a health professional. Home visits by health professionals to supervise the taking of medications or free transportation and meals often are provided to encourage patients to take part in this type of program.

* **sputum** (SPYOO-tum) is a substance that contains mucus and other matter coughed out from the lungs, bronchi, and trachea.

* **vaccine** (vak-SEEN) is a preparation of killed or weakened germs, or a part of a germ or product it produces, given to prevent or lessen the severity of the disease that can result if a person is exposed to the germ itself. Use of vaccines for this purpose is called immunization.

Resources

Organizations

American Lung Association, 61 Broadway, 6th Floor, New York, NY 10006. The American Lung Association offers information about tuberculosis and other diseases that affect the lungs at its website. Telephone 212-315-8700
http://www.lungusa.org

National Institute of Allergy and Infectious Diseases (NIAID), Building 31, Room 7A-50, 31 Center Drive MSC 2520, Bethesda, MD 20892. The NIAID, part of the National Institutes of Health, posts information about tuberculosis at its website.
http://www.niaid.nih.gov

U.S. Centers for Disease Control and Prevention (CDC), 1600 Clifton Road, Atlanta, GA 30333. The CDC is the U.S. government authority for information about infectious and other diseases. It provides information about tuberculosis at its website. Telephone 800-311-3435
http://www.cdc.gov

World Health Organization (WHO), Avenue Appia 20, 1211 Geneva 27, Switzerland. WHO posts information about tuberculosis and tracks TB cases worldwide on its website. Telephone 011-41-22-791-2111
http://www.who.int

Tularemia

Tularemia (too-lah-REE-me-uh), sometimes called rabbit fever, is an infection caused by bacteria that can be spread to humans by wild animals.

Do Rabbits Cause Rabbit Fever?

Tularemia is caused by the bacterium *Francisella tularensis* (fran-sih-SEL-uh too-lah-REN-sis). Most cases in the United States come from contact with infected rabbits and deer, although the bacterium also lives in other small mammals and birds, and it can be found in soil.

Tularemia bacteria enter the body through the mucous membranes*, the skin, the lungs, or the digestive system. There are seven different forms of the disease:

■ **Ulceroglandular tularemia** comes from handling an infected animal or from the bite of a tick or deer fly. An ulcer (an open sore) forms on the skin.

▶ *See also*
AIDS and HIV Infection
Pneumonia
Public Health

KEYWORDS
for searching the Internet and other reference sources

Biological weapons

Bioterrorism

Francisella tularensis

Rabbit fever

Tick-borne diseases

Zoonoses

*mucous membranes are the moist linings of the mouth, nose, eyes, and throat.

- **Glandular tularemia** causes symptoms similar to those of the ulceroglandular form but an ulcer does not form. The bacteria may enter the body through small cuts in the skin. Most cases of rabbit fever in the United States are glandular or ulceroglandular tularemia.

- **Oculoglandular tularemia** comes from touching the eye with infected fingers. The eye becomes red and painful and has a discharge.

- **Oropharyngeal tularemia** comes from eating the undercooked meat of an infected animal or from drinking water contaminated by the bacterium. It causes digestive system symptoms, such as vomiting or diarrhea.

- **Pneumonic tularemia** is caused by inhaling spores (an inactive form of the germ enclosed in a protective shell) in dust from a contaminated area into the lungs. Other types of tularemia also may spread to the lungs.

- **Typhoidal tularemia** affects many organs of the body. This rare form of the disease occurs without any previous signs of infection in any specific part of the body.

- **Septic tularemia** is a severe form of the disease that affects the whole body. Someone with this form may go into shock* and experience serious complications.

How Do People Contract Rabbit Fever?

People cannot catch tularemia from one another. Most cases in the United States occur when someone gets a bite from a tick or deer fly that has previously bitten an infected rabbit or deer. Those in contact with infected animals may be infected by the bacterium through small cuts on the skin. Hunters contract tularemia from handling or eating undercooked, contaminated meat. In rare cases, bacterial spores survive in the soil and are released into the air; people then breathe the spores into their lungs. Drinking contaminated water is another rare but possible way to contract the disease.

Is Tularemia Common?

Tularemia occurs in the United States, Europe, and Asia, mainly in rural areas. Tularemia is highly infectious, but in the United States fewer than 200 cases are reported each year (mostly from Texas, Arkansas, and Oklahoma). Some additional cases may not be recognized and reported.

Tularemia affects people of every age, sex, and race. In spring and summer months, it occurs most often in children who become infected when playing outside. In fall and winter, hunters are more likely to contract the infection.

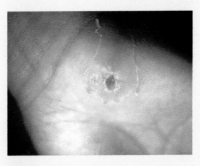

An ulcer associated with *Ulceroglandular tularemia*. This type of tularemia results from the bite of a tick or fly or from contact with an infected animal. *Custom Medical Stock Photo, Inc.*

*** shock** is a serious condition in which blood pressure is very low and not enough blood flows to the body's organs and tissues. Untreated, shock may result in death.

Is Tularemia the Next Anthrax?

It takes as few as 10 spores of the *Francisella tularensis* bacterium to infect someone with tularemia. The bacterium is hard to destroy and can be easily released into the air. For these reasons, experts on biological warfare fear that some groups might use tularemia as a weapon.

The United States stockpiled the bacteria during the 1960s but destroyed its stores in the 1970s at the order of the president. Russia, too, stockpiled and produced the bacteria through the mid-1990s.

There is no vaccine currently available in the United States. In the event of a bioterrorist attack, swift and widespread use of antibiotics could reduce the harmful effects of the disease.

* **lymph** (LIMF) **nodes** are small, bean-shaped masses of tissue that contain immune system cells that fight harmful micro-organisms. Lymph nodes may swell during infections.

* **pneumonia** (nu-MO-nyah) is inflammation of the lung.

* **respiratory failure** is a condition in which breathing and oxygen delivery to the body is dangerously altered. This may result from infection, nerve or muscle damage, poisoning, or other causes.

* **gastrointestinal** (gas-tro-in-TES-tih-nuhl) means having to do with the organs of the digestive system, the system that processes food. It includes the mouth, esophagus, stomach, intestines, colon, and rectum and other organs involved in digestion, including the liver and pancreas.

* **antibodies** (AN-tih-bah-deez) are protein molecules produced by the body's immune system to help fight specific infections caused by microorganisms, such as bacteria and viruses.

* **immunity** (ih-MYOON-uh-tee) is the condition of being protected against an infectious disease. Immunity often develops after a germ is introduced to the body. One type of immunity occurs when the body makes special protein molecules called antibodies to fight the disease-causing germ. The next time that germ enters the body, the antibodies quickly attack it, usually preventing the germ from causing disease.

What Are the Symptoms of Tularemia?

Symptoms of tularemia depend on the form of the disease. Most infected people have a red spot at the site of the insect bite or cut where the bacterium entered the body. This becomes an ulcer.

Other signs and symptoms appear within 1 to 14 days (most frequently in 2 to 5 days) and may come on suddenly. They can include extreme tiredness, muscle aches, fever, headache, sweating, chills, and weight loss. Lymph nodes* in the groin and armpits may become swollen.

People who contract tularemia from inhaled bacteria usually have pneumonia*-like symptoms, such as a dry cough, shortness of breath, or discomfort in the chest area. This form can progress to shock and respiratory failure*.

People who drink contaminated water or eat contaminated meat may experience nausea (NAW-zee-uh), vomiting, pain in the abdomen, diarrhea, sore throat, and sometimes gastrointestinal* bleeding.

How Can a Doctor Tell if a Person Has Tularemia?

Doctors use blood tests to check for tularemia. Some tests look for antibodies* to the *Francisella tularensis* bacterium. Doctors also may look for evidence of the bacterium in the blood, fluid from the nose and mouth, and lymph nodes. If the person has symptoms of pneumonia, a chest X ray will be taken.

How Is Tularemia Treated?

Tularemia responds well to antibiotics, and most people can receive treatment at home. Because tularemia is not contagious, people who have it do not have to be isolated.

In more severe cases, when the disease attacks the lungs or other organs, people may require hospitalization and closer monitoring.

Most people who receive treatment recover from tularemia. The septic and pneumonic forms of the disease can be life threatening, however. Symptoms of tularemia can last for several weeks. Most people do not experience any lasting damage from the disease and may develop some degree of immunity* to it.

Complications of tularemia can include pneumonia, meningitis*, osteomyelitis*, kidney problems, lung abscesses*, pericarditis (inflammation of the sac surrounding the heart), shock, and, rarely, death.

Is There Any Way to Prevent Tularemia?

In the past, laboratory workers at risk for contracting tularemia because of frequent contact with laboratory animals were vaccinated against the disease. In 2003, the vaccine is not available for public use in the United States while the Food and Drug Administration performs further studies.

The best way to avoid contracting tularemia is to prevent tick bites by using repellent and wearing light-colored clothing that covers arms and legs. It is wise to avoid contact with certain wild animals, such as rabbits. Experts recommend that hunters wear rubber gloves when handling animals and that all meat be thoroughly cooked. Swimming in or drinking water that might be contaminated should be avoided.

Resources

Organizations

American College of Emergency Physicians, 1125 Executive Circle, Irving, TX 75038. The American College of Emergency Physicians provides advice about avoiding tick bites in the article "Tick Bites— They're Not Just About Lyme Disease" posted at its website.
Telephone 800-798-1822
http://www.acep.org

U.S. Centers for Disease Control and Prevention (CDC), 1600 Clifton Road, Atlanta, GA 30333. The CDC is the U.S. government authority for information about infectious and other diseases. It has a web page explaining tularemia and how it can be used as a biochemical weapon.
Telephone 800-311-3435
http://www.cdc.gov

* **meningitis** (meh-nin-JY-tis) is an inflammation of the meninges, the membranes that surround the brain and the spinal cord. Meningitis is most often caused by infection with a virus or a bacterium.

* **osteomyelitis** (ah-stee-o-my-uh-LYE-tis) is a bone infection that is usually caused by bacteria. It can involve any bone in the body, but it most commonly affects the long bones in the arms and legs.

* **abscess** (AB-ses) is a localized or walled off accumulation of pus caused by infection that can occur anywhere in the body.

 See also
Bioterrorism
Meningitis
Osteomyelitis
Pneumonia
Tick-borne Infections
Zoonoses

U

Urinary Tract Infections

A urinary (YOOR-ih-nair-e) tract infection, or UTI, is an infection that occurs in any part of the urinary tract. The urinary tract is made up of the urethra*, bladder*, ureters*, and kidneys*.

What Are UTIs?

A UTI usually is caused by bacteria. The bacterium most often responsible for UTIs is *Escherichia coli* (eh-sher-IH-she-ah KOH-lye). Many kinds of *E. coli* bacteria normally are found in human intestines* (and the vagina in women), but sometimes they are able to make their way into the urethra. When this happens, the bacteria can spread up into other parts of the urinary tract and cause an infection. Other types of bacteria from the intestines and some viruses also can produce infections in the urinary tract. The bacteria *Chlamydia* (kla-MIH-dee-uh) and *Mycoplasma* (my-ko-PLAZ-muh) can cause UTIs as well, but these types of infections usually stay in the urethra or reproductive system.

The type of UTI that a person contracts depends on which part of the urinary system is infected with bacteria. When bacteria grow in the urethra and cause inflammation, it is called urethritis (yoo-ree-THRY-tis). If the infection involves the bladder, it is called cystitis (sis-TIE-tis). If infection has spread to the kidneys, it is called pyelonephritis (py-uh-lo-nih-FRY-tis).

How Common Are UTIs?

Urinary tract infections are very common: millions of people, especially women, have them every year. It is estimated that 1 in 5 women will have at least one UTI in her lifetime, and some women have them repeatedly. UTIs are not uncommon in children; by the time children reach their eleventh birthday, 3 in 100 girls and 1 in 100 boys will have had a UTI. Women and girls are at a higher risk of UTIs because the urethra is much shorter in a woman than it is in a man. A shorter urethra means a shorter distance for bacteria to travel to enter the urinary tract. Also, because the opening of the urethra is much closer to the anus* in females, if a girl has a bowel movement and any bacteria are left on the skin nearby, it is easy for them to invade the urethra.

Men may have UTIs too, but these infections usually result from something in the urinary tract that blocks the normal flow of urine from

KEYWORDS
for searching the Internet and other reference sources

Cystitis

Kidney infection

Pyelonephritis

Urethritis

Urology

* **urethra** (yoo-REE-thra) is the tube through which urine passes from the bladder to the outside of the body.

* **bladder** is a sac-like organ that stores urine before releasing it from the body.

* **ureters** (YOOR-eh-ters) are tube-like structures that carry urine from the kidneys to the bladder.

* **kidneys** are the pair of organs that filter blood and remove waste products and excess water from the body in the form of urine.

* **intestines** are the muscular tubes that food passes through during digestion after it exits the stomach.

* **anus** (A-nus) is the opening at the end of the digestive system, through which waste leaves the body.

The organs of the urinary tract, any of which may become the site of infection. ▶

Kidneys

Ureters

Bladder

Urethra

*kidney stone is a hard structure that forms in the urinary tract. This structure is composed of crystallized chemicals that have separated from the urine. It can obstruct the flow of urine and cause tissue damage and pain as the body attempts to pass the stone through the urinary tract and out of the body.

*prostate (PRAH-state) is a male reproductive gland located near where the bladder joins the urethra. The prostate produces the fluid part of semen.

*urinary catheters are thin tubes used to drain urine from the body.

the body, such as a kidney stone* or an enlarged prostate* in older men. In fact, anyone who has a problem with the structure of the urinary tract or the way it functions is more likely to have UTIs. Urinary catheters* can cause UTIs in either men or women because bacteria can enter the urinary tract more easily when a catheter is present. For this reason, UTIs can be a serious problem among patients in hospitals, where catheters are used frequently. UTIs are not contagious, which means that you cannot catch a UTI from someone who has one. *Chlamydia* and *Mycoplasma* bacteria, however, can be transmitted through sexual intercourse.

What Are the Signs and Symptoms of a UTI?

Some people may not have any symptoms of a UTI, but when the infection occurs, it usually brings with it a burning or stinging feeling during urination. People with UTIs may feel as if they have to urinate more frequently and more urgently than usual, but when a person does urinate, sometimes very little comes out. A UTI can make a person feel very tired or feverish; it also can produce a feeling of pressure in the lower belly in women and a sensation of pressure or fullness in the rectum* in men. The urine itself can be cloudy or have a bit of blood in it, and it may smell bad. If the bacteria spread to the kidneys and cause pyelonephritis, the person typically feels very ill, with fever, chills, nausea (NAW-zee-uh), vomiting, and sharp pain in the back or side.

How Do Doctors Diagnose UTIs?

If a doctor suspects that a patient has a UTI, he or she will ask about the person's symptoms to rule out other conditions. For example, an allergic reaction to a soap may cause irritation of the urethra that could lead to stinging when a person urinates, mimicking a UTI. The doctor may take a urine sample and then dip a special strip of paper into it, testing for infection-fighting white blood cells, protein, nitrates*, and blood, which can all be signs that a UTI might be present. The urine sample will be examined under a microscope for bacteria and types of white blood cells that might point to infection. To confirm the presence of a UTI, the urine sample will be cultured*. Any bacteria that grow are tested to see which antibiotics will kill them. This helps the doctor decide which medication will best treat the UTI.

If an infant has a UTI or if an adult or child has repeated UTIs, the doctor may want to see if there are any problems in the urinary tract that may be causing or contributing to the infections. The doctor may order tests (such as special X rays or ultrasound* images of the urinary tract) to take a better look at the shape and function of the kidneys, bladder, and ureters. If there are any problems, the patient may be referred to a urologist, a doctor who specializes in diagnosing and treating problems of the urinary tract. The urologist can examine the urethra and bladder with a cystoscope (SIS-tuh-skope), a special lighted tube with lenses that is inserted into the urethra.

What Is the Treatment for UTIs?

Once a doctor confirms that a bacterial UTI is present, antibiotics are prescribed, which usually clear up the infection. If the UTI involves the

*****rectum** is the final portion of the large intestine, connecting the colon to the anus.

*****nitrates** (NYE-trayts) are chemical substances that can be produced by the breakdown of proteins by certain bacteria.

*****cultured** (KUL-churd) means subjected to a test in which a sample of fluid or tissue from the body is placed in a dish containing material that supports the growth of certain organisms. Typically, within days the organisms will grow and can be identified.

*****ultrasound**, also called a sonogram, is a diagnostic test in which sound waves passing through the body create images on a computer screen.

375

*intravenously means given or injected directly through a vein.

*diabetes (dye-uh-BEE-teez) is a condition in which the body's pancreas does not produce enough insulin or the body cannot use the insulin it makes effectively, resulting in increased levels of sugar in the blood. This can lead to increased urination, dehydration, weight loss, weakness, and a number of other symptoms and complications related to chemical imbalances within the body.

*high blood pressure, also called hypertension, is a condition in which the pressure of the blood in the arteries is above normal.

*genital (JEH-nih-tul) refers to the external sexual organs.

*malformation (mal-for-MAY-shun) is an abnormal formation of a body part.

kidneys, this can be a more serious medical problem. Patients with a kidney infection usually need to be treated in a hospital. Antibiotics and fluids may be given intravenously* until fever disappears and the patient begins to feel better. Even if they have no symptoms, all men typically are treated if they are found to have a UTI, and so are women who are pregnant and those who have diabetes* or abnormalities of the urinary tract. Treatment is necessary in these cases because there is a higher risk of pyelonephritis. Young women who have bacteria in the urine but who do not have symptoms of a UTI usually do not need treatment.

A person taking antibiotics for urethritis or cystitis usually will feel much better soon after starting the medication. During the first few days of treatment, a heating pad can help soothe some of the lower belly pain that may come with UTIs. There are also medicines that ease discomfort during urination. It is important to remember that these medicines do not treat the infection; they treat only the symptoms of stinging and burning. Doctors advise people with UTIs to take all prescribed antibiotics, which usually are given for about a week. Taking all of the prescribed medication is necessary even if a patient begins to feel better right away. Stopping the antibiotics early can mean that the infection will come back, because all the bacteria may not have been killed. A person with pyelonephritis typically can expect a longer recovery time, possibly up to several weeks. It is very important that kidney infections be cured completely because they can lead to serious problems, such as permanent kidney damage, high blood pressure*, and even kidney failure later in life.

Can UTIs Be Prevented?

When it comes to preventing UTIs, practicing good hygiene is a major part of keeping bacteria from entering the urinary tract. It is wise for men and women to keep the genital*, urinary, and anal areas clean. It is recommended that women wipe from front to back, from the urinary tract opening to the anus, after going to the toilet.

Doctors advise that people who want to keep UTIs at bay drink plenty of water, which helps flush out the urinary tract. Going to the bathroom when a person feels the need to go, instead of holding urine in, also can help deter UTIs. Finally, some foods or drinks (such as acidic fruit juices, like orange juice or grapefruit juice; spicy foods; or foods or drinks that contain caffeine) can irritate the bladder; it is a good idea for a person with a UTI to avoid them if they cause irritation. Infants, children, and adults who have UTIs as a result of a malformation* or other problems in the urinary tract are at increased risk of contracting UTIs in the future. Their doctors may prescribe small doses of antibiotics to take every day for several months or longer to help prevent infections and possible damage to the kidneys over time.

Resources

Websites

Healthcommunities.com. Healthcommunities.com operates a website with links to many separate sites focusing on specific health concerns. The Urology Channel site has in-depth information about the parts of the urinary tract, urinary tract infections, and other urological conditions.
http://www.urologychannel.com

KidsHealth.org. KidsHealth is a website created by the medical experts of the Nemours Foundation and is devoted to issues of children's health. It contains articles on a variety of health topics, including urinary tract infections.
http://www.KidsHealth.org

▶ *See also*
Pinworm Infestation
Schistosomiasis
Sexually Transmitted Diseases

V

Valley Fever *See* Coccidioidomycosis

Varicella (Chicken Pox) and Herpes Zoster (Shingles)

Infection with the varicella zoster (var-uh-SEH-luh ZOS-ter) virus (VZV) causes the diseases varicella and herpes zoster. Varicella zoster belongs to the herpesvirus family* of viruses.

What Is Varicella?

This highly contagious disease is characterized by the appearance of crops of red, itchy spots on the skin. The spots progress to blisters and eventually develop crusts and heal. Primary (first-time) infection with varicella causes chicken pox. Usually someone who becomes ill with chicken pox will not have the disease again, because the body's immune system makes antibodies* that protect against chicken pox in the future.

After someone has chicken pox, the varicella virus stays inside the person's body for life. It has the ability to become dormant (inactive) and hide in nerve tissue. After many years, sometimes during a time of emotional or physical stress, varicella can reappear in the form of a disease called shingles, or herpes zoster. (Herpes zoster is not the same as the herpes simplex virus infection that causes cold sores and genital* sores.)

Although the varicella virus causes both chicken pox and shingles, the two have different symptoms and distinct rashes. Shingles usually affects people who are older than 50, although it can develop in people of any age, and its most common sign is a painful single band of red blisters in a small area on one side of the face or body.

How Common Is Varicella?

Chicken pox was once a rite of passage for nearly every child. It used to cause an estimated 4 million cases of illness, 11,000 hospitalizations, and 100 deaths each year in the United States. Today the varicella virus vaccine*, first used in the United States in 1995, has dramatically limited the number of people, especially children, who become infected with varicella. Even with the use of the vaccine, cases of chicken pox are not

KEYWORDS
for searching the Internet and other reference sources
Chicken pox
Herpesvirus family
Herpes zoster
Shingles
Varicella zoster virus

* **herpesvirus** (her-peez-VY-rus) **family** is a group of viruses that can store themselves permanently in the body. The family includes varicella zoster virus, Epstein-Barr virus, and herpes simplex virus.

* **antibodies** (AN-tih-bah-deez) are protein molecules produced by the body's immune system to help fight specific infections caused by microorganisms, such as bacteria and viruses.

* **genital** (JEH-nih-tul) refers to the external sexual organs.

* **vaccine** (vak-SEEN) is a preparation of killed or weakened germs, or a part of a germ or product it produces, given to prevent or lessen the severity of the disease that can result if a person is exposed to the germ itself. Use of vaccines for this purpose is called immunization.

Chickpea pox?

The word chicken pox may derive from *cicer*, the Latin word for "chickpea." A popular ingredient in salads and the base for spreads such as hummus (HUH-mus), chickpeas are round, buff-colored, and a bit larger than green peas. What is the connection to chicken pox? The pox blisters look a bit like chickpeas on the skin.

* **AIDS**, or acquired immuno-deficiency (ih-myoo-no-dih-FIH-shen-see) syndrome, is an infection that severely weakens the immune system; it is caused by the human immunodeficiency virus (HIV).

uncommon. The vaccine may not work in up to 10 to 15 percent of children, and older children and adults who have not had chicken pox or received the vaccine can contract varicella. Shingles is diagnosed in 600,000 to 1 million people in the United States each year.

Is Varicella Contagious?

Chicken pox is highly contagious. Most people who have never had chicken pox or been vaccinated will contract the disease if they come into close contact with someone who has it. Anyone with chicken pox can transmit the virus starting 1 to 2 days before the rash appears and will remain contagious until the pox blisters crust over. Varicella is less contagious when it resurfaces as shingles.

How Is It Spread?

Little bits of moisture, called respiratory droplets, that enter the air when someone coughs or sneezes can spread the varicella virus from one person to another. The fluid inside the pox blisters also can spread the infection. Because shingles blisters carry the varicella virus as well, it is wise for people with shingles to avoid contact with anyone, especially an adult, who has not had chicken pox. It is also best to avoid contact with pregnant women, newborns, and anyone whose immune system is weakened, for example, by HIV/AIDS*, certain kinds of cancers, or having had an organ transplant.

What Are the Signs and Symptoms of Infection?

Chicken pox   The signs of chicken pox usually appear 2 to 3 weeks after exposure to the virus and typically begin with fever, headache, and tiredness. The classic chicken pox rash starts as red spots on the face, chest, back, buttocks, and, less commonly, arms and legs. The spots quickly turn into blisters that break, oozing fluid and then crusting over. Chicken pox spots often pop up in crops, with several spots seeming to appear at once. New batches of blisters usually stop developing after the fourth or fifth day of illness. The rash ranges from mildly to severely itchy, and the number of blisters varies, too—some people have just a few, while others erupt with hundreds of sores.

Shingles   The first symptoms include an intense tingling, burning, or itching that is usually painful and occurs on only one side of the body. A rash of fluid-filled blisters on reddened skin appears next. The rash follows the path of the inflamed nerve tissue and looks like a streak or a band. It can last up to 2 to 3 weeks before healing completely and scabbing over. The pain of shingles usually subsides when the rash disappears, but it may last longer. Other symptoms, such as chills, fever, nausea (NAW-zee-uh), stomach pain, and diarrhea (dye-uh-REE-uh), may occur as well, although they are uncommon.

How Do Doctors Make the Diagnosis?

Doctors usually recognize chicken pox or shingles by their distinctive rashes. Laboratory tests on the fluid in blisters from either disease can help diagnose varicella infection. Blood tests to detect antibodies to the varicella virus can be used to determine whether a person is immune* to chicken pox.

What Is the Treatment for Varicella?

Because varicella is caused by a virus, it does not respond to antibiotics. Doctors advise infected adults and people with weakened immune systems, who are typically at greater risk of experiencing complications of chicken pox (such as pneumonia, nu-MO-nyah, which is inflammation of the lung), to be treated for a few days with specific antiviral medications, such as acyclovir (a-SYE-klo-veer), to control the infection. Preventive treatment also is recommended for people living in the same house with a person who has chicken pox. Children with chicken pox should not be given aspirin for fever, because of the risk of Reye syndrome*. A non-aspirin fever reducer such as acetaminophen (uh-see-teh-MIH-noh-fen) is recommended instead.

In general, the goal of chicken pox treatment is to ease the discomfort caused by itchy blisters. Cool compresses or lukewarm baths in water sprinkled with uncooked oatmeal or baking soda can soothe the skin and relieve itching. Over-the-counter antihistamines* also can help control itching. It is important to trim fingernails short, because scratching blisters can lead to skin infections if the scratching tears the skin. If shingles is recognized soon after its rash first appears it can be treated with oral (by mouth) antiviral medicine. This treatment can shorten the course of the disease and minimize pain.

How Long Does Infection Last?

Children usually recover from chicken pox within 1 to 2 weeks. Adults may be ill longer. Blisters from shingles typically clear up after 2 to 3 weeks, but nerve pain can linger for weeks or months, sometimes even years.

Are There Complications?

The most common complication of chicken pox is cellulitis (sel-yoo-LYE-tis), an infection of the skin caused by bacteria, such as streptococci (strep-tuh-KAH-kye) and staphylococci (stah-fih-lo-KAH-kye). Skin irritation from repeatedly scratching pox sores allows the bacteria to invade the skin. In some cases, varicella infection can spread to the lungs causing pneumonia. Newborn babies, teens, and adults are more likely to develop this complication. Even in healthy people, chicken pox pneumonia can be dangerous and may be fatal. Adults are also more at risk of other serious but rare complications, including liver and kidney disease and encephalitis (en-seh-fuh-LYE-tis, which is inflammation of the

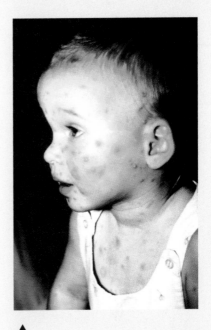

The majority of children in the United States contracted chicken pox until a vaccine, which became available in 1995, dramatically reduced the rate of infection. ©*John D. Cunningham/Visuals Unlimited*

* **immune** (ih-MYOON) means resistant to or not susceptible to a disease.

* **Reye** (RYE) **syndrome** is a rare condition that involves inflammation of the liver and brain, and sometimes appears after illnesses such as chicken pox or influenza. It has also been associated with taking aspirin during certain viral infections.

* **antihistamines** (an-tie-HIS-tuh-meens) are drugs used to combat allergic reactions and itching.

*cornea (KOR-nee-uh) is the transparent circular layer of cells over the central colored part of the eyeball (the iris) through which light enters the eye.

*immune globulin (ih-MYOON GLAH-byoo-lin), also called gamma globulin, is the protein material that contains antibodies.

*intravenously (in-tra-VEE-nus-lee) means given or injected directly through a vein.

► See also

Encephalitis

Herpes Simplex Virus Infections

Immune Deficiencies

Mononucleosis, Infectious

Pneumonia

Skin and Soft Tissue Infections

Staphylococcal Infections

Streptococcal Infections

Vaccination (Immunization)

brain). If a woman becomes infected with chicken pox early in her pregnancy, the virus can cause birth defects in the baby. In the final stages of pregnancy, a mother's chicken pox can cause a life-threatening infection in her baby. Left untreated, a shingles rash anywhere near the eye can spread to the eye. If the cornea* becomes involved, temporary or permanent blindness can result. More serious widespread infection from chicken pox or shingles can occur in anyone with a weakened immune system (such as someone who has HIV/AIDS).

How Can Varicella Be Prevented?

Since 1995, thousands of children and at-risk adults have been vaccinated against varicella. The American Academy of Pediatrics recommends that all children be vaccinated against chicken pox before 2 years of age. Older children and teens typically receive the vaccine, if they need it, at some point during a regular checkup with a health care provider. The vaccine prevents the disease in about 85 percent of vaccinated people. If people who have been vaccinated become infected with chicken pox, they usually have a milder case of disease. A single dose of varicella zoster immune globulin* (VZIG) can be given intravenously* to protect a person with a weakened immune system who comes into contact with varicella. VZIG contains antibodies to the varicella virus, and if it is given within 3 to 4 days of exposure to the virus, it offers temporary protection.

Resources

Organization

American Academy of Pediatrics (AAP), 141 Northwest Point Boulevard, Elk Grove Village, IL 60007. The website of the AAP offers information on varicella and the varicella virus vaccine.
Telephone 847-434-4000
http://www.aap.org

Website

KidsHealth.org. KidsHealth is a website created by the medical experts of the Nemours Foundation and is devoted to issues of children's health. It contains articles on a variety of health topics, including varicella.
http://www.KidsHealth.org

Warts

Warts are small, hard growths on the skin or inner linings of the body that are caused by a type of virus.

KEYWORDS
for searching the Internet and other reference sources

Condyloma

Flat warts

Genital warts

Human papilloma virus (HPV)

Plantar warts

Sexually transmitted disease (STD)

Verrucae

What Are Warts?

Warts are small areas of hardened skin that can grow on almost any part of the body. They are caused by human papilloma (pah-pih-LO-mah) viruses, or HPV. There are more than 100 different kinds, or strains, of HPV. Warts are usually skin-colored and bumpy or rough, but sometimes they are dark and smooth. The way a wart looks depends on where it is growing, and different kinds of warts appear on different parts of the body.

Common warts usually grow on fingers and hands, especially around fingernails. These warts usually have a rough, bumpy surface with tiny black dots, which are the blood vessels that feed the wart and allow it to grow. Flat warts are much smaller than common warts and are very smooth. This type of wart typically grows in little bunches on the face and legs; as many as 100 flat warts may grow together in one place. Common warts and flat warts generally are not painful except under certain circumstances, such as when the pressure of a pencil pushes against a wart on the finger while writing. Plantar warts, which grow on the bottoms of the feet, can be quite painful as a person walks on them, flattening them and pushing them back into the skin. Like a common wart, a plantar wart is covered with black dots marking the place of blood vessels.

Genital warts are small and pink, and they can grow one at a time or in bunches that make them look a bit like cauliflower. This type of wart can grow on the genitals*, the skin around the genitals, the rectum*, the buttocks, or in the vagina* or cervix*. Although most warts do not cause major health problems, genital warts may itch or bleed, and the ones caused by some strains of HPV are known to increase a woman's chances of developing cancer of the cervix.

Who Has Warts and Why?

About 1 in 4 people have common, flat, or plantar warts at some time in their lives. Children tend to have warts more often than adults do, and people who bite their fingernails or pick at hangnails may be more

* **genitals** (JEH-nih-tuls) are the external sexual organs.

* **rectum** is the final portion of the large intestine, connecting the colon to the anus.

* **vagina** (vah-JY-nah) is the canal, or passageway, in a woman that leads from the uterus to the outside of the body.

* **cervix** (SIR-viks) is the lower, narrow end of the uterus that opens into the vagina.

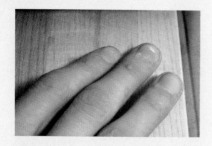

Warts commonly appear on the fingertips, where skin is more likely to be broken and susceptible to HPV infection. *Custom Medical Stock Photo, Inc.*

* **chronic** (KRAH-nik) means continuing for a long period of time.

* **pelvic exam** is an internal examination of a woman's reproductive organs.

* **Pap smear** is a common diagnostic test used to look for cancerous cells in the tissue of the cervix.

likely to have warts because tiny openings in the skin provide a way for HPV to enter the body. Someone with a weakened immune system, due to a chronic* illness or an infection, for example, also may be more likely to have warts. Warts are very contagious because HPV can pass easily from one person to another by contact. Genital warts spread through sexual intercourse. In fact, they are the most common viral sexually transmitted disease in the United States. In rare cases, a mother with genital warts can pass HPV to her baby during birth. The virus can cause growths on the baby's vocal cords or elsewhere in the infant's respiratory tract.

How Are Warts Diagnosed and Treated?

Health care providers can diagnose a wart by its appearance. It is important to have a professional examine the wart, because it is not always easy to know exactly what is growing on the skin or how to treat it. In the case of genital warts, a doctor also may screen a woman for cervical cancer by performing a pelvic exam*, including a Pap smear*. In some cases, warts eventually disappear on their own without any treatment. However, if a person has a lot of warts or if the warts are painful or seem to be spreading, there are several possible treatments.

Over-the-counter medicines containing salicylic (sah-lih-SIH-lik) acid often are used to remove common warts. The medicine can be painted on, or it may come in a patch that sticks to the wart. This type of treatment can take longer than others do, but it is painless. Cryotherapy, or freezing, is a typical treatment for common warts. A special chemical freezes the wart, and a scab develops as the skin heals. Cryotherapy may be used on plantar warts as well. These warts can be difficult to treat, because most of the wart is located beneath the surface of the skin. Electrosurgery can burn warts with a tool that uses an electric current; this type of treatment is used on both common and plantar warts. Chemical peels that contain acids are used to treat flat warts, which grow in such large bunches that the other types of treatments usually cannot be used efficiently. The chemicals are applied to the skin, and they eventually "peel" away the warts. Doctors also may use laser treatment to destroy any type of wart that proves difficult to remove. In some cases, doctors may give injections of interferon (in-ter-FEER-on), a substance that stimulates the body's immune system to attack the HPV causing the wart.

Genital warts require treatment from a doctor. To remove them, doctors may use cryotherapy, lasers, medicines that can be applied directly to the warts, or surgery. Once a woman has had genital warts, doctors may advise her to have Pap smears more often. In some cases, certain types of HPV infection can lead to cancer of the cervix, and a Pap smear will allow the doctor to find and treat the disease in its early stages.

Can Warts Be Prevented?

It can be very difficult for people to protect themselves from common, flat, and plantar warts, because they are so common and the virus spreads so easily. In addition, a person can come into contact with HPV many months or even a year before a wart grows big enough to see, so it is often impossible to know for sure where and how someone caught the virus. If a person has a wart, it is best for other people not to touch it. It is also advisable to avoid sharing towels and washcloths with someone who has a wart and to wear sandals at public showers or pools or in locker rooms, to avoid infection. It can be difficult to prevent genital warts, because skin-to-skin contact spreads them. Condoms may limit the spread of genital warts, but because some warts grow on the skin around the genitals and on the buttocks, a condom may not cover every one of them, making it still possible for the HPV to pass between sexual partners. Abstaining from sex with a person who has genital warts is the safest choice.

WORRIED ABOUT WARTS?

Warts have a long history in folklore, and the myths about them abound. Touching a frog, for example, has been thought both to cause and to cure warts. No one knows why certain unconventional treatments became popular; perhaps it is simply mind over matter. Among the many wart "remedies" are these, none of which has been proven to work:

- Put pebbles in a bag with a silver coin and then tie up the bag and throw it in the street. Whoever finds the money and keeps it will also keep the warts.

- Rub a dirty washcloth on the warts and bury it by the light of the full moon.

- Make the wart bleed. Put one drop of blood on seven grains of corn and feed it to a black hen.

- Apply a piece of raw meat to the warts and bury it. As the meat decays, the warts will disappear.

- Mix brown soap with saliva and make a paste. Apply it to the warts and leave on for 24 hours.

- Write a wish for your warts to disappear on a piece of paper, take it to the intersection of two roads, tear it up, and cast it to the winds.

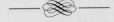

Resources

Organization

American Academy of Dermatology, P.O. Box 4014, Schaumburg, IL 60168-4014. The American Academy of Dermatology offers a fact sheet and general information about warts on its website. Information for young people can be found through the Kids' Connection at the website.
Telephone 847-330-0230
http://www.aad.org

Website

KidsHealth.org. KidsHealth is a website created by the medical experts of the Nemours Foundation and is devoted to issues of children's health. It contains articles on a variety of health topics, including warts.
http://www.KidsHealth.org

▶ *See also*
Sexually Transmitted Diseases

Skin and Soft Tissue Infections

West Nile Fever

West Nile fever is a viral infection that can result in inflammation of the brain, called encephalitis (en-seh-fuh-LYE-tis). The virus that causes it is spread to humans by infected mosquitoes.

What Is West Nile Fever?

West Nile fever (WNF) is caused by West Nile virus (WNV), which is part of the flavivirus family*. First discovered in Africa, WNV can infect animals and humans, although animals (mainly birds, but also horses, cats, and bats) are the primary hosts* for the virus.

Most of the time, people with WNF become only mildly ill. In some cases, however, WNF can develop into a life-threatening disease. If the virus passes into the brain, the infection can cause serious inflammation and complications affecting the nervous system. Of those infected, people older than 50 have the greatest risk of developing severe disease.

Do Many People Contract WNF?

WNF is found most frequently in Africa, the Middle East, Western Europe, and Asia. It was not found in the Western Hemisphere until 1999, when the first case appeared in the United States. Since then, presence of the virus has been documented in 39 states and the District of Columbia. WNF tends to occur more often in the summer and early fall, but the vast majority of cases likely go unreported because they cause only mild illness, if any.

* **flavivirus** (FLAY-vih-vy-rus) **family** is a group of viruses that includes those that cause dengue fever and yellow fever.

* **hosts** are organisms that provide another organism (such as a parasite or virus) with a place to live and grow.

Is WNF Contagious?

Generally, a person cannot contract WNF from another infected person or from an infected animal (transmission of the virus through a blood transfusion has been confirmed in some cases). Likewise, infected people cannot spread the virus to animals. Scientists think that the virus is transmitted almost exclusively by the bite of an infected mosquito. The chances of becoming ill with WNF actually are very small. Of all the mosquitoes in any area where infected mosquitoes have been found, fewer than 1 percent carry the virus.

The transmission cycle begins when a mosquito bites an infected bird and takes in blood that contains WNV. If the mosquito then bites a human, it can transmit the virus to that person. There is no evidence that humans can contract the disease by handling live or dead birds or any other animal that has been infected with the virus. Still, it is never a good idea to handle dead animals with bare hands; experts recommend that people always use disposable gloves and place the dead animal in a plastic bag when disposing of it.

How Do People Know They Have WNF?

The first symptoms of WNV infection are usually fever, headache, and body aches, sometimes accompanied by a rash and swollen lymph nodes*. Serious cases of the disease may cause more severe symptoms, including high fever, stiff neck, muscle weakness, convulsions*, confusion, paralysis*, and coma*. Very severe cases can result in death, but this is rare. Symptoms usually begin 3 to 15 days after infection.

How Is WNF Diagnosed and Treated?

If WNF is suspected, the first thing a doctor will do is take a history, which means asking a person about prior health, when symptoms began,

* **lymph** (LIMF) **nodes** are small, bean-shaped masses of tissue that contain immune system cells that fight harmful microorganisms. Lymph nodes may swell during infections.

* **convulsions** (kon-VUL-shuns), also called seizures, are involuntary muscle contractions caused by electrical discharges within the brain and are usually accompanied by changes in consciousness.

* **paralysis** (pah-RAH-luh-sis) is the loss or impairment of the ability to move some part of the body.

* **coma** (KO-ma) is an unconscious state in which a person cannot be awakened and cannot move, see, speak, or hear.

WEST NILE INVADES NEW YORK

In the summer of 1999, dead birds began appearing all over the New York metropolitan area. Public health officials were called in to find out why. They soon learned that the deaths were linked to the virus that causes West Nile fever, an infection that is spread by mosquitoes. Before 1999, West Nile fever had never been seen in the Western Hemisphere.

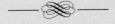

and recent travels and activities. This may help determine if the person might have been exposed to an infected mosquito. A blood test can confirm the presence of the virus.

For mild cases of WNF, there is no specific treatment. A doctor usually will recommend rest and over-the-counter medications, such as acetaminophen (uh-see-teh-MIH-noh-fen), to ease fever and aches. Severe cases of WNF may require hospitalization and more specialized care, such as intravenous (in-tra-VEE-nus) fluids (fluids given directly into a vein) to prevent or treat dehydration* in someone who is too sick to drink or who is vomiting. A person who is having trouble breathing may be put on a ventilator*.

How long WNV illness lasts depends on the severity of the infection. If a person has a mild infection, symptoms often will go away in about a week. Recovery from serious infection may take several weeks to months. Most people who are infected with WNV do not become very sick. Only about 1 percent of all infected people become severely ill. Of these severe cases, up to 15 percent are fatal. Elderly people have the highest risk of developing serious complications from the disease.

Can WNF Be Prevented?

There is no vaccine for WNF, so the best way to prevent the spread of the virus is to prevent mosquito bites. To do so, experts recommend that people avoid being outside at times when mosquitoes are most active (dawn, dusk, and early evening), and that they wear long sleeves and long pants and use insect repellent when outside. When using repellent, it is very important to follow the instructions on the package, especially for children.

In the United States, WNV often has been traced to areas where dead birds have been found. By tracking the disease and looking for patterns of infection, public health officials are better able to prevent future outbreaks. Experts advise people to contact the local or state health department if a dead bird is found in an area where WNV has been reported; a representative will collect the bird for testing.

Resources

Organization

U.S. Centers for Disease Control and Prevention (CDC), 1600 Clifton Road, Atlanta, GA 30333. The CDC is the U.S. government authority for information about infectious and other diseases. It provides fact sheets about West Nile fever at its website. Telephone 800-311-3435
http://www.cdc.gov

* **dehydration** (dee-hi-DRAY-shun) is a condition in which the body is depleted of water, usually caused by excessive and unreplaced loss of body fluids, such as through sweating, vomiting, or diarrhea.

* **ventilator** (VEN-tuh-lay-ter) is a machine used to support or control a person's breathing.

Website

KidsHealth.org. KidsHealth is a website created by the medical experts of the Nemours Foundation and is devoted to issues of children's health. It contains articles on a variety of health topics, including West Nile virus.
http://www.KidsHealth.org

▶ *See also*
Encephalitis
Zoonoses

Whooping Cough *See* **Pertussis (Whooping Cough)**

Y

Yellow Fever

Yellow fever is an infectious disease caused by a virus that is transmitted to humans by mosquitoes.

What Is Yellow Fever?

Yellow fever is a disease caused by yellow fever virus, a member of the flavivirus (FLAY-vih-vy-rus) group of viruses. The disease gets its name because it often causes jaundice*, which tints the skin yellow, and a high fever. Yellow fever also can cause kidney failure and uncontrolled bleeding, or hemorrhaging (HEM-rij-ing). Many cases produce only mild illness, but severe cases of yellow fever can be fatal. Once someone has survived the disease, the person will have lifetime immunity* against it.

Yellow fever afflicts both humans and monkeys and has been known since at least the 1600s. The disease is not spread by person-to-person contact. It is transmitted by several different species of mosquitoes; a person can contract yellow fever only from the bite of a mosquito that has bitten an infected person or monkey.

The disease once caused epidemics in the Americas, Europe, and the Caribbean, but at the beginning of the twenty-first century the disease occurs almost exclusively in South America and Africa. Each year, outbreaks lead to an estimated 200,000 cases and 30,000 deaths worldwide. Vaccines against the virus were developed in 1928 and 1937, and mosquito-eradication programs have made great progress in controlling the disease. The last recorded outbreak of yellow fever in the United States was in New Orleans in 1905. However, lapses in prevention programs in Africa and South America have allowed yellow fever to once again become a serious public health issue on those continents.

Are There Different Kinds of Yellow Fever?

Yellow fever occurs as three subtypes: epidemic (urban), intermediate, and jungle-acquired. Epidemic yellow fever spreads in densely populated areas of Africa and South America via the bite of *Aedes aegypti* (a-E-deez eh-JIP-tie) mosquitoes. Intermediate yellow fever occurs in Africa as the result of mosquitoes breeding in humid flat grasslands (savannahs) during rainy seasons, then infecting both monkeys and humans. In dry seasons, the virus can remain alive in unhatched mosquito eggs that are resistant to the heat.

KEYWORDS
for searching the Internet
and other reference sources

Aedes aegypti mosquito

Epidemic

Flavivirus

Mosquito-borne disease

Viral hemorrhagic fevers

* **jaundice** (JON-dis) is a yellowing of the skin, and sometimes the whites of the eyes, caused by a buildup in the body of bilirubin, a chemical produced in and released by the liver. An increase in bilirubin may indicate disease of the liver or certain blood disorders.

* **immunity** (ih-MYOON-uh-tee) is the condition of being protected against an infectious disease. Immunity often develops after a germ is introduced to the body. One type of immunity occurs when the body makes special protein molecules called antibodies to fight the disease-causing germ. The next time that germ enters the body, the antibodies quickly attack it, usually preventing the germ from causing disease.

391

Jungle-acquired yellow fever occurs mainly in South America when mosquitoes pick up the virus from infected forest monkeys and then transmit the disease to humans in jungles and rainforests. People who are regional settlers, soldiers, or agricultural or forestry workers are at greatest risk for this less common form of the disease.

How Do People Know They Have Yellow Fever?

After an incubation* period of 3 to 6 days, the yellow fever virus begins to produce symptoms. An early phase of disease occurs, which includes fever, headache, muscle aches, and vomiting. The infected person may have a slower heartbeat than that expected with a high fever. After a few days, most of the symptoms disappear. Many people recover from yellow fever at this point without complications. However, about 15 percent of patients develop a second, toxic phase of the disease, in which fever reappears and the disease becomes more severe. Inflammation of the liver occurs, along with jaundice, stomach pains, and vomiting. The mouth, nose, eyes, and stomach can bleed uncontrollably, with blood present in vomited material and bowel movements. The kidneys may begin to fail, and patients may go into a coma (an unconscious state in which a person cannot be awakened).

How Do Doctors Diagnose and Treat Yellow Fever?

Early stages of yellow fever can be easily confused with other diseases such as malaria*, typhoid fever*, and other hemorrhagic (heh-muh-RAH-jik) fevers and types of viral hepatitis*. Blood tests can detect whether a patient's body has produced yellow fever antibodies* to fight the infection. Doctors also will take a travel history to see if a patient recently has visited a country where yellow fever occurs.

No specific treatment exists for yellow fever. Care is geared toward treating complications of the disease. In serious cases, intensive care in the hospital usually is needed. Patients may be given fluids to prevent dehydration*, and blood transfusions* may be necessary if bleeding is severe.

Most people who contract yellow fever recover from the early phase of the disease within a week; those who progress to the toxic phase may take several weeks or longer to recover. About half of those who develop toxic phase symptoms die within 2 weeks; the other half may recover without significant long-term problems.

How Can Yellow Fever Be Prevented?

Vaccination against yellow fever is the single most important prevention measure, and it is a must for people traveling to countries where the disease is common. Most countries in which yellow fever occurs require a certificate proving that travelers have been vaccinated before they are allowed into the country. One dose of vaccine provides at least 10 years of immunity.

*incubation (ing-kyoo-BAY-shun) is the period of time between infection by a germ and when symptoms first appear. Depending on the germ, this period can be from hours to months.

*malaria (mah-LAIR-e-uh) is a disease spread to humans by the bite of an infected mosquito.

*typhoid fever (TIE-foyd FEE-ver) is an infection with the bacterium Salmonella typhi that causes fever, headache, confusion, and muscle aches.

*hepatitis (heh-puh-TIE-tis) is an inflammation of the liver. Hepatitis can be caused by viruses, bacteria, and a number of other noninfectious medical conditions.

*antibodies (AN-tih-bah-deez) are protein molecules produced by the body's immune system to help fight specific infections caused by microorganisms, such as bacteria and viruses.

*dehydration (dee-hi-DRAY-shun) is a condition in which the body is depleted of water, usually caused by excessive and unreplaced loss of body fluids, such as through sweating, vomiting, or diarrhea.

*transfusions (trans-FYOO-zhunz) are procedures in which blood or certain parts of blood, such as specific cells, are given to a person who needs them because of illness or blood loss.

Doctors recommend that infants under 6 months of age, pregnant women, people allergic to eggs (eggs are used in producing the vaccine), and people with weakened immune systems (such as people who have AIDS* or certain cancers) not receive the vaccine; these people are advised to delay visits to countries where yellow fever is endemic*.

Avoiding mosquito bites when traveling abroad reduces the risk of contracting yellow fever. To help prevent infection, experts suggest that travelers:

- wear long sleeves and pants
- avoid going outside when mosquitoes are active—at dawn, dusk, and early evening
- use mosquito repellent
- sleep beneath a mosquito net

Resources

Organizations

U.S. Centers for Disease Control and Prevention (CDC), 1600 Clifton Road, Atlanta, GA 30333. The CDC is the U.S. government authority for information about infectious and other diseases, including yellow fever.
Telephone 800-311-3435
http://www.cdc.gov

World Health Organization (WHO), Avenue Appia 20, 1211 Geneva 27, Switzerland. WHO provides information about yellow fever at its website.
Telephone 011-41-22-791-2111
http://www.who.int

* **AIDS**, or acquired immunodeficiency (ih-myoo-no-dih-FIH-shen-see) syndrome, is an infection that severely weakens the immune system; it is caused by the human immunodeficiency virus (HIV).

* **endemic** (en-DEH-mik) describes a disease or condition that is present in a population or geographic area at all times.

▶ *See also*
Dengue Fever
Hepatitis, Infectious
Malaria
West Nile Fever

Z

Zoonoses

Zoonoses (zoh-ah-NO-seez) are infections that humans contract from animals.

What Are Zoonoses?

Zoonoses are infections caused by parasites, bacteria, or viruses that are passed from animals to humans. Most people contract zoonotic (zoh-uh-NAH-tik) infections from animals with which they have a lot of contact, such as pets or farm animals. Wild animals and insects can be the source of disease, too, particularly for diseases spread by the bite of a tick, mosquito, or fly. Animals such as wild rodents and bats also can carry diseases that may be harmful to humans.

Zoonoses can cause minor or serious illness. In some cases, the organisms involved infect people, but they do not become ill. Other zoonoses can be very dangerous to people, especially anyone with an immune system weakened by age or illness.

Are They Contagious?

Most of these infections do not spread from person to person or do so only in rare instances. Usually they are spread from animals to humans in the following ways:

- from the bite of an infected insect
- through contact with an animal's feces* or urine, either through the mouth or by breathing in dust from dried feces
- from the bite or scratch of an infected animal
- from eating the meat of an infected animal

Some Examples of Zoonoses

Cat scratch disease A cat carrying *Bartonella henselae* (bar-tuh-NEH-luh HEN-suh-lay), the bacterium responsible for cat scratch disease, usually does not have symptoms, but if the bacteria are passed to a human through a scratch or bite, a person may experience skin sores, swollen and sore lymph nodes*, extreme tiredness, headaches, and fever. Antibiotics may be prescribed to treat the infection.

KEYWORDS
for searching the Internet
and other reference sources

Cat scratch disease

Hantavirus

Lyme disease

Plague

Psittacosis

Rabies

Toxoplasmosis

Trichinosis

* **feces** (FEE-seez) is the excreted waste from the gastrointestinal tract.

* **lymph** (LIMF) **nodes** are small, bean-shaped masses of tissue that contain immune system cells that fight harmful microorganisms. Lymph nodes may swell during infections.

Disease-causing Organism	Animal or Insect Carrier	Human Disease
Bartonella hensalae bacteria	Cats	Cat scratch disease
Chlamydia psittaci bacteria	Birds	Psittacosis
Mononegavirales virus	Mammals, including bats, raccoons, skunks, foxes, and coyotes	Rabies
Yersinia pestis bacteria	Fleas and rodents, including rats, chipmunks, prairie dogs, ground squirrels, and mice	Plague
Hantavirus	Rodents, including rats and mice	Hantavirus pulmonary syndrome
Borrelia burgdorferi bacteria	Ticks, deer, and mice	Lyme disease
Toxoplasma gondii bacteria	Cats and farm animals	Toxoplasmosis
Trichinella larvae	Bears, foxes, and other wild game; pigs and horses	Trichinosis

Psittacosis People who have contact with birds may be at risk for psittacosis (sih-tuh-KO-sis), also known as parrot fever. If a person inhales bird feces or urine particles while cleaning a bird's cage, he or she may develop symptoms of pneumonia (nu-MO-nyah, inflammation of the lung), such as fever, coughing, or chest pain. Antibiotics are used to treat psittacosis.

Rabies A virus that is carried in the saliva of infected animals can cause rabies when transmitted through a bite or, less commonly, through contact with saliva. Symptoms include fever, difficulty swallowing, delirium*, seizures*, and coma*. Death can result if the infection is not treated. Treatment includes intensive care in a hospital. A series of vaccinations* started at the time of a bite from a possibly infected animal can prevent the person from developing the disease. Many mammals, especially raccoons, bats, and dogs, may be infected with rabies, but human rabies is rare in the United States. According to the U.S. Centers for Disease Control and Prevention, there were no cases of rabies in humans in the United States in 2000. In many other countries, especially those in the developing world, rabies is much more common.

Plague   Plague (PLAYG) is a bacterial infection caused by *Yersinia pestis* (yer-SIN-e-uh PES-tis). Plague can be transmitted to humans through the bite of a flea that has become infected through contact with an infected rodent, such as a rat. The disease causes such symptoms as fever and swollen lymph nodes. In some cases the infection spreads through the blood and can infect the lungs. If this happens, plague can spread from person to person through coughing or sneezing. Plague was the cause of huge epidemics* in Europe and Asia during the Middle Ages, and it is still seen in many developing countries. It is seen in many developed countries too, including the United States, although not as many cases occur. The disease can be fatal if it is not treated with antibiotics.

Hantavirus   Rodents, such as mice and rats, may carry hantavirus (HAN-tuh-vy-rus). This virus can spread to humans when they inhale particles from rodent feces, saliva, or urine. People infected with hantavirus can develop hantavirus pulmonary (PUL-mo-nar-ee) syndrome (HPS), which causes such symptoms as fever, headaches, muscle aches, nausea (NAW-zee-uh), vomiting, diarrhea (dye-uh-REE-uh), abdominal* pain, and chills. In severe cases a person may experience shortness of breath and the lungs may fill with fluid. There is no cure for hantavirus infection, but people who have HPS typically are hospitalized in an intensive care unit, where they receive oxygen and other types of supportive care.

Lyme disease   *Borrelia burgdorferi* (buh-REEL-e-uh burg-DOR-fe-ree) bacteria inside an infected tick can cause Lyme (LIME) disease in humans after a tick attaches to the skin and feeds on a person's blood. Ticks pick up the bacterium by feeding on the blood of infected deer and mice, which serve as reservoirs for the organism. Lyme disease can produce a number of symptoms, such as extreme tiredness, muscle aches, and swollen, painful joints. At the site of the tick bite, some people develop a bull's-eye rash, a red rash surrounded by rings that resembles a bull's-eye target. A person with Lyme disease usually is treated with antibiotics.

Toxoplasmosis   Eating contaminated meat or having contact with the feces of an infected cat can put a person at risk for toxoplasmosis

* **delirium** (dih-LEER-e-um) is a condition in which a person is confused, is unable to think clearly, and has a reduced level of consciousness.

* **seizures** (SEE-zhurs) are sudden bursts of disorganized electrical activity that interrupt the normal functioning of the brain, often leading to uncontrolled movements in the body and sometimes a temporary change in consciousness.

* **coma** (KO-ma) is an unconscious state in which a person cannot be awakened and cannot move, see, speak, or hear.

* **vaccinations** (vak-sih-NAY-shunz), also called immunizations, are the giving of doses of vaccines, which are preparations of killed or weakened germs, or a part of a germ or product it produces, to prevent or lessen the severity of a disease.

* **epidemics** (eh-pih-DEH-miks) are outbreaks of diseases, especially infectious diseases, in which the number of cases suddenly becomes far greater than usual. Usually epidemics are outbreaks of diseases in specific regions, whereas worldwide epidemics are called pandemics.

* **abdominal** (ab-DAH-mih-nul) refers to the area of the body below the ribs and above the hips that contains the stomach, intestines, and other organs.

(tox-o-plaz-MO-sis). This zoonosis is caused by a parasite and can produce such symptoms as swollen lymph nodes, muscle aches, headaches, and sore throat in a healthy person and life-threatening brain infections in people with weakened immune systems, especially those who have HIV/AIDS*. If a pregnant woman becomes infected with the parasite, she can transmit the infection to her unborn baby, which can lead to a number of health problems in the child.

Trichinosis If people eat meat (especially pork products, such as sausage or ham) infected with the eggs of *Trichinella* (trih-kih-NEH-luh) worms, they can contract trichinosis (trih-kih-NO-sis), a disease that produces such symptoms as diarrhea, vomiting, and abdominal pain. Trichinosis can cause nerve and muscle damage as well as heart and lung problems. It can be treated with medication.

How Are Zoonoses Treated?

The treatment of a zoonotic infection depends on the specific disease, but many are treatable with prescription medications, such as antibiotics.

How Are Zoonoses Prevented?

Because household pets may carry zoonotic organisms, it is important to keep pets healthy and vaccinated to avoid infection. Some other ways people can protect against zoonoses include:

- having pets regularly examined by a veterinarian
- avoiding contact with stray, unfamiliar, or wild animals
- cleaning litter boxes daily and animal cages frequently to prevent the growth of bacteria and parasites
- having someone who does not have a weakened immune system and is not pregnant empty pet litter boxes, bathe pets, clean pet cages, and pick up pet feces
- cooking meat until it is no longer pink inside and the juices run clear
- washing hands with soap and warm water after handling animals and before eating
- clearing brush and other areas around the house where rodents might live
- not storing food or trash in an area where it could attract animals
- wearing long sleeves and long pants when outdoors, especially in wooded areas, to discourage tick and mosquito bites
- using insect and mosquito repellent
- examining the body and pets for ticks after spending time outside in areas where ticks are found

Resources

Organization

U.S. Centers for Disease Control and Prevention (CDC), 1600 Clifton Road, Atlanta, GA 30333. The CDC tracks various zoonoses, the areas where they occur, and how many people are infected at any given time. It offers information on specific zoonoses at its website. Telephone 800-311-3435
http://www.cdc.gov

Website

KidsHealth.org. KidsHealth is a website created by the medical experts of the Nemours Foundation and is devoted to issues of children's health. It contains articles on a variety of health topics, including cat scratch disease, Lyme disease, psittacosis, rabies, and other zoonoses. http://www.KidsHealth.org

▶ *See also*
Cat Scratch Disease
Chlamydial Infections
Hantavirus Infection
Lyme Disease
Plague
Rabies
Toxoplasmosis
Trichinosis

Bibliography

Ash, Lawrence R., and Thomas C. Orihel. *Atlas of Human Parasitology.* 4th ed. Chicago: American Society for Clinical Pathology Press, 1997.

Bakalar, Nicholas. *Where the Germs Are: A Scientific Safari.* Hoboken, NJ: John Wiley & Sons, 2003.

Barbour, Alan G. *Lyme Disease: The Cause, the Cure, the Controversy.* Baltimore: Johns Hopkins University Press, 1996.

Beers, Mark. *The Merck Manual of Medical Information.* 2nd ed. Whitehouse Station, NJ: Merck & Co., 2003.

Beers, Mark, ed. *Merck Manual Diagnosis & Therapy.* 17th ed. Whitehouse Station, NJ: Merck & Co., 1999.

Biddle, Wayne. *A Field Guide to Germs.* New York: Random House, 2002.

Breslow, Lester, M.D. *Encyclopedia of Public Health.* New York: Macmillan Library Reference Library, 2000.

Byers, Ann. *Sexually Transmitted Diseases: A Hot Issue.* Berkely Heights, NJ: Enslow Publishers, 1999.

Carter, K. Codell, and Barbara R. Carter. *Childbed Fever: A Scientific Biography of Ignaz Semmelweis.* Westport, CT: Greenwood Publishing Group, 1994.

Collins, James F. *Your Eyes: An Owner's Guide.* Englewood Cliffs, NJ: Prentice Hall, 1995.

Davies, Peter. *The Devil's Flu: The World's Deadliest Influenza Epidemic and the Scientific Hunt for the Virus That Caused It.* New York: Henry Holt, 2000.

Desalle, Rob, ed. *Epidemic! The World of Infectious Disease.* New York: The New Press, 1999.

Donnelly, Karen. *Leprosy (Hansen's Disease).* New York: Rosen Publishing Group, 2002.

Ebel, Charles. *Managing Herpes: How to Live and Love With a Chronic STD.* 2nd ed. American Social Health Association, 1998.

Edlow, Jonathan A. *Bull's-Eye: Unraveling the Mysteries of Lyme Disease.* New Haven, CT: Yale University Press, 2003.

Eynikel, Hilde. *Molokai: The Story of Father Damien.* Translated by Lesley Gilbert. New York: Alba House, 1999.

Fenn, Elizabeth A. *Pox Americana: The Great Smallpox Epidemic of 1775-82.* New York: Hill & Wang Publishers, 2002.

Frank, Steven A. *Immunology and Evolution of Infectious Disease.* Princeton, NJ: Princeton University Press, 2002.

Getz, David, and Peter McCarty. *Purple Death: The Mysterious Flu of 1918.* New York: Henry Holt and Co., 2000.

Gittelman, Ann Louise. *Guess What Came to Dinner? Parasites and Your Health.* New York: Avery Penguin Putnam, 2001.

Goldmann, David R., ed. *American College of Physicians Complete Home Medical Guide.* New York: DK Publishing, 1999.

Harvard Medical School Family Health Guide. 1st ed. New York: Simon & Schuster, 1999.

Hays, J.N. *The Burdens of Disease: Epidemics and Human Response in Western History.* Piscataway, NJ: Rutgers University Press, 1998.

Jones, Ann. *Looking for Lovedu: Days and Nights in Africa.* New York: Knopf, 2001.

Karlen, Arno. *Biography of a Germ.* New York: Random House, 2000.

Kolata, Gina. *Flu: The Story of the Great Influenza Pandemic.* New York: Touchstone, 2001.

Levy, Stuart B., M.D. *The Antibiotic Paradox: How the Misuse of Antibiotics Destroys Their Curative Powers.* Cambridge, MA: Perseus Publishing, 2002.

Mayo Clinic Family Health Book. 3rd ed. New York: Harper Resource, 2003.

McNeill, William H. *Plagues and Peoples.* New York: Random House, 1998.

Meyer, Andrea S., David R. Harper, and Robert R. Parmenter. *Of Mice, Men, and Microbes: Hantavirus.* San Diego: Academic Press, 1999.

Monroe, Judy. *Lyme Disease.* Mankato, MN: Capstone Press, 2001.

Newell, Mary-Louise, and James McIntyre. *Congenital and Perinatal Infections: Prevention, Diagnosis and Treatment.* Cambridge, UK: Cambridge University Press, 2000.

Oldstone, Michael B. A. *Viruses, Plagues, and History.* London: Oxford University Press, 2000.

Pasteur, Louis, and Joseph Lister. *Germ Theory and Its Applications to Medicine & on the Antiseptic Principle of the Practice of Surgery.* Amherst, NY: Prometheus Books, 1996.

Physicians' Desk Reference 2003. 57th ed. Montvale, NJ: Medical Economics Company, 2002.

Preston, Richard. *The Hot Zone: A Terrifying True Story.* New York: Random House, 1995.

Rahn, Daniel, and Janine Evans, eds. *Lyme Disease.* 5th ed. American College of Physicians, 1998.

Shnayerson, Michael, and Mark J. Plotkin. *The Killers Within: The Deadly Rise of Drug-resistant Bacteria.* New York: Little Brown & Co., 2002.

Sompayrac, Lauren. *How Pathogenic Viruses Work.* Boston: Jones and Bartlett Publishers, 2002.

Sompayrac, Lauren. *How the Immune System Works.* Boston: Blackwell Science, Inc., 1999.

Strauss, James, and Ellen Strauss. *Viruses and Human Disease.* San Diego: Academic Press, 2001.

Tierno, Philip M., Jr., PhD. *The Secret Life of Germs: Observations of a Microbe Hunter.* New York: Simon & Schuster, 2002.

Tucker, Jonathan B. *Scourge: The Once and Future Threat of Smallpox.* New York: Grove Press, 2002.

Turkington, Carol, and Jeffrey Dover, M.D. *Skin Deep: The Encyclopedia of Skin and Skin Disorders.* New York: Facts on File, 2002.

Vanderhoof-Foorschner, Karen. *Everything You Need to Know About Lyme Disease and Other Tick-borne Disorders.* New York: John Wiley & Sons, 1997.

Watts, Sheldon. *Epidemics and History: Disease, Power and Imperialism.* New Haven, CT: Yale University Press, 1999.

Zimmerman, Barry E., and David J. Zimmerman. *Killer Germs: Microbes and Diseases That Threaten Humanity.* New York: McGraw-Hill, 2002.

Zinsser, Hans. *Rats, Lice and History.* New York: Little Brown & Co., 1984.

Index

Volumes **1**, **2**, and **3** refer to the *Human Diseases and Conditions* base set; **S1** refers to the first supplement to the base set, *Behavioral Health*; **S2** refers to the second supplement to the set, *Infectious Diseases*.

Page numbers referring to illustrations are in *italic* type.

Volume numbers are shown in **bold**.

Concentration difficulties (continued)
attention deficit hyperactivity disorder (ADHD), **1:**103
chronic fatigue syndrome, **1:**206
depression, **S1:**133
post-traumatic stress disorder (PTSD), **S1:**278
unipolar depression, **1:**265
Conception, **3:**654
Concussions, **1:**232–235
amnesia, **1:**58
head injuries, **S1:**97
headaches, **2:**413
Condition, definition of, **1:**6
Condoms, **1:**28, **S1:**324
cervical cancer, **3:**893, **3:**894
gonorrhea, **2:**390
pelvic inflammatory disease (PID, **3:**656
sexually transmitted diseases (STDs), **3:**753, **3:**755, **S2:**341
Conduct disorders, **S1:**112–115
antisocial personality disorder (APD), **S1:**46
lying and stealing, **S1:**223
oppositional defiant disorder, **S1:**252
Conductive hearing loss, **1:**256–257
Condylomata acuminata, **2:**383
Cone-nose bugs, **S2:**361
Cones, **1:**228
Confusion
dementia, **S1:**127
heat stroke, **2:**432
hypertension, **2:**462
meningitis, **2:**563
multiple sclerosis, **2:**600
Rocky Mountain spotted fever (RMSF), **S2:**289–290, **S2:**296
schizophrenia, **3:**738
strokes, **3:**814
Congenital disorders. *See also* Birth defects
birth defects, **1:**69, **1:**126–130
bone malformation, **2:**362
fifth disease, **S2:**142
infections, **S2:**98–103, **S2:**115, **S2:**116
kidney disease, **2:**502
rubella (German measles), **2:**385–386, **S2:**101, **S2:**300
scoliosis, **3:**743
self-image, **S1:**140–141
syphilis, **S2:**338, **S2:**340
toxoplasmosis, **S2:**350
Congestion (stuffy nose), **S2:**21

Congestive heart failure, **1:**208. *See also* Heart, disease
Congo, Democratic Republic of the, **1:**201, **2:**320
Conjunctivitis, **1:**235–237, **3:**874, **S2:**103–105, **S2:**301
Connecticut, **S2:**218
Connecticut Clearinghouse, **2:**354
Connective tissue diseases, **1:**225
Consciousness, **S1:**115–117. *See also* Loss of consciousness
Constipation, **1:**237–239. *See also* Bowel movements
diverticulitis, **1:**295
endometriosis, **2:**334
hemorrhoids, **2:**440
incontinence, **2:**474
irritable bowel syndrome, **2:**492, **2:**493
lead poisoning, **2:**518
parasitic infections, **3:**650
soiling, **S1:**334–335
Constitutional growth delay, **2:**395. *See also* Growth
Consumption, **3:**875. *See also* Tuberculosis
Contact dermatitis, **3:**773
Contact lenses, **2:**612
Contact tracing, **3:**755
Contagious diseases, **S2:**9. *See also specific diseases*
Continence. *See* Urine/Urination
Contraceptives, **3:**655, **S1:**323–324. *See also* Birth control; Condoms
endometriosis, **2:**335
infertility, **2:**478
The Contractions (musical group), **1:**255
Contusions, **S1:**97
Conversion disorders, **3:**646, **3:**647, **S1:**117–119
hypochondria, **S1:**203
malingering, **S1:**225–226
as a somatoform disorder, **S1:**337
Convulsions. *See* Seizures
Cook Islands, 3
Cool mist therapy, **1:**242
Coordination difficulties, **2:**313, **2:**619
brain tumors, **1:**147
Huntington's disease, **2:**457
multiple sclerosis, **2:**600
tic disorders, **S1:**376–377
Copaxone, **2:**601
Coping. *See* Management
Copper, **1:**290
Copperhead snakes, **1:**134

Coprolalia, **3:**862, **S1:**377
Copropraxia, **3:**862, **S1:**377
Cor pulmonale, **2:**328
Coral snakes, **1:**134
Corn diet, **1:**288
Cornea, **1:**98–99, **1:**199, **2:**388
Cornett, R. Orin, **3:**790
Coronary arteries, **2:***417*, **2:**423. *See also* Heart, disease
Coronary heart disease, **2:**424. *See also* Heart, disease
Coronaviruses, **1:**215, **S2:**95
Corpus callosum, **S1:***10*
Corpus luteum, **1:**247, **2:**567
Cortés, Hernán, **S2:**225
Cortex, **S1:**231. *See also* Cerebral cortex
emotions, **S1:**164
sleepiness, **S1:**329
Cortex of the kidney, **2:***504*
Corticosteroids. *See also* Steroids
asthma, **1:**93–94
croup, **S2:**114
encephalitis, **2:**331
epiglottitis, **S2:**138
hair loss, **2:**407
hepatitis, **2:**447
hives, **2:**454
inhibiting immune response, **2:**469, **S2:**18, **S2:**176
lupus, **2:**540
systemic fungal infections, **2:**367
vitiligo, **3:**903
Corticotropin-releasing hormone, **1:**243, **3:**808, **3:**809
Cortical bone, **1:**158
Cortisol, **1:**23, **1:**243
Cushing's syndrome, **1:**242, **2:**400
post-traumatic stress disorder (PTSD), **S1:**278
stress, **3:**808, **3:**809, **S1:**341
Cortisone, **1:**182
causing osteoporosis, **2:**637
Cushing's syndrome, **1:**243
delayed puberty, **2:**396
Corynebacterium diphtheriae, **S2:**120. *See also* Diphtheria
Cosmetics, **2:**518
Cotton rats, **2:**410
Cottonmouth snakes, **1:**134
Coughing, **3:**675, **S2:**20–21
anthrax, **S2:**60
ascariasis, **1:**88
asthma, **1:**90–91
automatic reflex, **S2:**16
bloody sputum, **2:**534

418

Index

HIV (continued)
cervical cancer, **3:**893
coccidioidomycosis complications, **S2:**93, **S2:**94
cytomegalovirus, **1:**253
encephalitis, **2:**330, **S2:**130, **S2:**132
genital herpes, **S2:**167–168
hemophilia, **2:**436
hepatitis, **2:**444
immune deficiency, **2:**469, **S2:**17
lymphoma, **2:**549
medications for, **S2:**34
mother and child treatment, **S2:**35
pneumonia, **3:**677
sexually transmitted diseases (STDs), **3:**754, **S2:**310–311
syphilis, **S2:**341
trichomoniasis, **S2:**360
tuberculosis, **3:**876, **S2:**365
viral infections, **3:**899
Hives, **2:**453–454, **3:**773
HIVInSite, **S2:**59
Hoarseness
laryngitis, **2:**513, **S2:**203
lung cancer, **2:**534
Hodgkin, Thomas, **2:**547
Hodgkin's disease, **2:**547. *See also* Cancer; Lymphoma
shingles, **3:**756
systemic fungal infections, **2:**367
Hoffman, Dustin, **1:**112, **S1:***68*
Holter ECG monitor, **1:**310, **2:**421
Home-canned foods, **S2:**72
Homelessness, **1:**219, **3:**876, **S1:**197–199
Homeostasis, **1:**5
Homosexuality, **S1:**324
Honduras, **1:**201
Honeybees, **1:**133
Hong Kong, **1:**201, **3:**669
Hooker Chemicals and Plastics Corporation, **2:**337
Hookworms, **2:**454–456, **3:**650, **S2:**191–192, **S2:***193*
Hopkins, Gerald Manley, **3:**884
Hopkins Motor/Vocal Tic Scale, **S1:**386
Hormones, **1:**19, **1:**243
Addison's disease, **1:**23
anabolic steroids, **S1:**353
antidiuretic, **S1:**71
autoimmune diseases, **S2:**17
brain chemistry, **S1:**92–93

cancer treatment, **1:**175
corticotropin-releasing hormone, **1:**243, **3:**809
Cushing's syndrome, **1:**242
dwarfism, **1:**301
endometriosis, **2:**334
genetically engineered, **S2:**112
growth disorders, **2:**398–400
growth rate, **2:**395–396
hair loss, **2:**406
hypothyroidism, **3:**853
infertility, **2:**478
iodine, **1:**289
melatonin, **3:**781, **S1:**329
menstrual disorders, **2:**565, **2:**569, **2:**570
menstruation, **2:**567
obesity, **2:**625
pancreas, **1:**271
post-traumatic stress disorder, **3:**688, **S1:**278
proteins, **2:**581
sexual development, **S1:**319–320
sleep patterns, **2:**491
stress-related illness, **3:**808–809
testicular cancer, **3:**842
therapy for sex-change procedure, **S1:**186
therapy with, **2:**500, **3:**702
thyroid disease, **3:**850
urinary incontinence, **2:**474
uterine cancer, **3:**893, **3:**894
Hospitals/Hospitalization, **S2:**4
acquired pneumonia, **S2:**274
botulism, **S2:**73
detoxification unit, **1:**42
sepsis, complications, **S2:**308
The Hot Zone (Preston), **S2:**126
How and Why We Age (Hayflick), **1:**55
HPS (hantavirus pulmonary syndrome), **2:**410–411, **S2:**157–159
HPV (human papillomavirus), **2:**383–384, **S2:**249–250, **S2:**251, **S2:**383–386
cervical cancer, **3:**893
sexually transmitted diseases (STDs), **3:**753, **S2:***311*
as skin infection, **S2:**318
warts, **3:**905–906
HTLV-1 (human T-cell lymphotropic virus), **2:**547, **2:**548
Human bites, **1:**72

Human brain, **1:***2. See also* Brain
Human Genome Project, **S1:**190–191
Human granulocytic ehrlichiosis (HGE), **S2:**127
Human Growth Foundation, **1:**303
Human herpesvirus type 6 and 7, **S2:**298
Human lymphotrophic virus type 1 (HLTV-1), **S2:**251
Human papillomavirus (HPV). *See* HPV (Human papillomavirus)
Human parvovirus B19, **S2:**141
Human spongiform encephalopathy, **1:**239
Human tapeworms, **S2:**194. *See also* Tapeworms
Humidity, **2:**432
Humoral immunity, **2:**471
Hungary, **2:**411
Hunter, C. J., **S1:***353*
Hunter's syndrome, **2:**381
Huntington, George, **2:**457, **S1:**129
Huntington's disease, **1:**127, **2:**456–458
dementia, **S1:**128
genetic disorders, **2:**381
mental disorders, **2:**573
Huntington's Disease Society of America, **2:**458
Hydrocephalus, **1:**302, **2:**458–460
myelomeningocele, **3:**795
strabismus, **3:**800
Hydrocephalus Association, **2:**460
Hydrogen bonds, **2:***378*
Hydrogen breath test, **2:**512
Hydrophobia, **3:**666, **S2:**286
Hygiene, personal, **3:**738. *See also* Hand washing
Hyperactivity, **1:**102, **1:**103–104, **3:**662, **S1:**252. *See also* Attention deficit hyperactivity disorder (ADHD)
Hyperbaric oxygen chamber, **1:**126, **1:**180, **2:**375
Hypercalcemia, **1:**290
Hyperglycemia, **1:**277, **2:**467
Hyperinfection syndrome, **S2:**191
Hyperlipid disorders, **2:**420
Hyperpigmentation, **3:**772
Hyperpituitarism, **2:**399
Hyperplasia, **3:**704
Hypersomnia, **3:**778, **3:**780
Hypertension, **2:**418, **2:**460–465. *See also* High blood pressure
brain hemorrhages, **2:**439
hemorrhagic strokes, **3:**813
nephrosis, **2:**616

nosebleeds, **2:**620
strokes, **3:**816
Hyperthermia, **2:**355
Hyperthyroidism, **3:**850–851. *See also* Thyroid gland
constipation, **1:**238
secondary osteoporosis, **2:**636
Hypnosis, **S1:**200–202
and dissociative identity disorder (DID), **S1:**147, **S1:**148, **S1:**149
multiple-personality disorder, therapy for, **2:**597
therapy, **S1:**200–201, **S1:**368
Hypochondria, **2:**466, **S1:**202–203
malingering, **S1:**225–226
as somatoform disorder, **S1:**337
Hypogammaglobulinemia, **S2:**18, **S2:**175
Hypoglycemia, **1:**276–277, **2:**467–468
Hypopigmentation, **3:**772
Hypopituitarism, **2:**398–399
Hypoplastic anemia, **1:**64–65
Hypothalamus, **2:**355, **2:**396
circadian rhythms, **S1:**329
cortisol, **1:**243
and eating disorders, **S1:***158*
electroconvulsive therapy (ECT), **S1:**161
emotions, **S1:**164
response to stress, **S1:***341*
reticular activating system, **S1:**57
sexual development, **S1:**319
stress-related illness, **3:***808,* **3:**809
Hypothermia, **1:**218, **1:**219, **1:**220–222. *See also* Cold-related injuries
Hypothyroidism, **2:**400, **3:**851. *See also* Thyroid gland
as birth defect, **S1:**82–83
mental retardation, **2:**578, **S1:**238
lack of iodine, **1:**289–290
Hypovolemic shock, **3:**758
Hypoxia, **S1:**79
Hysterectomy, **2:**334, **2:**571, **3:**894
Hysteria, conversion disorders, **S1:**118
Hysteroscopy, **2:**570

I

Iatrogenic Creutzfeldt-Jakob Disease, **1:**240
Ibuprofen. *See also* Medications; Over-the-counter medications

Alzheimer's disease, **1:**54
causing nephritis, **2:**614
causing peptic ulcers, **3:**658, **S2:**161
fever, **2:**358
lupus, **2:**540
mononucleosis, **2:**589
Osgood-Schlatter disease, **2:**633
phlebitis, **3:**664
Iceland, **3:**797
Ichthyophobia, **3:**666
Id, **S1:**370
Identity crisis, **S1:**265
Idiopathic conditions, **1:**124
epilepsy, **2:**341
osteoporosis, **2:**636
precocious puberty, **2:**396
scoliosis, **3:**743
Iditarod Sled Dog Race, **1:**292
IgA deficiency, **2:**470, **2:**471, **S2:**174
IgE (immunoglobulin gamma E), **1:**45
Ileitis, **2:**482, **2:**483
Illness, definition of, **1:**5
Illusions, **S1:**195
Imaging tests, **S2:**28
Immediate families, **S1:**170. *See also* Families
Immigrants, **S1:**258
Immune deficiencies, **S2:**173–178. *See also* HIV (human immunodeficiency virus)
atypical mycobacterial infections, **S2:**238, **S2:**240
candidiasis, **S2:**147
cat scratch disease complications for patient with, **S2:**82
cytomegalovirus complications, **S2:**115
ehrlichiosis complications, **S2:**128
toxoplasmosis, **S2:**350
Immune Deficiency Foundation, **2:**473, **S2:**178
Immune globulins, **2:**443, **2:**444, **2:**472, **S2:**166, **S2:**227. *See also* Antibodies
gamma E, **1:**45, **1:**92
immunoglobulin A, **S2:**174–175
made up of proteins, **S2:**17
as part of immune system defenses, **S2:**14
rabies treatment, **S2:**287
tetanus treatment, **S2:**344
varicella zoster, **S2:**382

Immune system, **2:**470–471, **S2:**9, **S2:**13–16
abscesses, **1:**15
Addison's disease, **1:**23
allergies, **1:**43–45
alopecia areata, **2:**406
anemia, **1:**66–67
antibodies, **2:**475–476
bacterial infections, **1:**119
brain tumors, **1:**150
Chagas' disease, **1:**193
colitis, **1:**223
collagen vascular diseases, **1:**225
compromised, **S2:**11, **S2:**17–19
cytomegalovirus, **1:**253
fever, **2:**356
hepatitis, **2:**441
HIV (human immunodeficiency virus), **1:**28–29, **S2:***52*
immune deficiency, **2:**469–473
Legionnaire's disease, **2:**521
leukocytes, **1:**17
lungs, **3:**675
lupus, **1:**84
multiple sclerosis, **2:**599
psoriasis, **3:**705
responding to vaccines, **S2:**43
rheumatoid arthritis, **1:**82
shingles, **3:**757
skin conditions, **3:**773
stress-related illness, **3:**809
thrush, **3:**849
toxoplasmosis, **3:**869
tuberculosis, **3:**876
viral infections, **3:**899
vitiligo, **3:**902
Immunity, **S2:**9, **S2:**43, **S2:**82
Immunization, **2:**477. *See also* Vaccinations/Vaccines
Immunization Action Coalition, **S2:**122
Immunodeficiency, **2:**469–473. *See also* Immune deficiencies
Immunoglobulin A, **S2:**174–175
Immunoglobulin E (IgE) antibodies, **1:**45, **1:**92
Immunoglobulins. *See* Immune globulins
Immunology, **3:**785
Immunostimulants, **S2:**35
Immunosuppressant drugs, **2:**367, **2:**483
Immunotherapy, **1:**47
bladder cancer, **1:**137
kidney cancer, **2:**500
Impacted fractures, **1:**158

Index